PENGUIN BOOKS

THE NEW PREGNANCY AND CHILDBIRTH

Sheila Kitzinger is known and respected all over the world as the leading authority on women's experiences of pregnancy, childbirth and motherhood. As a social anthropologist she has studied antenatal care, birth plans, midwifery, induction of labour, episiotomy, epidural anaesthesia and crying babies in many different countries. She lectures in North and South America, Europe, Australia and Japan on the social and psychological dimensions of birth, parenthood and female sexuality. She has successfully campaigned to improve conditions for women prisoners, to give women the choice of water birth and birth at home, and to deepen the understanding of unhappiness after giving birth. As Honorary Professor at Thames Valley University she is developing further education for midwives.

Among her 30 books, Penguin publishes *Woman's Experience of Sex, The Experience of Childbirth, Breastfeeding,* and *Freedom and Choice in Childbirth.* She has also written *The Year After Childbirth, Ourselves as Mothers,* and *Becoming a Grandmother.*

Sheila Kitzinger is married to Uwe Kitzinger, former President of Templeton College, Oxford. They have five daughters and three grandchildren.

SHEILA KITZINGER

The New
Pregnancy and
Childbirth

NEW EDITION

*Black-and-white photography
by Marcia May*

Penguin Books

PENGUIN BOOKS

Published by the Penguin Group
Penguin Books Ltd, 27 Wrights Lane, London W8 5TZ, England
Penguin Books USA Inc., 375 Hudson Street, New York, New York 10014, USA
Penguin Books Australia Ltd, Ringwood, Victoria, Australia
Penguin Books Canada Ltd, 10 Alcorn Avenue, Toronto, Ontario, Canada M4V 3B2
Penguin Books (NZ) Ltd, 182–190 Wairau Road, Auckland 10, New Zealand

Penguin Books Ltd, Registered Offices: Harmondsworth, Middlesex, England

The New Pregnancy and Childbirth was conceived, edited and designed by
Dorling Kindersley Limited, 9 Henrietta Street, London WC2E 8PS

For the revised and expanded edition:
Project Editor Heather Jones
Senior Art Editor Cathy Shilling
Design Assistant Nathalie Hannequin
Production Controller Meryl Silbert
Senior Managing Editor Krystyna Mayer

Senior Managing Art Editor Lynne Brown
Additional colour photography Andy Crawford
Illustrations Joanne Acty, Karen Cochrane and Halli Verrinder

Pregnancy and Childbirth first published by Michael Joseph 1980
Published in Penguin Books 1986
Revised edition published by Michael Joseph 1989
Published in Penguin Books 1989
The New Pregnancy and Childbirth published in Penguin Books 1997
3 5 7 9 10 8 6 4

Reproduction by Colourscan, Singapore
Printed and bound in Singapore by Imago Publishing Ltd

Contents

Introduction **7**
Pregnancy week by week **10**

PREGNANCY • THE EARLY WEEKS
Finding out you are pregnant **18**   *Planning & preparation* **31**

PREGNANCY • PHYSICAL AND EMOTIONAL CHANGES
Life in the uterus **62**   *Forty weeks of life* **76**   *Expecting twins* **86**
Your baby's wellbeing **93**   *Your physical wellbeing* **116**
Emotional challenges in pregnancy **149**   *Becoming a father* **159**
Your changing relationship **164**   *Pregnant again* **170**

PREGNANCY • ANTICIPATING THE BIRTH
In tune with your body for labour **176**   *Windows into the uterus* **220**
The last few weeks **231**

THE EXPERIENCE OF BIRTH
What happens in labour **240**   *Different kinds of labour* **262**
Giving support in labour **277**   *Dealing with pain* **295**
Towards the medical control of birth **314**   *Gentle birth* **343**

YOU AND YOUR NEWBORN
The first hours of life **356**   *The baby who needs special care* **366**
Losing a baby **372**   *The first ten days* **381**
The challenge of new parenthood **396**

PHOTOGRAPHIC SEQUENCES
A hospital birth **54**
A home birth **256**
A water birth **284**

Useful reading **412**
Useful addresses **413**
Research references **415**
Glossary **420**
Index **426**
Acknowledgments **432**

Introduction

When I first started to teach and counsel pregnant women in the Sixties, there was little birth education around. For a small minority of women there were breathing and relaxation exercises taught by physiotherapists (who then had no special training for helping women in childbirth) and talks by midwives about "what to expect".

There was a handful of books written by the pioneers: Grantly Dick-Read, Kathleen Vaughan, Minnie Randall, Helen Heardman, Velvovsky and Lamaze. Although some discussed the fear of childbirth, there was nothing about the socially inculcated lack of confidence we felt in our bodies and in ourselves, nor the pressure on women by a powerful medical system to surrender themselves to it as passive patients. It seemed that all we could hope for was to put on as good a performance as possible and to be told "well done".

After the birth of my first child, when I started teaching for what is now the National Childbirth Trust, I remember talking to obstetricians from the former Soviet Union who had introduced psychoprophylaxis (a system of training for labour based on breathing techniques) into some of their bigger hospitals and were actually proud because "there is now no noise in the labour ward". It was supposed to be a great achievement – to silence women!

When psychoprophylaxis was first introduced in Britain from France, one woman told me that the day after a gruelling labour involving drugs and the use of forceps her childbirth teacher had shown up at her bedside and commented: "You didn't do too well!" In those days, if you needed painkilling drugs or help with the birth, you were made to feel that you had failed. The choice was between having doctors take over completely and putting on a solo performance without support or encouragement from professionals.

Remarkable changes have taken place since then – largely due to women in the childbirth movement who have joined together across continents. It is now acknowledged that women have a right to full and accurate information about their bodies and to participate in all decisions made about them. *The New Pregnancy and Childbirth* reflects the many changes that have come about because we refuse to remain ignorant of what doctors are doing to us. It is an expression of women's courage and growing self-confidence, and of the ways in which we have reached out to each other to explore and understand those experiences we have in common.

In order to take an active part in giving birth rather than submit passively to delivery, it helps to prepare yourself well in advance, understanding how to adapt to the work being done by your uterus, using breathing, relaxation techniques, changes of position, massage and focused concentration to "get in tune with" contractions. There is a good deal of practical material in the book on

The birth of a baby is a normal biological process. Yet it is more than that. Giving birth and caring for a baby is an act of love (opposite).

the various methods to do this. It is not just a matter of learning exercises. There is a harmony and rhythm about a natural labour: with the wave of each contraction you are swept on towards the birth of the baby in a pattern that transforms birth into a process greater than all its separate parts, one in which all the techniques you have practised are submerged by the total amazing experience.

The book describes the choices that are available so that you can decide how you would like to have your baby, the kind of setting and care you prefer, and how you wish your baby to be welcomed into the world. I include suggestions on talking with your doctor, how to ask about all the things that worry you and how you can share in the decisions about yourself and your baby. The book also sets out to give a map of the route through pregnancy and labour and out the other side, explaining who does what to you and why, and what happens when things are not straightforward. In writing the book I have used some of the words and phrases that you may see written on your medical chart or hear used by doctors or midwives, so that you will understand them when you meet them, but the main focus is on experiential aspects of birth – how it feels.

The book is threaded through with recognition of the father's importance to his partner and baby and suggestions as to how he can help most effectively during pregnancy, labour and the time after the birth. A baby is bound to change a couple's way of life, their feelings about each other, and the kind of partnership they have. The man, as well as the woman, often faces emotional challenges, and this is rarely acknowledged in our society. So another thing that I have done is to focus on the experience of childbirth for him.

Most new parents gain confidence and find it easiest to have "conversations" with their baby when there are no rules to be obeyed and no standards to live up to, when they can take the baby into bed with them and stroke, hold and cuddle their newborn as much as they wish. In this book I hope to show how a couple, or a woman alone, can create the kind of setting and atmosphere for birth, whether at home or in hospital, that nurtures relationships.

Pregnancy and childbirth are normal life processes, not illnesses. You feel the incredible surge of life moving inside you, the ripening of your body heavy with fruit deep inside it, and then at last the flood of vitality as labour starts and your uterus contracts in wave after wave, bringing your baby into your arms. It is exciting, awe-inspiring and deeply satisfying. At the same time, you grow up a bit, learn more about yourself and your partner, and develop understanding. I hope this book will help readers savour the intense reality of the experience of childbearing and enjoy it to the fullest.

NOTES TO THE READER

It is always difficult when writing about babies to know whether to use "he" or "she." I have mainly used a mixture of "he" and "she", since babies are people with their own budding personalities right from the start. I hope that the reader will not find this too awkward, and if there is a bias towards "she" in the text, note that my five babies were all girls, so it comes naturally to me.

Throughout the text all references to research findings are marked with an asterisk (*); this indicates that the works in which the research findings have been published are listed on pages 415–419, in order, under the appropriate page numbers.

AUTHOR'S ACKNOWLEDGMENTS

A number of people have contributed to this book, bringing their knowledge and special skills. I want to thank particularly Penny Simkin in Seattle, who read every word of the typescript, making many helpful suggestions. If there are any mistakes, they are not Penny's! She is meticulous and utterly committed to the cause of making birth better for women everywhere.

Kay Millar, Active Birth teacher in Oxford, has been superb, too. She oversaw all the exercise sequences taken in the photographic studio, ensuring that they were not only accurate but clear.

Marcia May took the wonderful photographs of birth. It is lovely to have a photographer who is so in tune with my beliefs.

Vreni Booth, who teaches movement classes based on the Feldenkrais method, has helped me rethink postnatal exercises in a constructive way.

Nicky Leap, the midwife in some of the birth photographs, is one of the most innovative thinkers and courageous practitioners in midwifery today. I value my discussions with Dr Michel Odent. They always stimulate lateral thinking, as he raises important questions that need to be answered. I am also grateful to Professor Lesley Page of Queen Charlotte's Hospital, London, for the many times that we have shared our thoughts about the future of midwifery, and its meaning for women and families.

In addition, I should like to thank Dr Iain Chalmers, former Director of the British National Perinatal Epidemiology Unit, now Director of the Cochrane Institute, for all the work he has done to base obstetric practice on scientific evidence rather than on medical "hunches", and to present the benefits and risks of different practices, so that women can make up their own minds about what they want. I have drawn heavily on the *Cochrane Library* for the new material in the book.

My birth activist colleagues, Beverley Lawrence Beech of the Association for Improvements in the Maternity Services, and Janet Balaskas, who created the Active Birth Movement, both contribute to my own vitality by their strength and energy.

In the writing of this book, I owe a great deal to my daughter, Tess, for her clarity of thinking, her understanding and her skills with the computer. As I write this we have her three-day-old baby, Josh, who was born at home, under water, as were her other two children, in an atmosphere of love and celebration.

Pregnancy week by week

This is a week-by-week guide to what may be happening to you and your baby throughout pregnancy. As different women's pregnancies develop at different rates, do not expect to be at exactly the same stage for the week described. Read the information for the two weeks either side, too. Since pregnancy is dated medically from the first day of your last period, this diary begins with what is termed the third week of a 40-week pregnancy, the week of conception.

WEEK 3

You have ovulated and an egg is travelling along one of the two fallopian tubes towards your uterus. During intercourse one of the millions of sperm that your partner has ejaculated has fertilized the egg while it is still inside the fallopian tube.

Your baby is now a cluster of cells that multiply rapidly as they continue on their journey along the fallopian tube.

WEEK 4

You have probably not noticed anything different, although some women have a strange, metallic taste in their mouths.

The fertilized egg has arrived in your uterus and, after floating in the uterine cavity for about three days, has embedded itself in the uterine lining. It is nourished from blood vessels in the lining of your uterus, and the placenta is beginning to form around it.

WEEK 5

You are beginning to think that you may be pregnant. Your period is late, but you cannot be sure, because you may feel as though it is about to start at any time. Your breasts are slightly enlarged and tender and you may find you need to pass urine more often than usual.

The embryo is approximately 2 mm (1⁄10 in) long and would be visible to the naked eye by now. Its spine is beginning to form and the brain has two lobes.

WEEK 6

You may be feeling nauseous first thing in the morning or when you are cooking a meal. Your vagina has become a bluish or violet colour. From the sixth day after your period was due it should be possible to find out by a urine test whether or not you are pregnant. Your uterus is now the size of a tangerine.

The baby has developed a head and trunk, and a rudimentary brain has formed. Tiny limb buds are starting to appear. By the end of this week the baby's circulation is beginning to function. The jaw and mouth are developing and ten dental buds are growing in each jaw.

WEEK 7

You may sometimes feel dizzy or faint when standing for a long time. Your breasts are noticeably larger and small nodules called Montgomery's tubercles may have appeared on the areolae, while your nipples may have become more prominent. Pregnancy can be confirmed by a vaginal examination.

The limb buds have developed rapidly and now look like tiny arms and legs. At the end of these limbs are small indentations that will later become fingers and toes. The spinal cord and brain are now almost complete and the head is assuming a human shape. The baby is now about 1.3 cm (½ in) long.

WEEK 8

You may find that you have "gone off" certain foods and that you fancy others that were not your favourite foods before. Many pregnant women can no longer drink alcohol, even if they previously enjoyed it, and a dislike of cigarettes or tobacco smoke is common. Your hair may seem less manageable than usual. You may also have a slight vaginal discharge.

The baby now has all its main organs in a rudimentary form. The eyes and ears are growing. The face is taking on a human shape, and the baby is just under 2.5 cm (1 in) long.

WEEK 9

You may notice a number of changes in your skin because of the pregnancy hormones now present in your system. Any wrinkles you have may become less obvious. Your gums may be softening because of these hormones, and you need to be especially careful about dental hygiene now and through the rest of the pregnancy. The thyroid gland in your neck may be more prominent.

The baby's limbs are developing very rapidly by this stage, and the fingers and toes are beginning to be defined on the hands and feet. The baby is already moving about gently to exercise its muscles, although you cannot feel it. At this point the baby weighs only about as much as a grape.

WEEK 10

Your uterus has expanded to the size of an orange, but is still hidden away within your pelvis. You should be wearing a bra with good support by now. If you buy a bra that fits your breasts but is adjustable to allow for later chest expansion, you may not need to get another size during the rest of your pregnancy.

The placenta, to which the baby is attached, begins to produce progesterone in a process that is completed by the end of the 14th week, when the progesterone produced is sufficient for the placenta to take over the function of the corpus luteum. The baby's ankles and wrists are formed, and fingers and toes are clearly visible. The baby has now grown to about 4.5 cm (1¾ in) long.

WEEK 11

If you have been nauseous during the last weeks, the sickness may gradually lessen from now onwards. The amount of blood circulating through your body has started to increase, and will go on increasing until about the 30th week. You should be thinking about arranging to attend childbirth classes, since they often get booked up early.

Your baby's testicles or ovaries have formed at this point, as have all of its major organs. These organs will not develop much further, although they will continue to grow inside the uterus. The baby is relatively safe from the risk of developing any congenital abnormalities from the end of this week.

WEEK 12

You will probably have your first antenatal visit this week. The doctor or midwife will be able to feel the uterus by external examination, as it has risen above your pelvis. Arrangements will be made for future appointments, probably once a month until you are 32 weeks pregnant.

The baby's head is becoming more rounded and its eyelids have formed. Its muscles are developing and it is moving about inside the uterus much more. It is now about 6.5 cm (2 in) long but still weighs only 18 g (½ oz).

WEEK 13

If you have had morning sickness this may have gone by the end of this week. From now on your uterus will be enlarging at a regular and noticeable rate.

The bag of water cushions the baby from bumps, keeps it at a constant warm temperature and enables it to move freely, turn its head, stretch and bounce around.

WEEK 14

You are less tired than you were at the beginning of pregnancy and probably feel fit and active. You may notice a dark line (the linea nigra) down the centre of your abdomen. This will begin to fade after the baby is born. Your nipples and the area around them are also starting to darken. Your uterus is the size of a large grapefruit.

The baby has eyebrows and a small amount of hair has appeared on its head. Its heart can be heard by ultrasound. The baby drinks some of the amniotic fluid and can pass urine. It is now receiving all of its nourishment from the placenta and measures about 8–9 cm (3¾ in) in length.

WEEK 15

Your clothes will now be getting too tight for you. It is best not to try to cram yourself into tight jeans. To cope with the increased amount of blood circulating in your body and the baby's need for oxygen, your enlarged heart has increased its output by 20 per cent.

The hair on your baby's head and brows is becoming coarser. If it has a gene for dark hair, the pigment cells of the hair follicles are beginning to produce black pigment.

WEEK 16
You feel butterflies in your tummy that might be the baby moving. Your waistline is now starting to disappear. If you have not already done so, book childbirth education classes. An "early-bird" class might be available to discuss diet, exercise, posture, emotions and health.

The baby is now completely formed. From now on its time in the uterus will be spent growing and maturing until it is able to survive independently. Lanugo (fine down) is starting to form all over the baby, following the whorled pattern of the skin. The baby is 16 cm (6¾ in) long and weighs nearly 135 g (5 oz).

WEEK 17
You may find you are sweating more than usual (due to the extra blood in your system) and also that your nose feels congested. This is common in pregnancy and will cease after the birth. Vaginal secretions may also increase.

The growing baby has by this stage pushed the top of the uterus to halfway between your pubic bone and your navel. From now on the baby weighs more than its placenta. It is probably aware of – and may even be temporarily startled by – loud sounds that occur outside your body.

WEEK 18
If this is your first baby, you may now start to become aware of the first prods and general signs of movement, which are definitely nothing to do with indigestion! At last you know that there really is a baby in there! Trouble with sleeping properly at night will be helped by increasing the number of pillows you use in order to support yourself.

Measuring about 20 cm (8 in) long, your baby is now beginning the process of testing its reflexes. Babies often move especially energetically during the evening and bounce around like a cork in water. As well as

20 weeks

24 weeks

28 weeks

kicking, the baby is now also grasping and sucking. Some babies find their thumbs while still in the uterus and are actually confirmed thumb-suckers even before they are born.

WEEK 19

Now is not too early to start practising deep relaxation and steady, rhythmic breathing. Set aside some time each day for this. You may notice that you are putting weight on your buttocks as well as your abdomen.

Buds for permanent teeth are forming behind those for the baby's milk teeth that have, by now, already formed.

WEEK 20

You will notice your baby being more and more active (often in the evenings), and you may even be able to see some of its movements. The growing uterus is pushing up against your lungs and pressing your tummy outwards. Your navel may suddenly pop out and stay that way until after the birth. Your chest (rather than breasts) has expanded and if you do not already have an adjustable bra now is the time to buy one.

The baby is now about 25 cm (10 in) long. Sebum from the sebaceous glands mixes with skin cells and begins to form the protective vernix, which clings to the lanugo all over the baby's skin, especially on the hairier parts of the skin and in the creases.

WEEK 21

You may start having heartburn (a form of indigestion that is felt as a burning sensation in the lower part of the chest). You may also bring up small amounts of acid fluid. Ask your doctor or midwife to recommend some appropriate antacid tablets.

The baby weighs just under 450 g (1 lb). It is still moving about freely in the amniotic fluid and can be felt kicking, sometimes high in your tummy, at other times low down.

32 weeks   *36 weeks*   *40 weeks*

WEEK 22

Your gums may be swelling because of the pregnancy hormones in your system.

The baby's fingernails are forming. It is settling into a regular pattern of activity and sleep. It is frequently most active while you are resting, and you may feel that you have a jumping bean inside you.

WEEK 23

The different parts of the baby can be felt (palpated) through your abdominal wall. You may feel a stitch-like pain at times down the side of your tummy; this is the uterine muscle stretching and the pain will probably go away after you have had a rest.

Braxton Hicks "rehearsal" contractions may be more noticeable at this stage, gripping and massaging the baby regularly. The baby's fingernails are almost fully formed.

WEEK 24

Another visit to the doctor or midwife – by now the baby's heart can be heard through a stethoscope or a special fetal trumpet. The top of your uterus (the fundus) now reaches to just above your navel.

The baby is growing rapidly – it is now about 32 cm (13 in) long and weighs over 0.5 kg (1 lb). Its vital organs are maturing but the lungs are unlikely to be sufficiently developed for survival outside the uterus.

WEEK 25

You may get cramps now and later on in your pregnancy. Avoid pointing your toes down. The baby may also be pressing against your bladder, causing you to want to pass urine.

The baby's bone centres are beginning to harden at this stage, and tiny veins are now visible through the baby's skin.

WEEK 26

You may notice streaks in your skin where it has been stretched from underneath. The marks will fade after birth.

When you speak your voice goes down into your body, and your baby can hear you. The baby's body is covered with fine, downy hairs and the skin is beginning to change: instead of being paper-thin and transparent, it is gradually becoming opaque.

WEEK 27

You will be putting on weight fairly regularly now until about the 36th week of pregnancy. It may be a good idea to start thinking about what to get for the baby and buy things now before you become so big that shopping becomes an unpleasant chore.

The baby's skin is very wrinkled, but it is protected and nourished by a layer of vernix.

WEEK 28

Colostrum may leak from your breasts. From now on you will probably be visiting the doctor every two weeks. If you are Rhesus negative, an antibody check is done.

Your baby's heartbeat speeds up when you speak and he or she can recognize your voice after birth. The baby is about 38 cm (14 in) long and weighs around 0.9 kg (2 lb).

WEEK 29

You probably feel as if all your internal organs are being crowded out by the baby. There is pressure on your diaphragm, liver, stomach and intestines.

By now the baby's head is more or less in proportion with the rest of its body.

WEEK 30

It is important to remember to maintain good posture when you are standing or sitting, even though the weight of the baby seems to be dragging you off balance.

The baby is probably very aware of the Braxton Hicks contractions, that are now coming at regular intervals, even when you do not notice them at all.

WEEK 31

You may now get very breathless when you climb stairs or exert yourself.

However breathless you feel, the baby is getting enough oxygen through the placenta. The baby now weighs 1.8 kg (4 lb). If the weather is hot or you have eaten a heavy meal the baby may be drowsy.

WEEK 32

At each health visit the doctor or midwife will feel the baby's position. At the same time, he or she will also assess the baby's rate of growth and check its heart.

The baby is 42 cm (16 in) long. It is perfectly formed but the fat reserves beneath its skin are only gradually laid down. If the baby were to be born at this time, it would still need to be cared for in an incubator.

WEEK 33

You may now be able to distinguish the baby's bottom from, for example, a foot or knee. You feel its movements more as prods and kicks – it may be too big now to swoop around in the amniotic fluid.

Your baby has probably adopted the most usual head-down ("vertex" or "cephalic") position, in which it will now stay until the birth. From now on, lying flat on your back may make you feel dizzy.

WEEK 34

The baby can differentiate between dark and light, and is bathed in a red glow when sunlight is on your tummy.

WEEK 35

You may have backache. This is because ligaments and muscles supporting the joints in the small of your back relax.

The baby's bottom presses against your diaphragm. At this stage of its development the baby measures approximately 44 cm (18 in) and weighs around 2.5 kg (5 lb).

WEEK 36

Clinic visits may be every week from now on. If this is your first baby, it will probably

Pelvic engagement Pelvis
A baby may engage in your pelvis at any time from six weeks before the birth. When you lie flat on your back the baby may not appear to be engaged, but as you sit up the baby's presenting part slips down into your pelvis.

Not yet engaged

Pelvis

Engaged

engage some time this week or soon after, and may have done so already. Your lump will settle lower down and you will find that breathing becomes easier, although you may also need to pass urine more often, and your sleep will be interrupted.

The baby is almost fully mature and any time now the presenting part may drop down into your pelvis ready for birth. It is about 49 cm (18 in) long.

WEEK 37

If you have chosen a hospital birth, you will have a chance to tour the birthrooms of the hospital in which you are to have your baby.

The baby is rehearsing its first breathing movements, although there is no air present in its lungs. In this way amniotic fluid actually passes into the baby's trachea, sometimes giving it hiccups!

WEEK 38

You may be aware that the baby moves less now and that, instead of whole body movements, there are only jabs from the feet and knees, and the strange, buzzing sensation inside your vagina as the baby's head moves against your pelvic floor muscles.

The baby may be putting on as much as 28 g (1 oz) a day at this stage.

WEEK 39

Your cervix is ripening in preparation for labour. You may feel heavy and weary and have strong Braxton Hicks contractions. The amniotic fluid is renewed every three hours.

The baby's bowels are filled with greenish-black meconium, excretions from the baby's alimentary glands mixed with bile pigment, lanugo and cells from the bowel wall – its first motion after birth.

WEEK 40

The long-awaited day is near, and you probably feel fed up with being pregnant. You may have slight diarrhoea.

The baby is about 55 cm (20 in) long. You feel sharp kicks under your ribs at one side or the other. The presenting part presses through the softened, partially opened, cervix. You will soon hold your child in your arms and at last be able to see each other face-to-face.

PREGNANCY

The early weeks

Finding out you are pregnant **18**

Planning and preparation **31**

Finding out you are pregnant

Some women are convinced that they are pregnant from the moment of conception; others have such irregular periods that a long gap in between does not alert them to the possibility of pregnancy. But for most women the first sign of pregnancy is a missed period.

Perhaps it is five days since the day when you expected it, but then you start wondering if your dates were wrong. Perhaps you usually make a note in your diary, but last time you forgot. You lie in bed, unable to sleep, trying to fix the dates firmly in your mind by finding some useful landmark, like your mother's visit or the end of a particular work assignment. Still another three days go by and the reality gradually dawns: you might be pregnant. You might not be, but it does seem quite possible that you are. When is it sensible to go to the doctor and how early can you know for certain?

When to diagnose

Until recently it was usual to visit the doctor after missing two periods. Nowadays there is a strong case for finding out if you are pregnant before two periods have been missed. It is during these few weeks, while the embryo is still no larger than a hazelnut, that the major organs of the body and the brain itself are being formed; the sooner you know that you are pregnant the sooner you can start caring for yourself and for the baby.

An early confirmation of pregnancy is also important if you take any medicines. You will want to avoid taking drugs that could harm the developing baby (see page 100). It can also be useful to know early for social reasons – you may be planning to go abroad or to move at the time the baby is due.

If there is any possibility at all that you may want to terminate the pregnancy, it is essential to diagnose pregnancy in the early weeks: a termination (abortion) at eight weeks is much safer and less upsetting than one after ten weeks.

How to diagnose

Pregnancy can now be diagnosed about two weeks after conception, on the day your period should have started if you have a regular menstrual cycle, although you are likely to get more accurate results if you wait at least another four days – which can be difficult if you are feeling anxious or excited. When you are pregnant, the embryo releases a hormone called human chorionic gonadotrophin (HCG) into your bloodstream. Minute traces of HCG will be present in your urine approximately six days after conception, but then the level builds up quite rapidly, doubling every two or three days until it reaches a peak about 60 days after conception – approximately 74 days after your last period started – when it begins to decrease. It is possible to detect the presence of this hormone in your urine or blood. Your doctor or midwife will take a urine or blood sample for analysis at a laboratory.

You may prefer to use one of the do-it-yourself pregnancy kits that are widely available (see below). Whichever method you choose, if at all possible test urine passed first thing in the morning, when you have not drunk anything during the night, since it is at this time that urine contains the highest concentration of pregnancy hormone.

Do-it-yourself tests There are a number of different kits on the market, and most involve mixing a drop or two of urine with the chemicals provided. If you are pregnant, the presence of HCG in your urine will, depending on the test, either prevent the mixture from coagulating (ring test) or change the colour of the chemical in the test tube or on the dipstick (colour test). Depending on the kit, you can use these tests when your period is between one and four days late, but you do need to be sure of when your period was due.

Occasionally a woman notices a little spotting (light bleeding) 10–12 days after fertilization. This is not really a period and the dating of pregnancy can start from your last actual period.

If the result is negative, but your period still has not arrived a few days later, do the test again. It is possible that you conceived later than you thought likely and that at the time of the first test there was not enough HCG in your urine to indicate that you were pregnant. If your periods are irregular or far apart, the chances of a false result are increased. After perhaps one conception in every ten, the fertilized egg does not manage to embed itself in the lining of the uterus. In this case, a pregnancy test will give a positive result, but a second test a few days later will produce a negative result. For this reason, some packs carry the recommendation that you always wait three to five days and then retest, and they include two tests in each pack in order for you to be able to do this.

"I wanted to find out myself, not get the news from the doctor. I wasn't sure I wanted this baby and didn't know how I'd react."

Going to the doctor or midwife A doctor or midwife will perform a blood or urine test and you will also be given an internal examination. He or she introduces two gloved fingers into your vagina as far as they will go, while pressing with the other hand into your abdomen where the top of the uterus lies. If it is more than six weeks since the first day of your last period they can feel the already softened lower part of the uterus, which is also slightly enlarged. The neck of the uterus, or cervix, which protrudes into the vagina, is felt as firmer than the lower part of the uterus, and it is about the same consistency as the tip of your nose. This internal change is known as "Hegar's sign". The examination may be uncomfortable but will not be painful. As the examining fingers are introduced, give a long, slow breath out through your mouth and continue breathing as slowly as you can.

DATING YOUR PREGNANCY

Once the pregnancy is confirmed it will be dated from the first day of your last menstrual period (LMP). If you cannot recollect this date with accuracy the doctor or midwife will probably ask you to make a guess at it. This means that from then on the length of your pregnancy is reckoned in terms of so many weeks, including the weeks from the beginning of your last period to the time when conception occurred. Since ovulation is most common midway between two periods, the usual medical way of dating pregnancy adds an extra two weeks to its length. The length of the average pregnancy is some 266 days from the date of conception: the doctor or midwife will therefore arrive at your expected date of delivery (EDD) by adding 280 days, or 40 weeks, to the first day of your last period. You may find that you pay your first visit to the clinic knowing that it is ten weeks since you conceived, but emerge from the consultation three months pregnant!

Since not all women ovulate halfway between two periods, the medical convention of adding on an extra two weeks is an artificial one, and an inaccurate method of working out when a baby is due. It is wise to think of the EDD as an approximate date rather than the day when you expect to go into labour.

If you have just stopped taking the birth control pill it is possible that your dates may be completely wrong. The period that immediately follows your last pill may not be followed by ovulation or you may have a slight spotting of blood which is not really a period. It may take several months to re-establish your natural menstrual cycle, and until then you cannot predict with any certainty when, or whether, you are going to ovulate. You might be a month or more out in your dates. This is obviously very important in estimating when the baby is due, especially since it could lead to labour being induced unnecessarily (see page 324). It is therefore advisable to wait for a clear three months after stopping the pill before trying to conceive; during this time you should use some other method of contraception.

CONCEIVING WHILE USING CONTRACEPTION

If you conceive with an IUD (intrauterine device or coil) still inside you, your chances of miscarrying are increased. It is therefore important to see your doctor quickly, as the IUD should be removed without delay if possible and this can only be done early in pregnancy. Sometimes doctors advise termination. This is certainly not necessary if you want the baby: even if it is by now too late to remove the IUD, many women deliver the IUD with the placenta after an uneventful pregnancy and birth.

WHEN IS YOUR BABY DUE?

This chart will help you to estimate the date your baby is due. Look along the columns at the figures set in bold type to find the first day of your last period. The date below it is 280 days later and is your estimated date of delivery (EDD). It is perfectly normal for a baby to arrive two weeks before or two weeks after this date.

January	1 2 3 4 5 6 7 8 9 10 11 12 13 14 15 16 17 18 19 20 21 22 23 24 25 26 27 28 29 30 31
Oct/Nov	8 9 10 11 12 13 14 15 16 17 18 19 20 21 22 23 24 25 26 27 28 29 30 31 1 2 3 4 5 6 7
February	1 2 3 4 5 6 7 8 9 10 11 12 13 14 15 16 17 18 19 20 21 22 23 24 25 26 27 28
Nov/Dec	8 9 10 11 12 13 14 15 16 17 18 19 20 21 22 23 24 25 26 27 28 29 30 1 2 3 4 5
March	1 2 3 4 5 6 7 8 9 10 11 12 13 14 15 16 17 18 19 20 21 22 23 24 25 26 27 28 29 30 31
Dec/Jan	6 7 8 9 10 11 12 13 14 15 16 17 18 19 20 21 22 23 24 25 26 27 28 29 30 31 1 2 3 4 5
April	1 2 3 4 5 6 7 8 9 10 11 12 13 14 15 16 17 18 19 20 21 22 23 24 25 26 27 28 29 30
Jan/Feb	6 7 8 9 10 11 12 13 14 15 16 17 18 19 20 21 22 23 24 25 26 27 28 29 30 31 1 2 3 4
May	1 2 3 4 5 6 7 8 9 10 11 12 13 14 15 16 17 18 19 20 21 22 23 24 25 26 27 28 29 30 31
Feb/March	5 6 7 8 9 10 11 12 13 14 15 16 17 18 19 20 21 22 23 24 25 26 27 28 1 2 3 4 5 6 7
June	1 2 3 4 5 6 7 8 9 10 11 12 13 14 15 16 17 18 19 20 21 22 23 24 25 26 27 28 29 30
March/April	8 9 10 11 12 13 14 15 16 17 18 19 20 21 22 23 24 25 26 27 28 29 30 31 1 2 3 4 5 6
July	1 2 3 4 5 6 7 8 9 10 11 12 13 14 15 16 17 18 19 20 21 22 23 24 25 26 27 28 29 30 31
April/May	7 8 9 10 11 12 13 14 15 16 17 18 19 20 21 22 23 24 25 26 27 28 29 30 1 2 3 4 5 6 7
August	1 2 3 4 5 6 7 8 9 10 11 12 13 14 15 16 17 18 19 20 21 22 23 24 25 26 27 28 29 30 31
May/June	8 9 10 11 12 13 14 15 16 17 18 19 20 21 22 23 24 25 26 27 28 29 30 31 1 2 3 4 5 6 7
September	1 2 3 4 5 6 7 8 9 10 11 12 13 14 15 16 17 18 19 20 21 22 23 24 25 26 27 28 29 30
June/July	8 9 10 11 12 13 14 15 16 17 18 19 20 21 22 23 24 25 26 27 28 29 30 1 2 3 4 5 6 7
October	1 2 3 4 5 6 7 8 9 10 11 12 13 14 15 16 17 18 19 20 21 22 23 24 25 26 27 28 29 30 31
July/Aug	8 9 10 11 12 13 14 15 16 17 18 19 20 21 22 23 24 25 26 27 28 29 30 31 1 2 3 4 5 6 7
November	1 2 3 4 5 6 7 8 9 10 11 12 13 14 15 16 17 18 19 20 21 22 23 24 25 26 27 28 29 30
Aug/Sept	8 9 10 11 12 13 14 15 16 17 18 19 20 21 22 23 24 25 26 27 28 29 30 31 1 2 3 4 5 6
December	1 2 3 4 5 6 7 8 9 10 11 12 13 14 15 16 17 18 19 20 21 22 23 24 25 26 27 28 29 30 31
Sept/Oct	7 8 9 10 11 12 13 14 15 16 17 18 19 20 21 22 23 24 25 26 27 28 29 30 1 2 3 4 5 6 7

It is possible to conceive while taking the pill if you miss one or more days when you should have been taking it, or if you have an upset stomach with vomiting so that you fail to absorb the hormones, or if you have been on antibiotics. If you do conceive but continue to take the pill for several months while pregnant, there is a slightly increased risk to the baby of congenital abnormalities, although the vast majority of women who have taken the pill while pregnant give birth to babies who are healthy and normal.

Sometimes a doctor prescribes pills containing the hormones oestrogen and progestogen in order to discover whether or not a woman is pregnant, the idea being that you take them and if you are not pregnant then your period starts. These types of hormone pill carry the same slight risk to the baby as the pill does: other diagnostic methods are therefore preferable.

PREGNANCY AND HIV INFECTION

If you are anxious that you or your partner has been exposed to the virus that causes AIDS (acquired immune deficiency syndrome), you may decide before you get pregnant, or in very early pregnancy, that you should be screened for it. The test does not identify the virus (the human immunodeficiency virus, or HIV) itself, but reveals whether antibodies to it are in the bloodstream. If someone has been infected, antibodies will be present. Even though that person may show no symptoms of infection, he or she can transmit the virus to someone else. A pregnant woman can infect her unborn baby, although 85 per cent of babies of HIV-positive mothers are born healthy. Most infections occur as the baby passes down the birth canal. Caesarean section seems to halve the risk of infection. But further research is taking place and your doctor may give you up-to-date information. Even if a baby has HIV infection at birth there is a slight chance that symptoms will not develop, and 6 per cent of babies born HIV-positive still have no symptoms at five years.

Before being tested you will have thought through the implications – social, emotional and physical – of getting a positive result. As one woman carrying the virus said: "The only difference between now and before is this piece of knowledge. And it's such depressing, unhappy knowledge, I find it quite paralyzing".* According to current research, anyone who is antibody-positive has a 10 to 30 per cent chance of developing AIDS within four years. Pregnancy affects the immune system, so it may trigger AIDS in a woman who is antibody-positive but who has had no previous symptoms. It is possible that she may develop the disease during pregnancy or soon after the baby is born.

Babies born to HIV-positive mothers always have antibodies. Some types of antibody, however, can enter the baby's blood without the child becoming infected with the virus, and if an HIV-positive woman is healthy during pregnancy, there is a good chance that her baby will lose inherited antibodies within 6 to 18 months. It may take more than a year, with tests every few months, to know for sure whether a baby is carrying the virus. Only about 22 per cent of antibody-positive newborn babies develop AIDS. If a woman has already given birth to an infected baby, there is a 66 per cent chance that her next baby will be infected, too. If she herself has AIDS the risk is still greater. An antibody-positive baby may have birth defects or a characteristic appearance with a very small head, box-shaped forehead, flat nose, blue eyeballs, widely spaced eyes and full lips.

Antibody tests may show up negative for three months following infection. It makes sense to have a second test 12 weeks after the first if you or your partner are at high risk of contracting the virus and if you are in very early pregnancy and are sure that you would want a termination if you were antibody-positive. No test is 100 per cent free from error. The "Western blot" – which is the most widely used test in North America and Britain – is 96 per cent accurate.

EARLY SIGNS OF PREGNANCY

Breast changes Even before your pregnancy is confirmed there may be early indications other than a missed period. Breast changes, in preparation for milk production, occur in the first weeks. The brownish circles round the nipples (the areolae) become darker and the little bumps on them (Montgomery's tubercles) more prominent.

If you are pink-skinned you may notice that the lacy network of blood vessels in your breasts has become much more obvious. Blue veins run over the breasts like rivers on a map. Your breasts may also feel tender and heavy. Women with small breasts may note an obvious increase in size very early on. If you have large breasts already you may not notice any size change at this stage.

Tiredness Enormous metabolic changes take place in pregnancy and your whole body has to adjust to the process of growing a baby. It is not surprising that you may feel tired and that you cannot carry on just as you did before. Many women complain of extreme tiredness during the first eight or ten weeks. But as your body adjusts to the pregnancy the fatigue vanishes and the middle months are often easy. If you are feeling tired it is only sensible to take the message from your body and go to bed early, have a rest at midday if you can or an early evening rest when you get home from work.

If it is your second (or third) pregnancy, you may find that you are constantly tired. Women who thoroughly enjoyed their first pregnancy say that the second one is much harder to cope with because they are exhausted by the non-stop pace of their first child's

The first physical changes of which you become aware may occur in your breasts. Veins may become more prominent and the areolae darker.

daily life. The only solution is to try to have at least a short time every day when you are free from domestic responsibilities. Even half an hour every evening when your partner attends to the child and the dishes can be relaxing if you are able to enjoy it to the fullest. (See pages 170–173 for more about second and later pregnancies.)

Nausea Another common sign of pregnancy is nausea. These waves of sickness often happen early in the morning, when your blood-sugar level is low, but they may also occur in the early evening or even at other times of the day. Some women just feel very sick, others actually vomit. Tiredness contributes to nausea, but so does an empty stomach: frequent small snacks of bland foods like dry biscuits or a banana may relieve the feeling. If you suffer from morning sickness, a cup of tea and a few crackers or dry toast immediately on waking may prevent it, or crackers alone may be better. A late-night snack may help, too. As a general rule, cut out all greasy fried foods, tobacco and alcohol. Avoid strong odours, especially cooking smells, exhaust fumes and perfume, and if nausea and vomiting are still bad, ask your doctor to prescribe an antihistamine, which is the drug most likely to be effective.*

Some women become really ill with vomiting (see page 135), although most stop feeling sick during the fourth month. Women who experience pregnancy nausea are less likely than others to have miscarriages. This can be a cheering thought. But nausea does not exist in all cultures; many societies have other illnesses and disabilities, or special dreams that they connect with pregnancy. Margaret Mead points out that in some societies of New Guinea boils are considered a typical symptom of pregnancy. Some Jamaicans do not acknowledge pregnancy until they have had a special fertility dream of ripe fruit bursting with seed. Dreams of this kind are characteristic of early pregnancy. It is as if all women need definite signs to link with pregnancy so that they can say, "I feel this, therefore I must be expecting a baby".

You may suffer from nausea for the first time in your second or third pregnancy. This is almost certainly the result of tiredness, and you may not relieve the nausea within three months unless you can somehow arrange to have more rest.

EMOTIONAL REACTIONS TO PREGNANCY
However much you want a baby, finding out that you really are pregnant can produce a flood of conflicting emotions: triumph ("We've done it!"), a sense of being trapped ("There's no going back – now what?"), fear ("Mum had an awful time having me – will I be able to stand the pain?"), apprehension ("Will we still love each other in the same way?") and doubt ("Will he still want me once my waist starts getting thicker?"). It is surprising how many women respond to their first pregnancy with shock and feel that it has happened "too soon", even though they very much want a baby

and have considered the matter carefully before stopping contraception. Confronted with the reality and the physical changes of pregnancy, they want to say: "Stop! I haven't prepared myself for this. Let's go back and start again."

If you discover that you are pregnant when you did not plan to be, you may also feel unfairly trapped. Yet, perversely, many women (for whom pregnancy is not a disaster) are aware of an odd pleasure that their fertility has triumphed over their conscious wish. Your partner may suspect that you wanted a baby all along and have not been "playing fair". Starting a baby under such circumstances can lead to conflict between you, because he may feel that you have not been open with him. Talk about it together: you need to understand each other.

Feelings about motherhood When you find out that you are pregnant you may actually have a crisis of self-confidence, feeling that you will be no good as a mother and have no maternal instincts. But mothering is a learned activity and little of it is purely instinctive. Moreover, for the first-time mother, who may never have handled a newborn baby, most of the learning goes on after the baby is born. The teacher is the baby. Even though you may not start as an expert, your baby will turn you into one.

Feelings about being on show You may feel suddenly that your most intimate relationship with the man you love is being publicly displayed, not just because you are pregnant and everybody knows, but because of the physical examinations and exposure at the antenatal clinic and the advice that people keep giving you. This sense of becoming public property may also be intensified by the obvious pleasure of your parents, who may have long been waiting for you to become pregnant.

Yet your body holds life. The wonder of that cannot really be understood by anyone else. You stand naked in front of the mirror and look for changes. You rest your hand on your tummy and wonder if you can feel the tiny seed of a baby beginning to grow inside you. You think back to when you made love and wonder which time it was that you conceived.

Feelings about your body If you feel on bad terms with your body as it starts out on the work of early pregnancy, arrange to attend some pregnancy exercise or dance classes if these are available in your area. Organizations that can help you are on pages 413–414. If these classes are not specially for pregnant women, let your teacher know that you are pregnant. Get out in the fresh air and walk. Buy a maternity swimsuit and swim regularly. Start doing the movements suggested on pages 124–125 a few times each day to pep up your circulation and increase vitality. In some countries massage is an anticipated and very pleasant part of being pregnant, so you

could go to a masseuse or your partner could learn how to massage you (see pages 186–194). This can be particularly useful if you are tense and find it difficult to release your muscles at will.

Your partner's feelings You are not the only person who has to adjust in pregnancy. Your partner does not have to cope with physical changes, but the emotional impact of a first pregnancy is no less real than your own, and the passage into fatherhood constitutes a major transition in his life. For a man this process is often delayed until several things have happened: the pregnancy has been officially confirmed; your figure has obviously changed; the baby has moved and he has felt it fluttering.

Emotions of joy, pride and wonder may be in conflict with other emotions of a more disturbing nature. There may be financial problems, which can cause a man to feel a sense of deep and burdensome responsibility for the new life that is coming.

A man, too, may feel trapped by pregnancy. Perhaps he felt that his relationship with the woman was intended to remain free and untrammeled by babies (especially if the couple have not discussed pregnancy and planned it together). His job may now assume importance not only in its own right, but because he feels an urgent need to be successful before the baby comes, as if it threatens his own powers of achievement. A man, too, may be frightened of birth and even of his partner's pregnant body, which can seem dangerous and not to be touched in case the baby is dislodged. He may feel that his own sexual desire is a terrible threat to the baby.

DISCUSSING YOUR EMOTIONS TOGETHER

It does not help to bottle up these emotions. If you pretend they are not there they become destructive. Anxiety has a positive function. It prods you to examine options, develop coping strategies, plan ahead, prepare yourselves emotionally and practically for the future. For example, you could avoid certain relatives until you feel you can cope with them. You may be able to arrange antenatal appointments together, so that your partner can meet the doctor or midwife and be present during the physical examination. Reading together about pregnancy and birth helps to replace ignorance with knowledge about the role a man can actively play in childbirth. Lying together in bed, cuddling and exploring each other's bodies is a way of communicating through loving touch and tenderness.

Pregnancy is not merely a waiting time. It is a time for working out together what you value in your relationship and what kind of world you both want to create for your child. This is not a question of making a nursery and buying things for the baby, but of helping each other to change from people who are responsible just for themselves into a mother and a father, with the new responsibility that parenthood brings. A man and a woman need to grow into parents. Then not only a baby, but a new family is born.

The realization that you are responsible for creating a new person may be awesome and sometimes overwhelming (opposite).

THE WOMAN ALONE

Pregnancy and childbirth are not easy when you have no partner to give you love and care. It is even more difficult once the baby is born to take complete responsibility for a new life. Yet many women have done this successfully and have reared happy, healthy children.

Talking about the single mother and the challenges she faces is in a way misleading, because women on their own bearing babies do not fall into one category any more than women with partners do. The reasons single women embark on pregnancy, and decide to go on with it, vary widely. Some continue with a pregnancy because they are unwilling or unable to face up to it and drift on hoping that it may go away. Others are bearing a much-wanted child "before it is too late". Others again loved the father of the child and hoped that the relationship would continue, but then found themselves rejected and bearing a child alone. There are also women whose men die while they are pregnant. And there are lesbian mothers who may have strong support from a female partner.

"Having Jane there made all the difference. She's had three children and understood exactly what I was feeling. She made suggestions, like thinking of my cervix opening during contractions, and helped by massaging the back of my neck with lavender oil and breathed with me when the going got difficult."

Whatever your reasons for having a child on your own, financial problems may loom large. Trying to combine a job with rearing a child, knowing that there is no one else to take over in time of need, can be difficult. It is important to anticipate and share the problems you will be coping with, and to seek counselling from people who understand them and who can put you in touch with other sources of help. Contact the organizations listed on pages 413–414 before you have your baby and see what they have to offer. They can help you cope with the practical difficulties such as housing, and sorting out which benefits you are entitled to. It is a good idea to book childbirth education classes (see page 176) as early as the third month. Many women delay until the last minute and find that classes are full. The Active Birth Centre and the National Childbirth Trust (addresses on pages 413–414) can tell you about the different classes, postnatal support and breastfeeding counselling available in your area.

Sometimes a man who is not a permanent partner is still willing to accept some of the responsibilities of fatherhood. It is quite common in an antenatal class to have couples who do not plan to marry or even stay together. Be frank with your antenatal teacher so that she has a chance to get to know you. It may be possible for you to arrange to see her privately for a session.

EMOTIONAL SUPPORT IN LABOUR

Think ahead to the birth and decide whether you would like to have a companion with you. Childbirth can feel very solitary if you do not have someone with you to encourage you and provide continuous emotional support. This person could be a good woman friend, a childbirth educator, a doula (a specific birth partner who is trained and experienced in supporting labouring women), a sister or your mother, or even a man friend who knows what birth is about and can give the right kind of help. Most hospitals allow companions in labour, although some restrict you to one person. Discuss the matter with your midwife and your antenatal teacher, and if necessary state your request in writing to the Director of Midwifery.

If there is no one who can be with you, discuss the subject in advance with your midwife. Say that you want someone with you throughout labour, and that you do not know anyone who can come with you; ask whether there is anyone – preferably someone you could meet beforehand – who could be with you. She may say that you will have a midwife and will not be left alone. But a birth companion is different and is simply there as a friend to give you emotional support and to remind you of your relaxation and breathing. If you are having your baby in hospital there may be a student midwife who can fill that role.

Suppose that you have to be without a companion in labour. Make the midwife your friend and ask her for help. Unfortunately there is still little continuity of care in many hospitals, and you may have to get to know two or three midwives, one after another – a lot to ask of someone in labour. On the other hand, sometimes one will stay on duty so that she can be with you until after the delivery.

MANAGING ALONE

If a man has been unwilling to accept responsibility or perhaps even acknowledge your pregnancy, you probably feel angry and resentful. One woman, who had been told she could never have a baby but who found herself pregnant, said, "I hadn't realized just how much his marriage was a going concern. Just when I most needed him I had to come to terms with the fact that he didn't want to break up his marriage and was devoted to his kids. My pregnancy was terribly embarrassing for him! I felt dreadfully on my own. I didn't hear from him through a large part of the pregnancy because it was the summer holidays and he went abroad with his family".

Another woman's husband left her when she was four months pregnant because he said he could not stand the idea of a third child. He had left her before for short periods and the baby was conceived during a reconciliation. Her great fear was that she would find him on the doorstep again, since she had been through so much emotional turmoil that she did not feel she could cope mentally with any more scenes. This led to a strained and difficult pregnancy followed by a prolonged labour and forceps delivery.

A university lecturer who had decided in advance that she wanted a baby but not a man said that her colleagues accepted this but that she found it difficult to tell her family: "Mother thought I was mad and said how could she ever let her friends know. I thought about them all at their coffee mornings and thought, 'Oh my God, I don't suppose she can.' I thought it would be hardest explaining to my 80-year-old grandmother but it turned out that she was the one who understood best". In fact, the woman's parents adjusted to the idea of her single motherhood after the baby was born and they became very proud grandparents.

Some women are rejected by parents, but one woman said: "In a way I rejected them and their values, by going ahead and having the baby". Even so, however "free" of your parents you may feel and however you delight in being independent of them, cutting roots like this can be extremely painful. You may feel guilty, even if you do not accept the social conventions which thrust feelings of guilt upon you. You may worry about imposing your views on your child, who will learn that in friends' houses there is a father as well as a mother.

The media tends to present single motherhood as a choice that many actresses and pop stars in their thirties or forties are making. Glamorous photographs accompany feature articles which give the impression that, like any other fashion accessory, a baby is the flavour of the moment. These women who are household names are not likely to be short of money and are able to employ nannies and other help. The decision to go it alone with a baby may result in many more practical difficulties for most of us.

Single mothers all stress that you do need help and must have the grace to accept it, for your child's sake as well as your own. There are the all-important questions of where you are going to live, what you are going to live on, whether you should and can go back to work, and if so, when. You must also then consider how you are going to retain any sort of mobility with a baby, how you will deal with the relationships between sex, motherhood and the other things you want to do, and how you are going to feel when things are difficult or impossible because of the baby. Many difficulties confronted by single women are the same as those faced by those with partners, but intensified because they are alone and unsupported. As one woman said, in order to go through with having a baby on your own, "you need to really want that child!"

Planning & preparation

Throughout history most babies were born at home. Maternity hospitals were first started for homeless women and were really extensions of the poor-houses. Many of the babies born in these hospitals were then put in foundling institutions. These first maternity hospitals were convenient centres for medical students to learn and practise obstetrics, but infection was rampant, since doctors conveyed bacteria on their hands from one patient to another, and many babies and mothers died. They were the most dangerous places in which women could possibly give birth.

Today, modern hospitals are no longer dangerous places to have a baby. Yet, despite very rapid advances and the tendency for most doctors to recommend a hospital birth, many women still feel a home birth would be the most appropriate for them.

WHERE WOULD YOU LIKE TO HAVE YOUR BABY?

Even before you are pregnant, or as early in pregnancy as you can, it is worth thinking about whether you would like to have your baby at home or in hospital – and if you decide on hospital, to discover whether you have any choices between hospitals. You can change your mind during pregnancy, but it is easier to switch from home to hospital than it is from hospital to home. So if you may want to have your baby at home you can keep your options open by saying this at the very beginning. If you discover that your GP is

"I'm considering the options open to me and am finding out about home birth because I'd like it to be as natural as possible."

discouraging and is not prepared to accept you as a patient, you can switch to another GP who does home births. But you do not need a doctor at all. You can write to the Director of Midwifery at your local hospital, say you are planning a home birth, and ask her to provide midwife cover. Midwives have a statutory duty to attend women in childbirth wherever they have their babies. Increasing numbers of midwives are really enjoying home births.

It is a good idea to make a list of things that are really important to you about the birth and the time immediately after, and to decide which environment best meets your requirements: home or hospital.

Hospital birth

Most women who decide to have their babies in hospital do so primarily because they are convinced it is the safest place. They want to be sure that all the skills and equipment of modern obstetrics are at hand for their baby's sake. For some women, especially those having their first child, giving birth is a frightening experience, a step in the dark, and they feel more secure in the knowledge that they are in the hands of a team who have been specially trained to cope with any possible emergencies that might arise. Often a woman who fears that her labour will be painful opts for a hospital delivery, knowing that there are certain painkillers that are available only in a hospital and not wanting to take the chance of finding herself in labour at home without any relief from pain when it is far too late to do anything about it.

Sometimes a woman may know and trust a particular obstetrician and want to be cared for by this person, while another woman wants to go to hospital because she feels she would probably benefit from a short period of release from the pressures of home and family. Occasionally a woman's partner would prefer her to go to hospital because he is very concerned about birth at home. He may just be frightened of being involved, but more frequently he is afraid that he might have to deliver the baby himself.

MEDICAL REASONS FOR HOSPITAL BIRTH

As well as those women who would prefer the security of hospital birth, there are those for whom it is advisable to give birth in hospital whatever their personal preferences. It is wise to consider hospital care if you have diabetes or a heart or kidney condition. Your doctor or midwife will have you admitted to hospital if you get pre-eclampsia (see page 139) or if you go into labour three weeks or more before your baby is due; you will probably be advised against home delivery if your baby is breech, since the baby may need some help with breathing immediately after birth (see page 366). There are really no absolutes, but there are certain factors that contribute to making childbirth a little more risky.

If you are over 40 and a first-time mother, for instance, labour may be longer than if you were younger, and many doctors would advise you to be in hospital so that you can have labour speeded up or get help with the delivery. Some doctors believe that all first-time mothers (primigravidas) should give birth in hospital because, they say, a labour is only normal in retrospect and there is always a small chance that even after a perfectly normal pregnancy you may have complications during the birth that will entail your being moved to hospital at the last minute for specialist care.

If you have had a haemorrhage with a previous labour, either before or after the delivery, you might want to choose hospital birth because you may need a quick blood transfusion if it happens again. (On the other hand, did you bleed because of aggressive intervention, and are you less likely to bleed if the labour progresses naturally?) The same goes for a retained placenta in a previous labour. Sometimes hospital interventions themselves contribute to the likelihood of birth complications.

If you are very short, under 1.55 m (5 ft 2 in), your pelvis may be a tight fit for the baby to get through, although many short women can and do give birth easily. Any other indications of disproportion,

For some women a one-to-one relationship with a midwife is an important element in choosing a home birth (opposite).

because of the way the baby is lying, for example, could also lead you to consider hospital birth. Three or more miscarriages are another reason for having the baby in hospital, because previous problems of this kind may mean that labour will present problems (although often everything is straightforward). If you have lost a baby because of a previous difficult birth, you will want to know that, if the baby should need it, intensive care is available at the hospital where you are giving birth. Doctors also advise mothers of twins to give birth in hospital, partly because they may come early and be of low birthweight and partly because the second twin sometimes gets stuck. But if both bodies are head down and full term, you may decide that home is the best place for the birth because you want to avoid any unnecessary intervention and know that you have the support of experienced and skilled midwives.

"The obstetrician was very pleasant. He told me they'd just had a baby three months ago. That made a lot of difference."

WHICH HOSPITAL?

There may be several choices of hospital in your area. You might have a choice between two large hospitals or between a large and a small one. A small hospital may actually be a GP unit or a midwife-run "cottage" type hospital.

The best way to find out what a hospital is like is to talk to other women who have given birth there within the last two years. If you do not know any, your local NCT branch will be able to put you in touch with some and an NCT or Active Birth teacher will be happy to discuss the alternatives with you.

CHOICES IN HOSPITAL CARE

If you have decided that a hospital birth is right for you, you will need to think about the alternatives available within the hospital system. There are two main kinds of maternity unit, a consultant unit or a general practitioner unit, as well as the Domino scheme.

Consultant units If you are having your baby under the NHS in a consultant unit, you are looked after by a team under the direction of a specialist. If the specialist is attached to a teaching hospital, medical students may also be involved in your care. If you are having the baby privately, the consultant sees you and contracts to attend your birth and deliver you if possible. It is your GP who refers you to a particular consultant in the hospital. You are not normally asked whether you have any preferences, but you can in fact choose your consultant, provided you make your request early enough in your pregnancy. GPs do not like their patients changing from one consultant to another, mainly because of the administrative difficulties this involves, so it is best to ask around and find out from other mothers about the practices of different consultants and then to discuss this with your GP before your case is referred.

Teaching hospitals and general hospitals in which consultant units are based, tend to have a great deal of technologically advanced machinery and are to be recommended especially for pregnancies where the baby may be "at risk" and where it is vital to keep a careful eye on mother and baby. If there is any indication that the baby may be born before term and be of very low birthweight, birth should be in a unit with a neonatal intensive care unit, equipped with all the sophisticated technology and manned by specially skilled staff to give your baby the best attention possible.

GP units In a GP unit, which may be a small cottage hospital or a ward inside a larger consultant unit, you stay under the care of a GP and the midwives who work with that particular practice. The GP may not be your usual family doctor since not all of them are trained in obstetrics. Your doctor may pass you on to another GP for obstetric care or you can find one yourself who, you feel, understands and sympathizes with the style of childbirth you would like. These units are for low-risk care where it looks as if everything is going to be straightforward. By the time you are ready to give birth, you usually know the midwife who will deliver you and consequently feel more relaxed. GP units far away from consultant units do entail some extra risk, however, and you should only be booked into a hospital of this kind if no complications are expected.

The Domino scheme Some hospitals offer an alternative to the consultant unit in the Domino scheme, in which community midwives bring their own patients into hospital and deliver them themselves. The midwives then go home with the mothers after they have had a rest following childbirth, which may be anything from a few hours to a day and night, depending on the wishes of the mother and the state of her and her baby. Your GP will be able to tell you whether Domino operates in your nearest big hospital.

LOOKING OVER THE HOSPITAL

Some Directors of Midwifery are happy to arrange for you to look over the hospital where you are to give birth before you book in. If it is not the usual practice to do this in a hospital, get in touch with the antenatal out-patients sister and ask if you can talk to whoever runs childbirth classes. There is probably a visit by the antenatal class to the labour and delivery suite and you may be able to go too (see page 183). You can also write to the Director of Midwifery asking about the things that matter most to you.

When you see the hospital, bear in the mind that people matter more than the architecture and interior decoration. Do you get a sense of a warm, caring atmosphere or do the staff seem brusque? The attitude of the doctors and nurses towards you and your child's birth is one of the most important factors in making hospital birth a rewarding experience.

The birth room

Until recently birth rooms were organized exclusively for the comfort and convenience of doctors and midwives, instead of the woman having the baby. In many hospitals that has changed and there are birth beds and other equipment that enable the woman to sit upright, kneel, squat and stand with something solid to grip on to. But obstetric practice often limits women's opportunities to move about and get into different positions. If you have had an epidural or are harpooned to an intravenous drip or electronic fetal monitor – or both – it may be almost impossible to move at all. In England and Wales 87 per cent of hospitals state that women can choose their own positions in childbirth, but in effect 74 per cent of women are in a reclining position.* This is often because of obstetric interventions, such as having an intravenous drip set up and being tethered to an electronic fetal monitor, which keep women in bed and leave them with little or no choice of position.

Women who can remain upright in the first stage of labour have less pain, so need fewer pain-relieving drugs, and dilate faster than those women who are lying down. Their babies' heart rates are also more likely to fall within the normal range.*

"I got stuck flat on my back last time I was in labour and felt trapped. This time it was much better as I was able to move about; I felt in control, and it was so much easier to handle the pain."

In the second stage being upright also results in less pain, fewer drugs, easier pushing, fewer tears, more normal vaginal births and, in fact, a more positive birth experience.* When you look around the hospital take special note of how you could use ledges at different heights and furniture in the birth room to give you support and move your pelvis. Ask for a bean bag to flop over or lean against, or take one into hospital, if it is not already provided.

Hospitals may now also offer a rocking chair for the first stage and a birth stool and squatting bar to grasp in the second stage. Some have elaborate birth beds or chairs that can be switched to almost any position. These may look impressive, but the important thing is to have the equipment under your own control, not someone else's, and to be free to move your pelvis.

Whatever happens, the equipment is less important than you. It should not be allowed to dominate or restrict what you do during birth. Look critically at whatever is on offer and think how you may want to use it, if at all. A sculptural design is not helpful if it limits your movements. One problem with sitting on a rigid chair or stool for a long time, especially one with back support that limits the pelvic movements you can make, is that you may develop swelling around your vulva and the circulation of blood may be impeded, so that you bleed more heavily with the birth.* When it comes down to it, the best physical support may come from other human beings holding you while you do whatever you want to do at the time.

Another item of equipment that may be available is a birth pool. Most hospitals in Britain have a pool nowadays, although in many it is used for labour, rather than birth. Seize the opportunity to use it, if only during the first stage of labour. It gives extraordinary relief from pain and a more private, personal environment for your labour. In larger pools you can move freely, and there is plenty of room for you to give birth in the water.

If a pool is not available in your hospital, you can rent a portable pool and take it with you into hospital. Discuss this with the midwife at the antenatal clinic. Details of places from which you can hire pools are given on pages 413–414.

Home birth

While hospital birth remains the standard way to have a baby, there is a small but steady increase in the number of women who decide to have their babies at home. Most women who have a baby at home after a previous hospital birth say that they enjoyed it much more and feel that it must have been much pleasanter for the baby. Some opt for home births because they want to give birth in a familiar, comfortable, non-medical environment, surrounded by their own possessions, in the home they have created with their partner. They want to be able to make their own decisions, to give birth in their own way and behave spontaneously, without being forced into the role of patient and having to conform to hospital rules and regulations. They also want to avoid having to change rooms and move from a bed to a delivery room, and to be able to adopt any position they find comfortable. In your own home you are in charge and the midwife and doctor and his or her assistant are familiar and welcome guests in your home.

For some women, this continuous relationship and co-operation with just a few helpers is extremely important.

"My eight-year-old daughter made a birthday cake for the baby while I was in the first stage of labour and we celebrated afterwards with the cake, champagne and lemonade."

Some women say that since birth is an act of love, personal and intimate, it should take place in one's own environment, without unnecessary observers, among friends in a loving atmosphere. They want to know that the father of the baby or a close friend can be present, can take an active part, and can give emotional support through the labour. Some would like the father to "catch" the baby himself. Most hospitals allow fathers to be present for labour and delivery nowadays, but they are sometimes sent out for some procedures, just when the labouring woman feels she needs her partner most.

Often a woman would like to ensure that her baby has a "gentle birth" and that he or she is welcomed into the world with tenderness, without the machinery and bright lights that are often inevitable in hospitals.

A midwife gets to know her client during the pregnancy and routine checks are part of an ongoing relationship (right).

Your blood pressure is less likely to be raised when you are happy and relaxed (below).

"BONDING" OCCURS NATURALLY

Evidence of research on "bonding" between mother, father and baby points towards the importance of the time immediately following birth for the couple to get to know their baby and feel it belongs to them and that they belong to it. In some hospitals separation immediately after the child is born is still arbitrarily imposed on new parents, time for cuddling is either restricted or denied, and routines take precedence over the emotional unfolding that heralds the birth of a family.

Many women also suspect that medical intervention is often unnecessary and that they will have a better chance of giving birth naturally and without drugs at home. They believe that full awareness of what is happening to them is a valuable experience and that drugs can be harmful to their unborn babies. After a previous difficult hospital birth, one pregnant woman said: "I was determined to have a natural birth this time. Last time I had the whole works, and finished up with an epidural and a forceps delivery. I can't help thinking that if I let things take their own time and keep walking around, and can relax and use my breathing and feel comfortable in my own home, with the people I love around me, my body will know what to do".

If you already have other children, you may be concerned that they should see giving birth as a normal, happy part of life and not as a surgical operation that entails your going off to hospital. Birth is a family affair and the baby should belong to the whole family. Some women hope that the other child or children can be involved in the labour, and some would like them present at the birth. This is difficult or impossible to arrange in most hospitals. Some mothers who have never left their toddlers worry that separation from them will lead to emotional and behavioural problems in the older child, and this just at a time when the new baby puts in an appearance. There are also those mothers who just find it impossible to get someone to look after their family while they are away in hospital. It is sometimes stated that women having their fourth or subsequent babies should always give birth in hospital, but if all your previous pregnancies and labours have been straightforward, there is no additional risk with a fourth or fifth birth and some definite advantage in giving birth at home where the other children can also be involved.

Some doctors are reluctant to give their approval to your having a home birth once you are actually pregnant, even though they have seemed flexible earlier. For example, one woman said that her doctor had agreed to a home birth for her third child "in principle" before she was pregnant but then "did her best to change our minds. She did not really seem to understand that there was absolutely no one who could come to look after our other children, and that I would not have my husband with me if the baby was not born at home . . . There were many occasions when I was

UNDERSTANDING YOUR MEDICAL RECORD

It can be very confusing to try to decipher your medical record, and some of the abbreviations may suggest alarming abnormalities. Here are some of the abbreviations most likely to be used. You can ask your doctor or midwife to explain any that you do not understand. Two-way communication is vital in a working partnership.

Abbr/term	Full title/Name	Meaning of abbreviation
Para 0		The mother has had no previous birth.
Para 1 (or 2)		The mother has had one (or two) previous births.
Para 2 + 1		The mother has had two previous births plus a miscarriage (or termination) before 28 weeks.
LMP	Last menstrual period	Date of first day of last menstrual period.
EDD/EDC	Expected date of delivery	Expected date of delivery or expected date of confinement.
Alb	Albumin in urine	Your urine is analyzed for the presence of sugar, which may be a sign of diabetes, and albumin (protein) which can be a sign of pre-eclampsia. When sugar is present, it is noted as a percentage. Two per cent is a large amount. Ideally albumin should not be present at all. There are occasional traces of sugar and albumin in a normal pregnancy.
Hb	Haemoglobin	Haemoglobin is an oxygen-carrying substance present in red blood cells. If your haemoglobin level is lower than 10.5 per cent, or your hematocrit (see below) is below 32 per cent, you may be considered to be anaemic and be prescribed iron. Because of the greater quantity of circulating blood, most healthy pregnant women have reduced haemoglobin.
Hct	Hematocrit	Hematocrit is the percentage of red blood cells in the blood.
Fe	Iron	This means that you have been prescribed iron.
BP	Blood pressure	This is the pressure inside the arteries as the blood is pumped from the heart. The pressure that is built up every time the heart beats is called systolic pressure. Between beats the heart muscle relaxes and the pressure drops. This lower level is called diastolic pressure. Systolic pressure is the upper figure on your card, diastolic pressure the lower. The lower figure is more significant than the upper one. A woman is considered to have moderately high blood pressure, hypertension, if it exceeds 140/90 when measured on more than one occasion.
FHT	Fetal heart tones	The number of fetal heartbeats per minute.

Abbr/term	Full title/Name	Meaning of abbreviation
H/NH	Heard/not heard	This usually refers to the fetal heart.
Oedema	Swelling	Part of your weight gain is due to water retention, causing puffiness in the feet and ankles, hands, and vulva. A great deal of fluid retention may be a sign of pre-eclampsia, but it can be perfectly normal.
Fundus	The top of the uterus	As the baby grows, the fundus is pushed up to just above your navel at 22 weeks and under your ribs at 36 weeks. But when the baby drops down into the bony pelvis ready for birth the fundus is lower again. You can find your own fundus and chart its position week by week through your pregnancy. Lie on your back with your tummy bare and, with the sides and palms of your hands, feel around the hard top of your uterus, pressing against what feels like a wall of muscle.
Cx	Cervix	The neck of the uterus, which softens, shortens, and opens during birth.
PP	The presenting part of the baby	This is the part which is down at the bottom of the uterus and likely to be the first to press through the opening cervix if you are at the end of pregnancy. In the last few weeks the doctor or midwife may note the presentation precisely, so that you can get an idea of exactly what part of the baby is in the cervix.
Vx/Vtx	Vertex	This indicates the baby's position is head down, as it should be.
Ceph	Cephalic	This also indicates that the baby's position is head down.
Long L	Longitudinal lie	The baby is lying parallel to your spine.
LOA LOP ROA ROP	Left Occipito Anterior Left Occipito Posterior Right Occipito Anterior Right Occipito Posterior	These terms all refer to the position (anterior or posterior) of the crown of the baby's head (occiput) in relation to your body (right or left). Therefore ROP means that the baby's head is to your right and back.
RSA	Right sacrum anterior	This is the most common breech presentation.
Eng/E	Engaged	This is written on your card when the baby's head has dropped down into your pelvis, which can happen any time from about six weeks before you go into labour until after you have actually started.
T	Term	The doctor or midwife writes this on your card when it is estimated that you are right at the end of your pregnancy and the baby is ready to be born.

reduced to tears on my arrival home. If I had been less determined, or if my husband had not been so supportive, I should have given in". If you are concerned that this might happen to you, you could contact the organizations on pages 413–414.

CHANGING CHILDBIRTH

The early 1990s brought new health service policy concerning childbirth. A Government-commissioned report entitled "Changing Childbirth" is now official policy. The first principles are that "the woman must be at the focus of maternity care, in control of what is happening to her. Women can "choose where her babies are born and their right to make this choice should be respected".* The aim is that every woman can get to know one midwife, who ensures continuity and helps her plan the kind of care she would like. In many cases a midwife, not a doctor, is the one who has access to beds so that she can admit her own patients without having to go through a doctor.

One-to-one midwife care is being introduced in some hospitals, and is worth asking about. It has many advantages. When a midwife gets to know her client well and does not have to flit from one task to another with different women, a woman in labour needs fewer pain-relieving drugs. If she does have them, they may work better. She is less likely to need an epidural and has fewer interventions, such as being tethered to a fetal monitor. She is also less at risk of episiotomy and more likely to have an intact perineum. Women who have this kind of care feel more positive about the birth, their own preparedness and how well they manage. In fact most who have a personal midwife say that birth was "hard work but wonderful".*

Whether or not you are able to get one-to-one midwifery care, the UK Central Council for Nursing, Midwifery and Health Visiting instructs midwives that women must have choice: "Practice must . . . be sensitive, relevant, and responsive to the needs of individual patients and clients".* Suppose you want to use a birth pool for instance: "Water birth", the UKCC says, "must fall within the duty of care and normal sphere of the midwife, who has responsibility to develop her skills and give the right kind of help".

You cannot make accurate choices without accurate information. The Midwives Information and Resources Centre, together with the NHS, now produce "informed choice" leaflets. Each leaflet is published in two forms; one is intended for professionals, the other for pregnant women. The professional version gives more information and includes all the research references, so that if you can get hold of that version you will probably find it the most useful. Topics include alcohol in pregnancy, blood tests for congenital abnormalities, ultrasound in pregnancy, the place of birth, support in childbirth, positions in labour and delivery, epidural analgesia, monitoring the baby during birth and bottle-feeding versus breastfeeding. You can ask your GP, midwife, or hospital clinic for these free leaflets.

Antenatal care

One ingredient of a happy birth is good antenatal care, so that you are confident that you are healthy and the baby starts life under the best possible conditions. But the care you give yourself is probably more important than the care you receive from professionals. It also includes learning how to cope with stress in everyday life and understanding how to work with your body. You do not need to attend classes until you are five or more months pregnant, but it is worth thinking about the different classes available and perhaps beginning a few exercises earlier than this.

Antenatal care has progressed piecemeal since the 19th century and we do not really know which elements in the entire package are valuable for all women, which are best kept for those at special risk and which might be discarded altogether. It is common for confusion to occur about whether a baby is growing well inside the uterus, for example, and many women are told that there is intra-uterine growth retardation when, in fact, it turns out that everything is fine. In spite of this, good medical care during pregnancy every now and then can make all the difference between life and death for the baby – and even, very occasionally, for the mother, too.*

Unfortunately, in the antenatal clinic waiting for appointments is usually a fact of life. It is a good idea to take a book or needlework, or make friends with other expectant mothers attending the same clinic to keep each other company.

Some couples come together and many clinics actually encourage fathers to be there but sometimes this is not expected and fathers may be asked to remain in the waiting room. If, however, it is important to you that you both talk to the doctor or midwife and that your partner be involved in the pregnancy, not only the birth, it is worthwhile being quietly but firmly persistent to get what you want. Think through beforehand any questions or worries that you may have. Many women find it easier to write down their questions so that they will not forget to ask in the rush. If there is anything you particularly hope for concerning the way in which you have your baby, ask the doctor or midwife if it can be noted on your record.

Many tests in pregnancy, the value of which has been taken for granted in the past, are now being questioned. Multi-centre research is taking place to determine whether they do what they are assumed to do or even if they do more harm than good. This is the only way to discover which are useful and which should be discarded. If there is justifiable uncertainty about a screening procedure or other intervention and you are invited to take part in a randomized controlled trial, consider all the implications seriously. You have the right to be fully informed about any research in which you are taking part; you can consent or refuse, and can leave the study if and when you wish.

ROUTINE TESTS

Most women see their doctor or midwife once a month until they are 32 weeks pregnant. At this stage you will be seen every two weeks and in your final month will be given weekly appointments.

During a typical visit you may be weighed before you see the doctor. While your baby is growing, you will probably be putting on weight fairly steadily (see page 94).

At the first antenatal visit the midwife or doctor may listen to your heart. Heart sounds change during pregnancy, and a heart murmur may be detected. This is usually perfectly normal.

Your blood group is determined at your first visit and a test is done to check whether the baby might develop Rhesus disease (see page 113). Your blood is automatically tested for syphilis and you may be offered amniocentesis (see page 226). At each visit your blood pressure and urine will be tested and your weight, the height of the fundus and the fetal heartbeat (as soon as it is audible) will also be checked. You may be offered screening for spina bifida and Down's syndrome (see pages 220–223). Regular blood tests are done for anaemia (see page 143). However, what was once treated in pregnancy as "anaemia" is usually a normal drop in haemoglobin due to plasma volume expansion. A pregnant woman has about 40 per cent more blood flowing in her body. It used to be thought that women's haemoglobin levels must be kept high during pregnancy

Having a vaginal examination

You may be examined vaginally early in your pregnancy. If you are more than six weeks pregnant the midwife or doctor will be able to detect a slight enlargement and softening of the uterus. The embryo is well protected and cannot be dislodged by the examination.

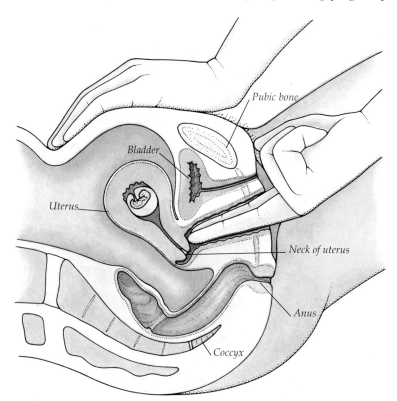

Pubic bone

Bladder

Uterus

Neck of uterus

Anus

Coccyx

by giving iron supplementation. But women whose haemoglobin concentration *does* fall are more likely to go to full term and to have babies of good birth weight. If haemoglobin concentration fails to fall there is a marked increase in the incidence of low birth weight and pre-term birth.*

In fact, a woman who is pregnant is better able to absorb iron from food. If you drink orange juice instead of tea or coffee, both of which inhibit absorption of iron, your body will make good use of the iron which is naturally present in the food you eat.*

An ultrasound scan (see page 223) may be suggested at any time during the pregnancy. The use of ultrasound at around 16 weeks is routine in most hospitals. However, you can refuse if you do not want one. In late pregnancy a single scan can show the size of the baby's head in relation to your pelvic outlet. If you have a series of scans at different sessions, an estimate can be made of the baby's rate of growth and expected date of delivery.

At the first antenatal visit you may have a vaginal examination. At most subsequent visits the uterus and baby will be felt by abdominal palpation, not by a pelvic examination. As this is done, you should give a long breath out and release your tummy completely, then go on breathing slowly, releasing more on each breath out. This makes it easier to determine how the baby is lying and is much more comfortable for you than when you are tense.

The examining hands feel first for the distance between your pubic bone and the baby and then the top of the uterus. This process is called fundal palpation. The hands move down the sides of the baby so that by late pregnancy the back and limbs can be felt. The part of the baby that is positioned over the cervix is said to be "presenting". The doctor or midwife turns to face your feet and presses his or her hands downwards and from side to side to determine whether the baby's head, buttocks, or any other part, is presenting. The next manoeuvre tends to be uncomfortable but is quickly performed. Facing you again, one hand is spread wide and presses in above your pubic bone to feel the exact position of the presenting part in relation to the pelvis.

In late pregnancy, take the opportunity to find out how your baby is lying and discuss anything that may be worrying you. Become aware of fetal movements and tell your caregivers about any distinct change in their frequency or how they feel.

Talking to doctors

Some people have doctors with whom they quickly feel at ease and experience little difficulty discussing their own requirements. However, the expectant mother and her doctor are more likely to meet in a system in which time is at a premium and sometimes one or both of them finds it difficult to avoid a formal relationship with all that this implies of authority and subordination.

Being pregnant is a physiological process. It also involves a kind of emotional journey into being a patient. And as if all this were not enough, it propels you into new kinds of social relationships. Some of these are with the professionals you encounter during your pregnancy. So, as well as having to understand the changes taking place in your own body and your emotions, you may have to develop new social skills to create a satisfactory dialogue with those who care for you and your baby. This is especially the case when you meet different doctors and midwives at each clinic visit and others again when in labour. The lack of continuity in care is one of the main criticisms that women have made about childbirth in hospital.*

Some women feel very vulnerable emotionally when they are pregnant, and cannot help crying under pressure, even though (or perhaps because) it is the last thing they *want* to do. You are not abnormal if you feel intense surges of emotion that are difficult or impossible to control, but you may feel at a disadvantage in an interview with a doctor when you want to ask for something or talk about the kind of birth you are hoping for.

This possibility is a good reason for having your partner or a close friend or relative with you on such occasions. It is important, of course, that you discuss your wishes thoroughly with this person first. You may find it useful for him or her to play "the devil's advocate" and act out an imagined encounter so that you have some practice in discussing the subject and can develop a strategy. Do not make the mistake of anticipating opposition from hospital staff; you will probably be pleasantly surprised. But do be prepared to give carefully thought-out reasons for what you want.

See that you are well briefed about the matters you want to discuss. Today there is a good deal of published research on emotional and sociological aspects of maternity care, for example, and many papers on the technology of modern obstetrics and the active management of labour (see page 329) are published in medical journals. It will help if you have a clear idea of some of the most important statements. If you are attending childbirth education classes, you can ask your teacher to help. The National Childbirth Trust produces leaflets and books,* and the Informed Choice leaflets published by MIDIRS are chockfull of up-to-date information.

PREPARING YOUR QUESTIONS

Since questions may go out of your head when you have a chance to ask them (pregnancy amnesia is a well-known phenomenon), and because some doctors seem to concentrate on the lower end of your body to the exclusion of you as a person, it is a good idea to jot down subjects on paper. Hospitals vary in their routine interventions. You may not want some or all of them, and it is best to state your preferences as early as possible. On the other hand, you may want an intervention that would not usually be given but is probably available if you make a special request. Your list could include

In childbirth classes *you learn different positions and movements to help you give birth actively (opposite).*

47

questions concerning the use of ultrasound in pregnancy. You can find more about that on page 223. You may also want to explore doctor's policy on induction and augmentation of labour, routine enemas or suppositories, intravenous drips, electronic fetal monitoring, episiotomy, forceps (see page 334) and Caesarean section. You could ask about the policy concerning drugs for pain relief and epidural (see page 309) and enquire whether you will be able to keep your baby with you day and night. It may also be important for you to know whether there will be a special midwife to help with breastfeeding, and to know her name in advance. Be specific in your requests, to avoid any misunderstandings later on.

Sometimes the clinic is so crowded that you feel reluctant to take up anybody's time with your questions. Even so, it is probably worth saying that you have made a note of things you would like to discuss and ask whether it is convenient that day, or, if not, whether you can arrange to have some time to talk at the next visit. There is no need to be apologetic about wanting further information or asking for help to achieve the kind of birth you would like. After all, you are not just a baby-producing machine!

During the interview make sure you sit in a relaxed way, check that fingers and toes are unclenched, and breathe out just before speaking for the first time. Make eye contact and address the doctor by name or ask his or her name if you do not know it.

When a woman is feeling nervous, she tends to pitch her voice too high. Modulate it so that it does not sound too demanding. You might also smile nervously without realizing it. This can be confusing for the doctor, who then thinks that you are happy about something when you are not. Or it may be that the doctor unconsciously smiles because he or she is concerned to get you to accept another point of view and is sugaring the pill; your spontaneous reaction may then be to smile back, giving the doctor the idea that you are content when in fact you are not.

Avoid aggression and state your requests clearly and concisely. If you lose your temper, you may be classified as difficult or neurotic. If you encounter opposition or are made to feel that you cannot know what is in your best interests, restate your wishes firmly and give the reasons for them. It is a good idea to include requests that are not top priority, so that there is a possibility of compromise on some matters. Belligerence provokes further opposition. Tell your doctor instead how happy or disappointed you are. Always try to give "I" messages rather than "you" messages. Say "I prefer . . ." or "I'm unhappy about . . ." Be assertive in a pleasant way. You may not have any medical knowledge about your body, but you know a great deal about it all the same, since it is you who lives in it. If a woman acts as if she expects to be bossed around, it is more likely that she will be. Some doctors think it is enough to have a chat with you when you are lying flat on your back with your knickers off. You can say that you would like to talk clothed and face-to-face. If a test or intervention is proposed that you do not want, either now or during childbirth, simply say, "No, thank you," and repeat it if necessary. If this seems too difficult, practise speaking out in less threatening situations, perhaps with your colleagues at work or with members of your family, for instance. Complain in a shop that has sold you shoddy goods, tell guests who are still hanging round your home at midnight that it is time you went to bed, or send back bad food in a restaurant.

You may want to take notes of the conversation you have with your doctor, and can always say: "I'd like to think more about that; may I just make a note of it?" However, you should be careful not to imply that you are cross-examining the doctor and writing down any answers in preparation for a later attack. Make it clear that you are listening closely by "playing back" the important statements: "Do you mean . . . ?" "So you are saying that . . . ?" and rephrase whatever has been said as accurately as you can. You can sometimes add to your remark the implications that you think such a statement entails. By clarifying a point in this way you may be working towards modifying it. For example, if the doctor says, "I never allow husbands to remain if I have to give the patient a vaginal examination or do a forceps delivery because they only get in the way", you might ask: "Are you saying that it is dangerous for a husband to stay because he might affect your judgment?" Few experienced obstetricians would say that the presence of a husband could affect their professional judgment, and the doctor might reply by telling you a story about men who have fainted. In response to this you could say: "I take it you feel happier about a man who stays calm and who gives emotional support to his wife?"

"I'm not used to being assertive but my doctor was OK about it and we've had some lively discussions."

If your interview has gone badly, you can consider changing your doctor, or alternatively, if there is more than one in your area, the hospital where you are to have the baby. But it is best to give yourself a couple of days to simmer down and think it over calmly before finally deciding. You can write a letter explaining your reasons for seeking other care; it is a good idea to send copies to the Manager if it concerns a hospital. But such drastic measures are usually unnecessary, and you will find that you can open up the possibility of getting the kind of childbirth you want by other means. There is always a price to pay for being submissive. A woman avoids conflict but afterwards frequently feels that birth was something done *to* her, not something she did herself. Women who have suffered a sense of complete powerlessness in birth may go on feeling this long after the baby is born. It often leads to their feeling incompetent with the baby, too.

Good communication means that, if for medical reasons you do not get all you had hoped for in terms of care and advice you can still take an active part in decision-making. And it may be that you will improve conditions for other women.

Making your birth plan

Here are some of the questions you might like to consider in constructing your birth plan. Some may not be relevant to you and you may wish to include others, but this list should get you off to a good start.

Q Who would you like to have with you during labour and at the birth? Do you want to place a limit on the number of people caring for you?

Q What is your top priority while in labour? Is there anything that matters to you apart from the safety of your baby and yourself?

Q Do you want to put yourself unreservedly in your caregivers' hands and leave them to get on with it, or do you want to be kept fully informed of all developments and to share in any discussions and decisions made?

Q How do you plan to cope with the pain you are likely to experience during labour?

Q Are there any things you would like to have in the birth room with you, for example, pictures, familiar objects, candles, aromatherapy essences, music or equipment to give you physical support and enable you to get into comfortable positions?

Q Have you any special requests about the birth itself, such as having the lights in the birth room dimmed, receiving or avoiding an episiotomy, and the way in which the baby is delivered?

Q Is there anything that is important for you to be able to do during labour, such as using a shower, tub or birth pool, being able to adopt upright positions and move your pelvis, using alternative methods of pain relief, or being free to make a lot of noise?

Q What are your thoughts about common medical procedures that may be used during labour, such as artificial rupture of the membranes, hormone stimulation of the uterus, electronic fetal monitoring, an intravenous drip, pain-relieving drugs, restriction of positions and movements and the active management of labour?

Q Do you want the third stage of labour to be speeded up with a hormone injection and controlled cord traction immediately after the birth, or would you prefer the afterbirth to be delivered physiologically?

Q Have you any special requests about the hour following birth, for example, keeping your baby in bed with you and in skin-to-skin contact, or being left alone with your partner and your baby to enjoy a little privacy? Would you like the pediatrician to examine the baby in your presence?

Q In the 24 hours after birth how much time would you like to spend with your baby, for example would you like to keep her in bed with you, in a cot beside your bed, or in the nursery for some or most of the time? Are you happy to be woken up at night in order to feed your baby or would you rather be left to sleep?

Q How do you intend to feed your baby? If you plan to breastfeed, are you willing for your baby to be given supplementary formula, dextrose or water, or do you want him or her to have breast milk only?

Q What other things are important to you after the birth, for example, if you have a boy do you want him to be circumcised or not, and would you like your partner to be able to stay with you both overnight?

MAKING YOUR BIRTH PLAN

A birth plan is a list of your priorities and wishes for the birth and the time immediately afterwards. It is best constructed after you have met your caregivers and discussed your options with them, but early enough for you to negotiate any modifications in hospital protocols or a midwife's standard practice. One copy is clipped to the doctor's notes and you keep another copy yourself.

If you have had a baby before you will be pretty clear what is most important to you about the care you receive. If you work in the health services yourself, or have listened to other women's accounts of birth with the same caregivers or in the same hospital, you may also have a clear idea of exactly what you want and do not want. This may include the kind of setting in which you wish to give birth, and the general style of birth you prefer – high-tech, epidural or drug-free and mobile, for instance.

Some people think the idea of a birth plan is ridiculous because no one knows in advance how birth is going to be. That is true. But if you were setting off on safari, or even on a picnic when you were not sure how the weather would turn out, you would plan for alternatives. It is the same with birth. You know what you want, and you also know what you want if things do not turn out exactly as expected.

Doctors and midwives do not have to be burdened with patients' trusting reverence, and many nowadays prefer women to think through what they want and to make choices. There are still caregivers who feel threatened by birth plans and see them as undermining their authority and expertise, like the obstetrician who said he could not stand "backseat drivers". Yet when women become utterly dependent on those caring for them it can be more threatening than open confrontation, for if things go wrong and a baby is damaged or dies, total faith then often turns to litigation. It is almost invariably those who put their unquestioning trust in an obstetrician who sue for malpractice – not women who accept responsibility, weigh the pros and cons of different kinds of care, and make decisions for themselves. It is also sometimes suggested that making a birth plan shows lack of trust in the doctor or midwife. But at best it is something you do *together*. It enables your caregiver to learn about you at the same time that you learn about him or her. It can be a positive part of your developing relationship, and can contribute a lot to it. Those who oppose the idea of birth plans often urge women to be nice to their doctors in order to get what they want. But being nice is often not enough. The kind of doctor who brushes aside a request for "natural childbirth" by saying, "Of course you can give birth naturally. All birth is natural", or who tells you, "You can hang from a chandelier as far as I'm concerned", is likely to want you harpooned to a fetal monitor, and may be knife-happy, too. Stating your wishes in writing and confidently affirming expectations gives you a greater chance of having what you want than playing the part of the obedient patient. Birth plans are a vital part of an active approach to labour as a spontaneous process in which a woman's body knows how to act without anyone having to "manage" it. Yet they can equally well be used if a woman is certain that she wants an epidural or is convinced that induction is a good thing to have if she goes a week "overdue".

What to include in your birth plan Some things will be simple and straightforward: for example, points such as "I should like to hold the baby immediately, skin to skin" . . . "I would like to be helped to lift the baby out of my own body." These may already be standard practices for your midwife or doctor. Other choices may be more complicated and entail further discussion. As an example, if the early stages of labour are long drawn out, what, if any, interventions might be proposed and which would you prefer? With the method of active management of labour, which is increasingly popular in hospitals all over the world, every woman whose cervix fails to dilate one centimetre every hour has her uterus stimulated artificially by hormones that are introduced through an intravenous drip into her bloodstream. The principle behind this treatment is that no labour should be allowed to exceed 12 hours. The Irish obstetricians who devised this system of management say it is what women want, that women like to know that the baby will be born by eleven a.m., or six p.m., or whatever. They also say that it reduces the need for Caesarean section, a claim that recent research with 2000 in Great Britain has been unable to substantiate.*

"Working on a birth plan helped me and my partner sort out what was most important and discuss it with the midwife."

In the hospital in Dublin where this method was first introduced, each woman also has her own special midwife who stays with her. Meta-analysis of clinical data and randomized control of trials of active management show that it is not hormone stimulation but the presence of someone who gives one-to-one care and stays with the mother throughout labour and birth that makes Caesarean section less likely for women who have this treatment.* You may welcome the whole package of active management if it is available. Or you may want only specific elements, to be sure for instance that you have a midwife who does not disappear at the end of a shift, but stays with you until you have given birth. And you may want to add that you would like to get to know the midwives before you go into labour, so that you have a chance to talk to whoever your personal caregiver might be. You may also want to have a "doula" present. This is a woman who is trained and experienced in providing encouragement, reassurance, non-medical advice and physical comfort throughout labour and birth. She also gives support to the father or other partner. You can find out about the possibility of having a doula if you contact the National Childbirth Trust (address on page 414).

There may be certain interventions you want to avoid entirely, if possible. For many women episiotomy, the cut to enlarge the vaginal opening as the baby is being born, is one of these. There is ample research now to show that a woman is most comfortable afterwards when she has been helped to give birth gently without a cut or tear. So you may want to find out the episiotomy rate and to ask specifically for help from someone who is good at delivering without damage to the perineum. Research also shows that most tears are small ones – first or second degree – and that they heal better than episiotomies. So you can state in your birth plan that you would like to avoid an episiotomy, would prefer a tear if an intact perineum proves impossible, and that, whatever happens, you do not wish an episiotomy to be performed without giving your consent first. On the other hand, you may have no preferences and just want whoever is assisting with the birth to get on with it.

When you are constructing your birth plan it helps to have an idea of normal practice in the hospital and with the caregivers you have chosen. In Great Britain there are wide variations in routine practices between different areas of the country. If you live in the North-east Thames region, for example, you have a 74 per cent chance of a normal birth, whereas if you live in the West Midlands that is reduced to 67 per cent. On Merseyside there is a 17 per cent rate for Caesarean section, but in Trent that rate is only 13 per cent. In Scotland 90 per cent of babies are delivered by forceps, but only 5 per cent are in North-east Thames. In the North-west Thames region 33 per cent of women have epidurals, but only 17 per cent do on Merseyside. Northern Ireland still has an induction rate as high as 35 per cent, whereas in the West Midlands it is only 15 per cent.*

Keep your birth plan concise, no longer than two pages. Retain one copy yourself and have it ready with the other things you need to take to hospital with you when labour starts. Make sure that whoever is going to be your birth companion also knows what is in it. Birth plans are not set in tablets of stone. Think of your plan as an expression of your individuality and a way of describing the sort of person you are, so that if a doctor or midwife meets you for the first time in labour they will get a good idea of how you want to be treated and the things that matter most to you. Use your birth plan as part of a developing dialogue with the people caring for you.

A hospital birth

Louise's first labour was long and she was worried that her second labour would be long, too. But it is usually quicker the second time around if the baby is in a good position.

This labour lasts four and a half hours, and Louise needs no drugs for pain relief. She is wired to an electronic fetal monitor. Electrodes strapped to her abdomen record the strength of uterine contractions and her baby's heart rate, and these are registered on the chart emerging from the monitor.

There has been a shift change and another midwife is caring for her now (below). She has started to push, sitting well supported by foam-rubber wedges, and is getting hot, so the midwife turns on an electric fan.

After a while Louise finds it difficult to push sitting on her coccyx and feels she needs to get into a forward leaning position. She decides to turn on to her hands and knees, which she finds more comfortable. Her perineal tissues fan out easily as the baby's head presses through. The midwife supports the head, then holds the baby under the shoulders as she lifts her out.

The baby is delivered between her mother's legs. The midwife clamps and cuts the cord, and then places the baby in her mother's arms. She has no episiotomy, and only a small labial tear, which the midwife sutures immediately. Her baby weighs over 4 kg (9 lbs) – much heavier than the first. Afterwards the midwife says, "She coped brilliantly with her breathing. Her partner rubbed her back and encouraged her and she chose different positions, including kneeling, in order to help the baby's descent".

PREGNANCY

Physical and emotional changes

Life in the uterus **62**

Expecting twins **86**

Your baby's wellbeing **93**

Your physical wellbeing **116**

Emotional challenges in pregnancy **149**

Becoming a father **159**

Your changing relationship **164**

Pregnant again **170**

Life in the uterus

In the first days of pregnancy life is budding in cells far smaller than a pinhead. Because everything is happening on such a minute scale, it can be difficult to accept the reality of a baby growing deep inside you. Even when you begin to believe in your pregnancy, other people remain unaware of it. It can seem as if an explosion has taken place without anybody noticing, or as if all the colours have become more brilliant but everyone else is carrying on as usual. The chance meeting of one out of four hundred million sperm with a ripe and vibrant egg has resulted in a dramatic series of events, conducted on a scale so miniature that you cannot feel the astonishing life process unfolding inside you, even though you know it is happening.

FERTILIZATION

At birth the ovaries of every baby girl contain almost 500,000 potential single-cell eggs, but they do not ripen until the menstrual periods begin. Each cell that ripens into an egg is nourished by

Sperm

nearly 5,000 other eggs that will never themselves ripen. From your first period until the menopause, when your periods stop, you may carry up to 4,000 ripe eggs; each month between 100 and 150 begin to ripen, but usually only one a month reaches maturity and is capable of being fertilized. The frequency with which eggs are produced and released is determined by hormones, which interact regularly in the menstrual cycle.

This cycle lasts for about a month, and begins when a hormone released by the pituitary gland stimulates an ovary to start ripening an egg. As the egg matures, the ovary releases oestrogen into the bloodstream. This stops the pituitary gland's production of hormone, so no more eggs ripen. It also makes the uterine lining change and thicken in anticipation of the egg, which bursts out of the follicle (a capsule bulging on the surface of the ovary) about midway through each

A sperm fertilizes the ovum, penetrating the outer membrane.

cycle. It is then drawn by the fingered tentacles of the fallopian tube into its long canal, which is about the thickness of a ballpoint refill.

The egg itself is a minute speck. It is barely visible to the naked eye, yet when it meets with a still more minuscule sperm it has the potential to develop into a human being. The follicle (also known as the corpus luteum) that held the egg begins to produce progesterone, which carries on the work that the oestrogen has

Ovulation cycle

New follicle

Egg released

Ovary
An external view of one of the pair of ovaries of a fully grown woman.

Inside the ovary
A section through an ovary showing the stages of development of the follicle during a menstrual cycle.

The menstrual cycle
While a follicle is developing in the ovary, the uterus is building up a lining of coiled arteries and glands. If the ripe egg released from the ovary is not fertilized, the uterus sheds the lining (menstruation) and the process begins again.

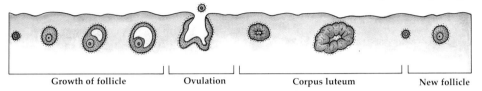

| Growth of follicle | Ovulation | Corpus luteum | New follicle |

Days

Uterine cycle

In pregnancy the lining continues to thicken

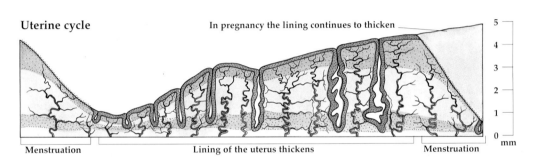

5
4
3
2
1
0 mm

Menstruation   Lining of the uterus thickens   Menstruation

been doing. If the egg is not fertilized within a few days, the follicle dries up and the progesterone level falls dramatically. As a result of this drop in progesterone level, the uterine lining decomposes, and a menstrual period occurs.

Even while bleeding is going on, the menstrual cycle renews itself: the pituitary gland is stimulating the ovary into ripening a new egg. But if the egg is fertilized, the follicle does not shrivel up, the progesterone level does not drop and the uterine lining continues to thicken, so that you do not have a period.

The usual pattern is that the ovary on one side releases an egg one month, the one on the other side the next. Sometimes one ovary becomes especially active for a few months. Occasionally only one ovary is functioning. If part of a fallopian tube or an ovary has been surgically removed the other one usually takes on the work of both.

Sperm are so tiny that 30,000 of them placed side by side would just stretch across a bottle top. A man ejaculates hundreds of millions of sperm every time he has an orgasm. After intercourse, a mere 2,000 of these survive the journey up the vagina to the fallopian tubes, and only one can fertilize a ripe egg, which immediately puts up a chemical barrier to keep all others out. Each sperm is shaped like a tadpole with a long, lashing tail; a healthy sperm is highly mobile. The head is rounded and holds the gene-carrying nucleus.

The female reproductive organs

When a woman ovulates, the released egg from one of the two ovaries is immediately drawn into a fallopian tube, where, if intercourse has taken place, it may be fertilized by a sperm. The fertilized egg embeds itself in the lining of the uterus. If the egg is not fertilized, it is shed, along with the lining of the uterus, down through the opening in the cervix and out of the vagina: this is menstruation.

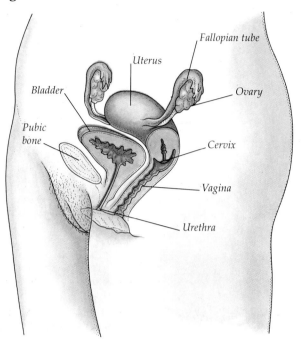

The male reproductive organs

Sperm mature in both testes, which are enclosed within the scrotum. They travel up through each vas deferens, where they are stored temporarily. When a man is sexually aroused, his penis becomes erect and the outlet from the bladder into the ejaculatory duct is closed, leaving it free for the sperm. The sperm entering the ejaculatory duct are accompanied by secretions from the seminal vesicles, Cowper's glands, and the prostate gland. About a teaspoon of the fluid (semen), containing millions of sperm, is ejaculated from the urethra at orgasm.

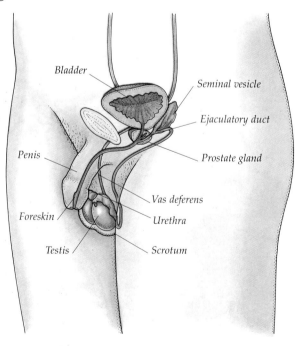

When a sperm meets the egg it burrows its way deep into it and its nucleus fuses with the nucleus of the egg. It is at this moment that the parents' genes, or units of inheritance, first meet.

Genetics

Inside the nucleus of every body cell – with two exceptions – there are 46 chromosomes, making 23 pairs. The two exceptions are the egg cell and the sperm cell, which have 23 chromosomes each instead of 46. Chromosomes are rodlike structures shaped like Egyptian hieroglyphs, each containing thousands of genes.

When the nucleus of the sperm cell fuses with the nucleus of the egg, each chromosome – and each gene inside each chromosome – unites with its opposite number. The newly fertilized cell now contains 46 chromosomes, like every other human cell. The physical characteristics of the future person are determined, and the cell can start to develop into a human being.

BOY OR GIRL?
Out of the 23 pairs of chromosomes in every human cell, one pair determines the person's sex. The two sex chromosomes in a female cell are known as XX, and the two in a male cell as XY. Since the egg and the sperm cell contain half the usual number of chromosomes, every egg cell contains 22 chromosomes plus one sex chromosome, which is an X. Every sperm cell contains 22 chromosomes plus one sex chromosome, which can be either an X or a Y.

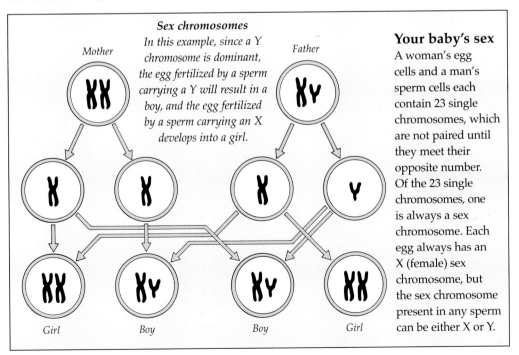

Sex chromosomes
In this example, since a Y chromosome is dominant, the egg fertilized by a sperm carrying a Y will result in a boy, and the egg fertilized by a sperm carrying an X develops into a girl.

Mother

Father

Girl   *Boy*   *Boy*   *Girl*

Your baby's sex
A woman's egg cells and a man's sperm cells each contain 23 single chromosomes, which are not paired until they meet their opposite number. Of the 23 single chromosomes, one is always a sex chromosome. Each egg always has an X (female) sex chromosome, but the sex chromosome present in any sperm can be either X or Y.

The sex of the baby depends on these differences between sperm cells. If the egg is fertilized by a sperm with an X chromosome, the union of the two sex chromosomes will result in XX, a girl. If the egg is fertilized by a sperm with a Y chromosome, the union of the two sex chromosomes will result in XY, a boy. There is usually a 50/50 chance that a boy or a girl will be conceived; statistically it appears that as women grow older and also as they bear more children, the chance of having a girl is slightly increased.

Although the baby's sex is determined by the sex chromosome carried by the sperm, it is also partly a consequence of the environment into which that sperm is received. Natural alkalinity or acidity of the secretions in your reproductive tract makes it easier for some sperm to survive their long journey than for others. Traditionally an acid medium has been thought to increase the chances of having a male child, and an alkaline medium a female child; because of this people have douched with acid or alkaline solutions before intercourse, but there is little evidence that this significantly affects your chances of producing one sex or the other.

DOMINANT AND RECESSIVE GENES

When a Y chromosome meets an X chromosome, the Y chromosome dominates to produce a boy. Similarly, when a gene encounters its opposite number one always takes precedence. A baby receives half of its genes from each parent. If a gene for brown eyes from one parent meets a gene for blue eyes from the other, the gene for brown eyes will always prevail. This does not mean that a child of one brown-eyed and one blue-eyed parent will always have brown eyes. But the gene for brown eyes is known as *dominant,* the one for blue eyes as *recessive.* So someone with brown eyes who has received a gene for blue eyes from one parent retains the blue-eye gene as a recessive gene. If he or she should have a child by another brown-eyed person also with a recessive gene for blue eyes, there is a one in four chance that both parents will pass on their recessive genes for blue eyes to produce a blue-eyed child.

This ability of two brown-eyed parents to have a child with blue eyes is a simple example of the way in which heredity introduces diversification with each generation.

DEFECTIVE GENES

Occasionally genes are defective, but since healthy genes are usually dominant over faulty ones, your baby's normal development is almost always assured. Some defective genes are carried by the sex chromosomes, and then the children of one sex only are affected. Colour-blindness, for instance, is carried by some women in one of their two X chromosomes; since the normal gene in their other X chromosome is dominant over the faulty one they do not suffer from colour-blindness. But if a boy inherits an X chromosome with a faulty gene he has no other X chromosome with a healthy gene to

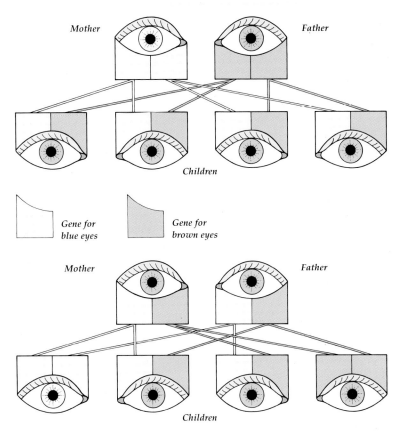

Mother · Father

Children

Gene for blue eyes

Gene for brown eyes

Mother · Father

Children

Dominant and recessive genes
When several different genes are found on a pair of chromosomes, the cell takes instructions from only one, the dominant gene. This masks those of the other, the recessive gene. For a recessive gene to succeed, a child must inherit from its parents two copies of the recessive gene.

Blue or brown eyes?
If both parents have one gene for brown eyes and one for blue, each child has a three in four chance of having brown eyes.

dominate it, so he is colour-blind. This is how colour-blindness is transmitted through alternating generations of affected boys and carrier mothers. Haemophilia is passed on in the same way.

If you are anxious about the possibility of your children inheriting any diseases or handicaps from your family or your partner's, tell your doctor before you become pregnant, if possible. Failing that, as soon as your pregnancy is confirmed ask to talk to a genetic counsellor. There is a genetic counsellor in every teaching hospital who can tell you the mathematical chances of bearing a child with a disability and the tests that can be carried out (see pages 220–230). If it is discovered that you are carrying an abnormal child, your pregnancy can be terminated *if you wish*. Nobody has to agree to termination of pregnancy even under these circumstances.

The beginning of pregnancy

The genetic make-up of the future child is decided at the moment of fertilization. But conception is a process, not a split-second event. Immediately after it has been penetrated, the egg starts to divide. It divides repeatedly as it is swept along the fallopian tube to the uterus, which it reaches seven days after leaving the ovary. By then it is a ball of cells, called a blastocyst, like a tiny blackberry but hollow in the centre. The blastocyst floats in the cavity of the uterus until about the tenth day, when it embeds itself into the uterine lining. Some blastocysts do not manage to root themselves into the wall of the uterus, and are swept out with the next menstrual period. Conception is complete only when the blastocyst has successfully nested into the wall of the uterus. You have not yet missed a period.

IMPLANTATION

The cells now number hundreds. The blastocyst releases enzymes that penetrate the lining of the uterus, causing the tissues to break down and the blood and cells – on which the blastocyst can feed – to seep out. It is a kind of nourishing soup. The quality depends on the state of the lining of the uterus. Sometimes this is not rich enough to maintain the pregnancy and there is a miscarriage, which resembles a late and heavy period, without your ever realizing you have been pregnant. An inadequately nourishing uterine lining is one cause of infertility.

EARLY DEVELOPMENT

During the second week of the fertilized egg's life, the cells become differentiated. One set becomes the amniotic sac, an envelope of salty fluid in which the baby will later grow. Another cluster develops into the yolk sac from which the embryo can make blood corpuscles. Yet another group becomes the placenta (see page 70). In between these structures are other rapidly developing cells which will form the baby. These cells are at first just an embryonic disk, but

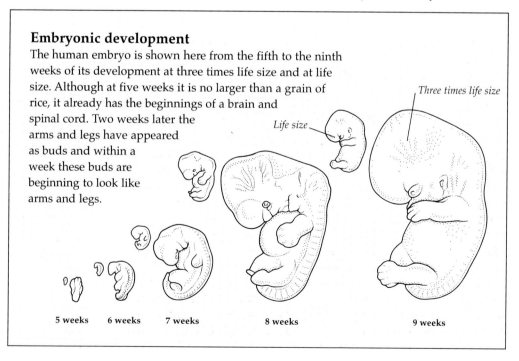

Embryonic development

The human embryo is shown here from the fifth to the ninth weeks of its development at three times life size and at life size. Although at five weeks it is no larger than a grain of rice, it already has the beginnings of a brain and spinal cord. Two weeks later the arms and legs have appeared as buds and within a week these buds are beginning to look like arms and legs.

Three times life size

Life size

5 weeks   6 weeks   7 weeks   8 weeks   9 weeks

they grow lengthways in the third week until there ⌐
tail end, with a yolk sac attached by a stalk to the middle
At this point you are about one week past the date v.
expected your period to come. Although you are not sure, p
you suspect that you might be pregnant.

Six weeks pregnant It is three or four weeks after the meeting of
sperm and egg, and about two weeks since you missed your period.
According to the medical method of dating pregnancy (see page 20),
you are about five or six weeks pregnant. The cluster of living cells
has now developed into an embryo: there is a neck and a head with
rudimentary eyes and ears, a brain and a heart that is already
beating, although it has only two chambers instead of the four that
will develop shortly. There is a bloodstream and a digestive system,
kidneys and a liver, and tiny buds that will become arms and legs.

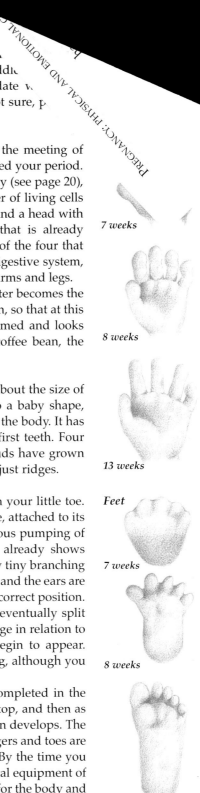

7 weeks

8 weeks

13 weeks

Feet

7 weeks

8 weeks

13 weeks

   A rod of cells develops – the notochord – which later becomes the
spine. The embryo develops from the head end down, so that at this
stage the lower part of its back is as yet barely formed and looks
more like a tail. In fact, while now the size of a coffee bean, the
embryo closely resembles a miniature sea horse.

Seven weeks pregnant A week later the embryo is about the size of
a baby broad bean. Its body has plumped out into a baby shape,
although the head is at a strange angle in relation to the body. It has
nostrils, lips and tongue, and even the buds of its first teeth. Four
chambers have developed in the heart. The limb buds have grown
into arms and legs, although the hands and feet are just ridges.

Eight weeks pregnant The baby is still smaller than your little toe.
It floats in the amniotic sac like an astronaut in space, attached to its
life-support system. The heart has started the vigorous pumping of
blood that will continue for a lifetime. The brain already shows
through skin as thin as waxed paper, revealing every tiny branching
blood vessel beneath. The jaw is not yet fully formed and the ears are
slung low and have not yet been moulded into their correct position.
The eyes are covered by an intact skin, which will eventually split
to become the eyelids. The head of the embryo is huge in relation to
its body. The limbs elongate; elbows and knees begin to appear.
Even now the baby is trying out some gentle kicking, although you
cannot feel any movement inside you.

   All the organs and features of the embryo are completed in the
course of the next month. The face grows from the top, and then as
the lower parts form the neck is elongated and a chin develops. The
nose and outer ears are completely constructed. Fingers and toes are
visible, although webbing stretches between them. By the time you
are 12 weeks pregnant (see page 71) the basic physical equipment of
the embryo is in working order. The head is still big for the body and
the limbs small; few muscles are working yet. All the internal organs

have formed and some of them are functioning. The genitals have developed, but it is not yet easy to tell yet what sex the baby is. The umbilical cord has started to circulate blood between the embryo and the group of membranes attached to the wall of the uterus. It is at this stage that the embryo begins to rely on these membranes for nourishment and the placenta starts to function. From now on the baby is known as a fetus, and the rest of its time in the uterus is spent on growth and maturation.

The placenta

In the early weeks of pregnancy one cluster of cells begins to develop into the placenta, which is an organ grown especially to nourish the baby and to excrete its waste products. The outside layer of this cell cluster develops into a membrane with hundreds of tiny roots that penetrate the uterine tissues.

Your blood does not flow directly into the baby at any stage of pregnancy. It passes across the tissues on the maternal side of the placenta and the baby's blood passes back across the tissues on the other side. The two bloodstreams are separated by the membrane; chemical substances can be diffused from one bloodstream to the other through the membrane, but the bloodstreams themselves normally never mix. (Some fetal blood cells do cross the placenta, but usually without any significant effect.) The baby can thus have a different blood group from yours, while still taking its nourishment from your blood. In just the same way the baby's waste products are passed back through the placenta into your bloodstream, to be filtered and excreted by your kidneys.

Although the baby makes breathing movements, it does not really breathe inside you: it takes its oxygen from your blood and passes back carbon dioxide. The oxygen diffuses through the membrane into its blood in the same way that oxygen from the air passes through the lining of your lungs. The placenta therefore works rather like a coffee filter: the coffee grains never enter the pot, but substances from them filter into it.

Changes in the constituents of your blood as a result of stress, illness, or any toxic substances that you might absorb will affect the quality of the substances that flow through the membrane. Blood takes only half a minute to flow from the baby's heart to the placenta and back again to the baby's heart. The flow of blood through the placenta in the fourth month of pregnancy is about 27.5 litres (8 gallons) a day, and by the end of pregnancy 330 litres (100 gallons) of blood are passing through the placenta each day.

As the placenta starts to function, it gradually takes over responsibility for production of a range of hormones, including oestrogen and progesterone, from the glands that normally secrete these hormones. Oestrogen and progesterone control most of the changes in your body during pregnancy. The oestrogen stimulates the growth of the uterus and the development of new uterine blood vessels, and also causes the milk glands in your breasts to develop so that you can feed the baby. The progesterone prevents the uterus from contracting strongly and endangering the baby during pregnancy, and thus holds off the start of labour until term. When the baby is ready to be born, the progesterone level drops. By this time the uterus has become exquisitely sensitive to the level of oestrogen in the blood, so that when the placenta reduces its output of progesterone, the oestrogen takes over, initiates labour and ensures that the uterus contracts strongly right through to the end of the third stage.

The growing baby

At 12 weeks The fetus has a large head and small, rounded rump; the sex organs are distinguishable although as yet incomplete; the eyes are closed, the retina showing dark and round through translucent skin. Toes and fingers are formed; the arms are the right length in proportion to the body and the nails are beginning to grow.

Fetal circulation

This simplified diagram shows how blood that travels along the umbilical cord towards the fetus has received oxygen from its mother through the placenta. Before reaching the fetal heart, it mixes with some of the deoxygenated blood that has already circulated through the fetus. This travels through the heart and is pumped up into the head and around the body, becoming less oxygenated. To obtain more oxygen, it returns to the placenta via the heart again, most of it bypassing the lungs. At birth the blood vessels around the baby's navel are automatically sealed off and the baby's circulation rapidly adapts to self-survival, with the lungs taking over the vital function of oxygenating the blood.

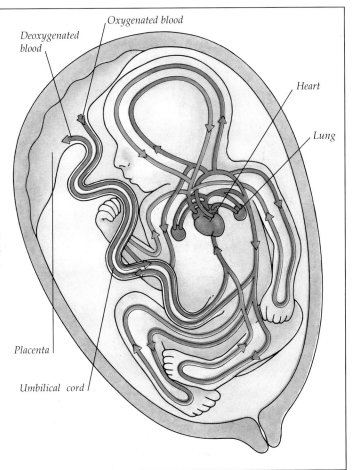

Oxygenated blood

Deoxygenated blood

Heart

Lung

Placenta

Umbilical cord

The ribs and spine are just starting to harden into bone and the baby is moving vigorously. You cannot yet feel these movements, but it is kicking, curling its toes up and down, rotating its ankles and wrists, clenching and unclenching its fists, pressing its lips together, frowning and making other facial expressions. The baby is also swallowing the amniotic fluid, gurgling it from its mouth or passing it out through its bladder. There is still plenty of room in the uterus, so the fetus can swoop and undulate in its own enclosed sea.

At 16 weeks Although the baby is growing rapidly, it could still nestle easily into a teacup. Its face is developing specifically human features, although the chin is still small and the mouth wide in comparison. The eyes are huge, closed and spaced far apart. The baby is covered with a fine down, called lanugo. This is the earliest stage at which you may first become aware of movements. At first these feel like butterflies or little fish zigzagging about in bursts of activity, but soon they are unmistakably the kicking and lunging movements of a live being deep inside your body.

At 20 weeks The baby is half as long as it will be at delivery and about as heavy as a medium-sized Spanish onion (250 g or 8 oz). You could still hold it in the palm of your hand. The closed eyes are bulbous, because the face has not yet plumped out. Hair on the head is starting to grow and there are delicate eyebrows. The baby's movements are becoming more complex and it may be sucking its thumb.

You will probably notice that there are times when your baby is asleep and times when it moves very actively (often when you have just settled down to go to sleep yourself). This seems to be partly because when you lie down it is easier for the baby to move. When moving around you also automatically rock the baby in your pelvis, so when you are busiest the baby is often asleep.

At 24 weeks The baby is about the length of your telephone receiver (32 cm or 13 in). It is covered with vernix, a creamy substance that protects its skin inside the uterus and prevents it from becoming waterlogged. The vernix sticks to hairy parts and many babies are born coated with it. Your baby may respond to loud noises and to music, especially to the brass section of an orchestra, and leaps around. The sound wave patterns of babies' cries and of adult speech can be recorded by spectographs. The spectograph of a baby's first cry can be matched with that of its mother's speech. This is so even if the baby is born in the seventh month. The baby has been listening to its mother's voice and has learned her speech characteristics.

At 28 weeks The fetus is now considered legally viable; if it is born it must be registered as a birth. If the fetus dies it is now legally considered to be a stillbirth rather than a miscarriage. With modern intensive care a baby at this stage of development has a 60 to 70 per

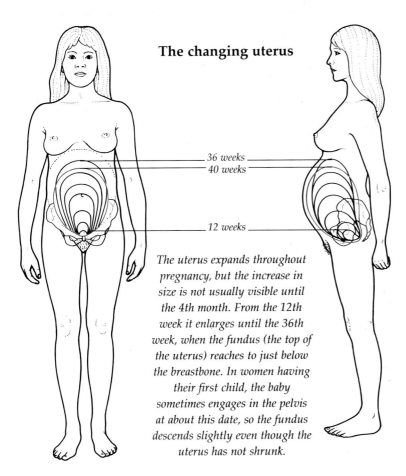

The changing uterus

36 weeks
40 weeks

12 weeks

The uterus expands throughout pregnancy, but the increase in size is not usually visible until the 4th month. From the 12th week it enlarges until the 36th week, when the fundus (the top of the uterus) reaches to just below the breastbone. In women having their first child, the baby sometimes engages in the pelvis at about this date, so the fundus descends slightly even though the uterus has not shrunk.

cent chance of survival and this figure can be even higher in some hospitals. The main problem encountered is usually that the baby's lungs have not yet developed bubbles of surfactant, the substance that prevents the complete collapse of the lungs between each breath. Another problem is that there is still only a very little fat under the baby's skin, and so that its temperature control mechanisms cannot yet work efficiently.

The baby has virtually filled all the available space in the uterus. Most babies turn upside down at some point during the seventh month and then seem to fit more comfortably.

By now you may be able to distinguish the baby's bottom from a foot or a knee. When you lie in the bath you can enjoy watching the baby swivel from one side of your abdomen to the other. Foot and knee movements are more jerky than whole-body movements and hands produce soft flutters like sea anemones moving. It is at this stage that other people may be able to feel the baby kicking when they place a hand on your abdomen. Throughout later pregnancy you will find that you can often anticipate the periods of most hectic movement; many babies are at their most energetic between eight and eleven in the evening.

At 32 weeks By the eighth month the baby lacks only some lung surfactant and a good layer of insulating fat before it is ready to be born. Movements are vigorous: the prods coming from the feet are so energetic that they may make you catch your breath. Every now and again the baby may jerk spasmodically in what can be a rather alarming manner; some women worry that their babies are having seizures. But it is usually an attack of hiccups, brought on perhaps because the baby has been gulping amniotic fluid.

At 36 weeks At some point between 36 weeks and term (which is around 40 weeks from the first day of your last period) the baby will probably descend into the pelvis with its head firmly fixed like an egg in an egg cup. It is then said to be "engaged"; this is a good sign and one indication that the baby can pass through the pelvic cavity without difficulty. Once your baby has engaged you can often feel the head like a coconut hanging between your legs. It is not comfortable to sit down suddenly on a hard chair and you may also feel sensations in your vagina like mild electric shocks (see page 231).

When you are examined lying flat on your back, the baby's head may not seem to be engaged. But if you sit up, the head engages.

After the baby has engaged, its larger body movements tend to be more limited; you will probably feel only the kicking of legs and feet, the action of the head as it uses the pelvic floor as a trampoline and the fainter movements of the arms. Although the movements change in type no day should pass without some lively indications from the baby of its presence (see page 237).

The last weeks may be tiring and involve tedious inaction. The baby is three times as heavy at birth than it was at 28 weeks. It weighs anything from 2.5 to 5 kg (5½ to 11 lbs), and is between 44 and 55 cm (18 and 22 in) long. It is now ready for its extraordinary journey to life.

Patterns of growth
Babies do not all grow at exactly the same rate. One baby may weigh nearly twice as much as another, yet both be normal. A steady increase in your weight during pregnancy is reassuring because it suggests that the baby is growing well. Many women, however, experience a plateau in weight gain at some stage of their pregnancy, only to put on more weight again by the next antenatal check-up. It can be terribly worrying when intrauterine growth retardation is suspected (IGR). Ways of detecting IGR are notoriously inaccurate, and it is overdiagnosed. One study revealed 2.5 false positives (that is, it was recorded that the babies were not growing well enough) for each one correctly diagnosed.*

The quickening
The moment when a woman first becomes aware of her baby's movements used to be very important. It even had a special name – the quickening. Italian paintings celebrated the meeting between

Elizabeth, who was pregnant with John, and her sister Mary, pregnant with Jesus. When the two women reached out to each other Mary's baby "leapt within her".

For centuries pregnancy had little social acknowledgment before quickening occurred and abortion was exclusively a matter for women. Only after quickening was the baby considered to be a "life". Only a woman knew when it had taken place. It was her personal experience. Neither medicine, church, nor state controlled that.

Today doctors claim "bonding" can be achieved via ultrasound, and after the scan at 16 to 18 weeks many women are handed a photograph of a spotted image of the baby. There are no studies to show whether women "bond" better if they have a scan. There have been studies of the effect on pregnant smokers who see their babies on the ultrasound screen, and it has been found that they do not reduce their smoking after a scan. So it cannot be said with certainty that ultrasound promotes bonding.* Whether this happens probably depends on the quality of communication during the scan. A woman should have a chance to discuss what she sees with the obstetrician or radiologist, and what the baby looks like and what it is doing.

You may treasure a photograph of the ultrasound image. It is proof that there really is a baby, that it has tiny limbs, feet and hands, and is even sucking its thumb. On the other hand, it may not feel quite right. It may seem like an intrusion. Women somehow bonded with their unborn babies long before ultrasound was invented. They did not need the external image because they cherished the internal reality – the bumps, twists, turns and kicks that assured the mother that she cradled life within her, and that were part of the continuing communication between her and her unborn baby.

It is thrilling when you first feel your baby move. But it is more than that. It is the start of a journey shared by a pregnant woman and her unborn child in which they are – quite literally – in touch with each other. You carry on an intimate conversation. Sometimes you press your hand firmly over the baby's back and the rapid movements are stilled. You have soothed your baby. You massage around where the baby lies and it is as if you are playing together – the baby rolls, dips and dances in response. You exercise on all fours and the baby drops away from your spine, cradled by the muscles of your abdominal wall. It seems that it is joining in the exercises. As the weeks pass your baby can hear the rumblings of your digestive system, the steady beat of your heart and noises from the outside world – the vacuum cleaner, the bark of a dog and the zoom of an aircraft, music, television and radio programmes, the chattering of children and your voice with its modulations of mood and intensity, changing rhythms and pitch, speaking, singing, whispering, calling and humming. By the 24th week the baby is starting to listen to and learn the sounds of language. A woman who listens to her baby, knowing that her baby is listening to her, too, is already "bonding" with her child months before she holds her newborn in her arms.

Forty weeks of life

The next ten pages show different stages of the development of a baby from the moment of conception to its last week in the uterus. The illustration below shows the five-day journey of the egg along the fallopian tube, where it is fertilized, to the uterus.

The growth of the cell cluster

  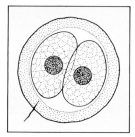

1 One of the sperm that has arrived in the fallopian tube penetrates the ripe egg.

2 The head of the sperm separates from the tail and approaches the egg's nucleus.

3 The chromosomes of the two nuclei pair off to create a two-celled egg.

The uterus and fallopian tubes

Nestling deep inside the pelvis between the bladder in front and the intestines at the back, the uterus is cupped by springy pelvic floor muscles (see page 118). The fallopian tubes branch out at either side, ending in fronds – like those of a sea anemone – which hold the ovaries.

Ovum may meet sperm here...   *Fallopian tube*   *...or here*

A ripe egg is released from the ovary

The egg is ready for fertilization for only 12–24 hours. A sperm burrows its head into the egg. The sperm's tail drops off. The egg absorbs the sperm. In three days there is already a cluster of 32 cells, and in five days a cluster of 90 cells.

Ripe ovum | *Ovary*   *Fertilized ovum embeds itself in uterine lining*

Uterus

4 *The two cells divide as the egg continues its journey along the fallopian tube.*

5 *As the cells continue to divide they gradually get smaller and smaller.*

6 *On about the fifth day the egg reaches the uterus and loses its jellylike coating.*

7 *Six or seven days after fertilization the egg embeds itself in the uterine lining.*

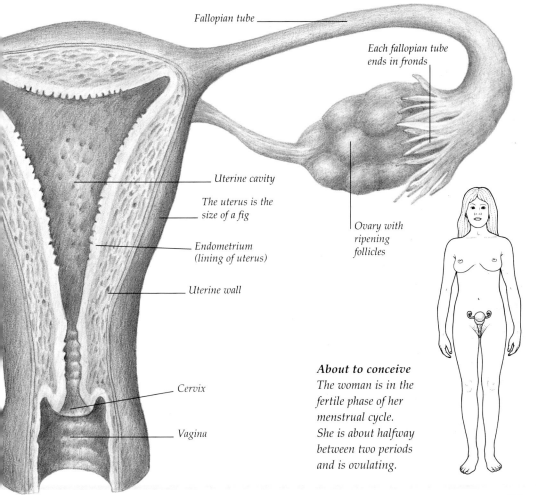

Fallopian tube _____

Each fallopian tube ends in fronds

_____ Uterine cavity

The uterus is the size of a fig

Endometrium (lining of uterus)

_____ Uterine wall

Ovary with ripening follicles

_____ Cervix

_____ Vagina

About to conceive
The woman is in the fertile phase of her menstrual cycle. She is about halfway between two periods and is ovulating.

77

Eight weeks pregnant

The baby is just under 2.5 cm (1 in) long. The bones of its arms and legs start to harden and it makes slight movements, still too feather-light for the mother to notice. The face is developing. Some time during this week the baby starts to open its mouth and the upper palate forms. The lower jaw is taking shape, with muscles that will enable the baby to suck and chew. The sound-perceiving mechanism of the ear has now developed.

Uterine lining

Uterine wall

Uterine cavity

Amniotic sac

Developing umbilical cord

Developing placenta

Embryo

Mucous plug

Cervix

Vagina

The embryo in the uterus

Pregnant!
The uterus is still hidden inside the pelvis. The pregnancy is dated from the first day of the woman's last period – before she conceived.

Twelve weeks pregnant

The baby is now just over 5 cm (2 in) long. It has developed sexual organs that later will show whether it is male or female. Its head is more rounded and it is no longer so top-heavy: it is about two-thirds the size of the body. The eyes are widely separated in a broad face. The jaws have 32 permanent tooth buds and the baby is starting to suck. It is already exercising the muscles that will be used in breathing after birth.

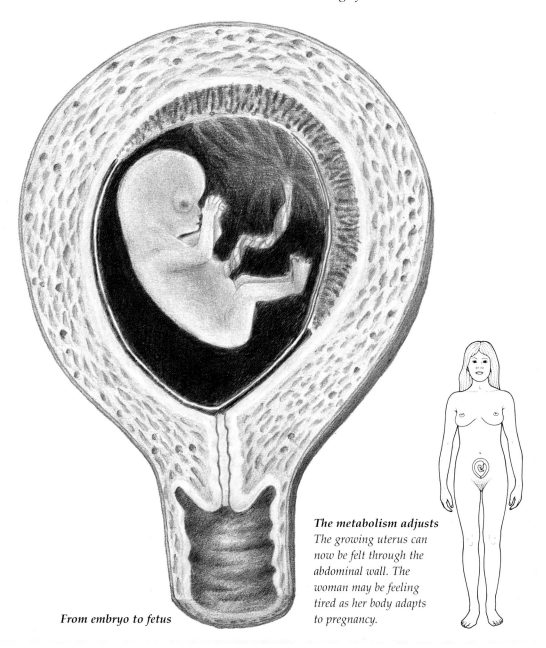

From embryo to fetus

The metabolism adjusts
The growing uterus can now be felt through the abdominal wall. The woman may be feeling tired as her body adapts to pregnancy.

Twenty weeks pregnant

The baby's rapid rate of growth slows down a little at this stage. It is about 25 cm (10 in) long from head to toe. The legs are the right length in proportion to the body and there are miniature toenails and fingernails. The baby kicks, twists, jumps and somersaults. Hair on the baby's head and delicately etched eyebrows have appeared and there is fine, downy hair called lanugo over much of the body.

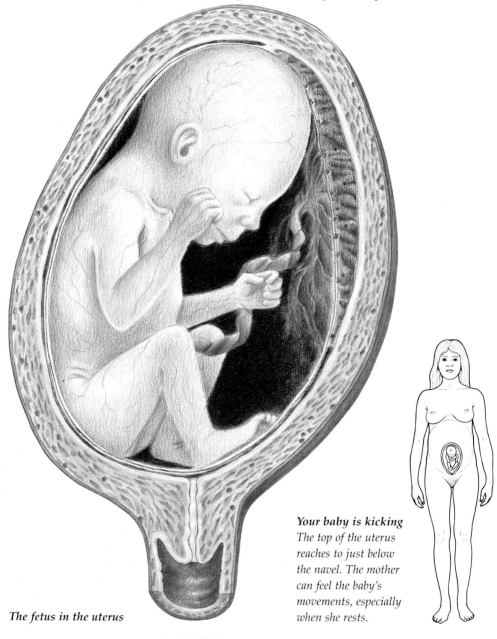

The fetus in the uterus

Your baby is kicking
The top of the uterus reaches to just below the navel. The mother can feel the baby's movements, especially when she rests.

Twenty-four weeks pregnant

The baby is thin and the skin is wrinkled. A network of veins and arteries shows through the translucent skin. The face is now fully formed and the eyes are rather prominent because fat pads have not yet built up in the cheeks.

The fetus and the uterus are growing

Mid-pregnancy
The fundus is in line with the top of the hips and the mother may be gaining 225 g to 450 g (½ lb – 1 lb) a week.

Thirty-six weeks pregnant

There is no longer enough room in the uterus for the baby to move about freely. It has settled into one position and the main movements the mother feels are jabs from the arms and legs. By now the skin is smooth and peachlike and the body has plumped out. When the baby is awake, the eyes are open and it is aware of strong light flowing through the tissues of its mother's abdominal wall. If it is born at this time, the baby has an excellent chance of survival.

The baby turns head down in the uterus

Four weeks to go
*The top of the uterus
reaches its highest point,
just below the breastbone.
The mother may feel heavy
with her pregnancy and
feel it is going on for ever.*

Forty weeks pregnant

The baby is now about eight times bigger than it was at three months, when all its vital organs were formed, and has increased in weight approximately 600 times. Most of the lanugo has dropped off, although there may still be some down the centre of the back, in front of the ears and low on the forehead. The fingernails extend beyond the fingers and may need cutting at birth so that the baby does not scratch his face.

The baby is ready to be born

Impatient for the great day
*The uterus has moved down a
little into the pelvis, so the
fundus has dropped slightly.*

Expecting twins

Finding out that you are going to have twins usually comes as a shock. Some women suspect quite early in their pregnancy that this will be the case, especially if they have had a singleton pregnancy with which they can compare this one. If you are a fraternal twin (see below), you are about twice as likely to give birth to twins yourself as are other women. The chances of having fraternal twins depend on heredity, age, race and the number of children you have already had. Although fraternal twins often skip a generation, the chances of their occurring in successive generations are high. The frequency of identical twins seems independent of these variables.

MIXED FEELINGS
However, if nothing has led you to suspect that you are carrying more than one baby, it can be very upsetting to be told, after an ultrasound scan or an antenatal visit (see page 43), that suddenly all

---

How twins are conceived

Normally conception occurs when one egg released from a woman's ovary is fertilized by one sperm from a man's testes. Seven out of ten pairs of twins are the result of the woman releasing two eggs, which are then fertilized independently by two different sperm (fraternal twins).

Usually the two eggs then implant and develop separately in the uterus. Less commonly, one egg fertilized by one sperm divides, resulting in two developing babies with the same inherited characteristics (identical twins). Often this division occurs after implantation in the uterus.

Identical twins
Monozygotic or identical twinning takes place after, rather than at, fertilization, and it often occurs after implantation in the uterus. As a result the twins almost always share a placenta although each has its own cord and bag of water.

Fraternal twins
Dizygotic or fraternal twins have separate water bags and cords, and separate placentas. Occasionally the two eggs implant close together in the uterus, so that the placentas become fused and it looks as if there is only one.

Monozygotic (one-egg) or identical twins

...*divides*

...*and splits into two*

One ovum is fertilized

Dizygotic (two-egg) or fraternal twins

Two ova are fertilized   ...*two individuals develop*

your expectations of birth and the time afterwards need readjusting. If you are to be a mother for the first time, the natural apprehension you originally felt about the labour and how you would cope with a new baby is greatly increased. Added to this you wonder how you will manage two babies at the same time in all their noisy reality – two mouths to feed, two nappies to change each time, two babies to bathe, two loads of clothes to wash, two budding personalities who will need your love and attention.

One woman, who was dismayed on hearing that she was expecting twins, said that she never really veered from this attitude throughout her pregnancy. During a hospital stay in her eighth month of pregnancy, she took the opportunity of watching mothers who had just given birth to twins, and felt that all her worries were justified, since they seemed to have such trouble in managing two babies. However, shortly after her twins were born, she was able to comment on the "totally unexpected delight of being able to breast-feed both, often simultaneously". She did admit, though, that it was hard work at first and that "the intense joy and delight the babies now give has only come as we have got to know them".

Positions of twins in the uterus

Twins fill the available space in the uterus more quickly than a single baby, so they may adopt the positions in which they will be born at an earlier stage.

The pictures below show fraternal twins (with two placentas), but the same positions apply to identical twins (with a single placenta).

This presentation, with both twins in the cephalic or head down position, is the most common. It is also the most straightforward: birth should present no special complication.

When one twin is head down and the other head up the breech baby is often born second. The first baby opens up the birth canal so that the breech baby can usually be born vaginally without difficulty.

If both babies are breech the risk of complications will be evaluated in advance. Caesarean section may be performed in preference to a vaginal delivery.

When one baby is lying transversely and the babies are large, a Caesarean section will be carried out. If the babies are not large, it is usually possible to turn the second baby after delivery of the first.

Sometimes a woman is unhappy to discover that she is expecting twins because she has been planning a home birth and this may no longer be possible. Doctors and midwives usually advise hospital birth for twins, since the chances of a complicated delivery, especially for the second twin, are increased and it is possible that the babies will be premature and underweight. If you are going to term, however, and both babies have grown well and are head down, you may decide on a home birth after all.

Alternatively a woman may be overjoyed to find that she is going to have twins. Perhaps she had wanted more than one child, but was not particularly enjoying her pregnancy and certainly not looking forwards to another. Suddenly she discovers that she can have two children for the price of one pregnancy and labour!

GETTING ADEQUATE REST

The first thing to accept is that a pregnancy with two babies tumbling about inside can be more of a strain than an ordinary pregnancy. The risk of developing pre-eclampsia (see page 139) is higher; the babies are more likely to be born pre-term, and they may not be very strong. Because they have to share the space in the uterus and the nutrition available through the placenta, twins are often of low birthweight. You will feel better if you have regular rest times and frequently go to bed early. You need help with housework and cooking and someone who will, at least occasionally, bring a delicious meal to your bed. If you already have other children, it is worth making an effort to find some motherly (or fatherly) person who can look after them for an hour or so each day so that you can relax without feeling that you will be needed in a minute. Many obstetricians require women pregnant with twins to get more rest. However, there is no evidence to support the value of total bed rest in twin pregnancies.* If you are able to plan ahead for your pregnancy you may be able to reorganize your life well enough to allow you to take an adequate amount of rest at home.

There is no need to be an invalid. Plan things you can do in bed: read, write, sew, learn a language, take up a craft you have always wanted to try your hand at. If you think about the extra demands made on your body by a multiple pregnancy you will realize that your whole system has to adjust to the babies' needs. Such an adjustment involves widespread metabolic changes; there is also extra pressure put on your digestive organs and on your diaphragm and lungs, as well as stress on bones (on your lower ribs, which tend to splay out, and on your spine, for example). Your muscles, too, will have to cope with much of the stress of a twin pregnancy, especially your tummy muscles, your pelvic floor and the muscles of legs, feet, arms, shoulders and back, which have to support the extra weight and do the work of lifting and coping with your body mechanics. Above all there is a general crowding out that may well make you feel very full and heavy.

Your babies may look like two peas in a pod but they have distinct personalities (opposite).

So rest will help your body adjust to the increased demands made on it by a multiple pregnancy. And the rest that helps most is rest taken before you become exhausted and irritable and *before* you feel that you cannot carry on a minute longer.

LYING COMFORTABLY

You may find it very uncomfortable to lie flat. Your heavy uterus is pressing on major blood vessels in that position, too, so, both for your own comfort and for the blood supply to the babies, lie either well propped up or in the "three-quarters-over" position. Prop your breasts with one pillow and put two under your upper knee if this feels good. Even more so than with a singleton pregnancy, special back supports may be needed in the last few weeks. A large bean bag may feel comfortable; and so might a contour pillow used with other pillows, two firm foam wedges or the kind of cushion that is sold for making it more comfortable to read in bed. Whatever you choose, try to get something solid that will support the exaggerated curve of your lower spine.

POSTURE AND EXERCISE

Sensible body mechanics are also more important when you are expecting more than one baby (see pages 120–122). Learn how to counteract the effect of the enlarged and heavy uterus by standing straight and tall, with tail tucked in. Aim to balance on the balls of your feet rather than going flatfooted and waddling like a duck, which is only too easy to do when you are overtired. Above all, learn how to get up from a lying-down position by rolling over, if necessary kicking off with your foot and hand against solid objects, and then rising on to all fours.

Pelvic-floor toning activity (see pages 118–119) is very important throughout, whether you are carrying one baby or two; with twins it will be especially vital after the birth, as the muscles around the vagina have been stretched by the extra weight of two babies.

"I've never been keen on exercises, but I like the idea of keeping muscles toned by activity, having a body that's alive."

It is a good idea in any case to do these movements from early pregnancy, before there is any appreciable change in weight, as muscle tone is really best built up before there is any particular stress on the muscles.

If your pelvic-floor muscles are under a great deal of strain, you can do these movements while lying on the floor with your lower legs raised on a chair. In this position weight is not pressing on the pelvic muscles and it is easier to feel what is happening there. In advanced pregnancy, however, when the babies are low down, it may be impossible to use this position. Try letting your pelvic muscles "dance" when sitting propped up with pillows.

You will probably be aware of the babies moving a great deal inside you. Your abdomen feels like a basket full of puppies. It can be difficult to sleep and you are often awakened by all the internal activity. Practising release from tension and letting muscles relax all over your body can help enormously. Some mothers worry that with all this movement the babies are in danger of harming each other. They can certainly shuffle each other up a bit, but each one is sealed off in its own bag of waters, and this also means that each baby bobs around like a cork in a glass of water. The fluid cushions the babies from shock and allows free movement until the very last weeks of pregnancy, when the pelvic girdle cradles the babies so closely that you may feel only small movements.

DIET AND NUTRITION

For a detailed discussion of diet in pregnancy, see pages 93–100. The demands made on your body by a twin pregnancy require an even more careful attention to diet than is necessary in a singleton pregnancy. Aim for a nutritious diet with plenty of salads and fruit and only those foods that are of positive value to yourself and the babies. Cut out ice creams, sickly doughnuts, cakes and biscuits. The easiest way to do this is to convince yourself how awful these foods really are and to think instead of rich, golden hunks of cheese, glowing fruit salad, a peach that melts in the mouth, jade-green watercress, rosy apples and a luscious, long glass of milk.

To save labouring over a hot stove have at least one raw food meal a day, which will give you a good supply of vitamins. You may like to buy some new cookbooks that concentrate on salads and fruit and stimulate your imagination. If you normally eat white bread and cereals, now is the time to switch to wholewheat bread and flour, brown rice and whole grains. Eating like this will help you after the babies come, too, as you cannot feel full of vitality if you are poorly nourished and weighed down with "junk" foods.

The more tired you become the more you may feel that you cannot be bothered about preparing nutritious meals and shopping for food. But your health depends on your having a good diet and not skimping on protein, vitamins and minerals. Is there any chance of getting help with groceries? Could someone else shop for you? Or could you and your partner or a friend do it together in bulk, loading up a car? (But do not lift boxes and bags into the boot yourself or attempt to unload them!) If you have to shop unaided, use a shopping trolley and avoid carrying bags. There is probably a shop in your area that will deliver to your home provided that you order enough at one time. If you live in the country, a village shop may do this when they know you are expecting twins. Or could your partner take a neighbour who has no car to the supermarket, so that she can help do your shopping?

Your baby's wellbeing

Looking after yourself in pregnancy, from the very first weeks, is probably more important for the welfare of your baby than anything else you can do. It ensures that you provide the best possible environment for the developing baby – and, equally important, it gives you the best chance of being healthy and full of vitality, ready for the birthday and the first stages of motherhood.

Nutrition

Your baby depends on what you eat and drink for adequate nourishment in the uterus. It used to be thought that provided the expectant mother had a "sensible" diet there was no need to give her any advice about what she should eat, because the fetus would always take what it needed. There were certain "do nots", the most important of which was "do not eat for two". However, such a vague instruction led to the unfortunate result of large numbers of women going through pregnancy on inadequate diets.

Then research revealed that when pregnant women have an inadequate diet, their babies may die or be born in poor health, and the women themselves may have difficult pregnancies and labours, as well as subsequent illness after delivery.* If a woman is nutritionally deprived, her baby is deprived, too; she is more likely to have a miscarriage and, if the pregnancy is maintained, her baby is more likely either to be born prematurely or to be of low birth weight because it has not received sufficient nourishment in the uterus. Research has also revealed that poor nutrition in the latter part of pregnancy can affect a child's brain development.*

However, further research has shown that sometimes too much emphasis has been placed on having huge quantities of food and a great deal of animal protein. Metabolic changes in pregnancy mean that most women can make better use of the food they eat, and this increased efficiency extends into the period of breastfeeding, too.* So there is no need to worry about whether you are having the right diet, to take vitamin pills and mineral supplements routinely or to feel you ought to be eating foods you dislike just because you are told that they are good for the baby.

Women often develop food intolerances in the first weeks of pregnancy. They cannot digest food they liked before. The modern emphasis on good nutrition in pregnancy can make women who are suffering from nausea and vomiting feel very anxious about depriving their baby of essential foods. In many traditional cultures it is believed that the baby asks for the foods it wants and rejects others, and that it is important to give a pregnant woman exactly what food she fancies because it is her baby speaking through her.

Take time to enjoy food during pregnancy and eat plenty of fresh fruit and vegetables (opposite).

93

Vomiting is one way in which your body refuses food with which it cannot cope. If you are experiencing nausea it is best to trust your feelings and eat only what you fancy. Do not worry that you are not having a "balanced diet". In a few weeks you are likely to enjoy a much wider range of foods again. If you have a very restricted diet take vitamin supplements to ensure that you supply the nutritional elements necessary for your baby's development.

WEIGHT GAIN

It is quite normal to put on between 9 and 13.5 kg (20–30 lb) during pregnancy. Some women put on more, with no ill effects. Do not assume that because your baby will weigh only 3 to 4 kg (6¼–8½ lb) at birth, the rest of the weight you put on is fat. Consider the weight of the placenta, membranes and amniotic fluid, the increase in size of the uterus and breasts and the increase in volume of your blood. Fluid retention also accounts for a substantial weight gain in some women. All these things return to normal after the birth.

Since different women gain weight at different rates it is impossible to be dogmatic about how much weight you should put on. Medical opinion is that "arbitrary weight restriction is potentially harmful to both mother and baby".* If you start your pregnancy underweight you and your baby may benefit from a bigger weight gain than the woman who starts pregnancy overweight. It is most unwise for any woman to try to remain slim in pregnancy, and an attempt to keep your figure might result in the eventual loss of your baby. However, if you start pregnancy overweight, you are likely to put on more weight than a woman who is not fat at the onset of pregnancy, and also to suffer from high blood pressure and urinary tract infection.*

WEIGHT GAIN IN PREGNANCY

Since most women gain weight at different rates it is impossible to say how much weight you should put on. However, if you are seriously overweight or underweight this may lead to complications during pregnancy and labour.

Proportions of weight gain

Your total weight gain in pregnancy is made up as follows:

Weight of baby	38%
Weight of placenta	9%
Weight of amniotic fluid	11%
Increase in weight of uterus and breast	20%
Increase in weight of blood	22%
Total weight gain	**100%**

Timing of weight gain

0–12 weeks	0%
12–20 weeks	25%
20–30 weeks	50%
30–36 weeks	25%
36–40 weeks	0%

So you can assume that if, for instance, you are 30 weeks pregnant, the weight you have gained in pregnancy will be about 75% per cent of your total weight gain.

One way of checking to see whether you are putting on superfluous fat during pregnancy, which you will then be left with after the birth, is to measure your upper thighs each week, keeping an accurate record of the measurement. This is an excellent way of recording any increase in your own body fat as distinct from the weight you are gaining as a result of the pregnancy. The upper thigh measurement should stay about the same, although fluid retention may increase it slightly in the last weeks of pregnancy.

PROTEIN

Women who are not pregnant are recommended to have 46 g (1½ oz) of pure protein a day for optimum health. When you are pregnant you may benefit from about twice as much protein as this. The foods that are rich in protein are lean meat, fish, beans, nuts, brewer's yeast, milk, yoghurt, cheeses and other dairy products.

All proteins are made up of chemical substances – called amino acids – in different combinations. Animal or "first-class" proteins contain all the amino acids necessary for the protein to do its body-building work; vegetable proteins, which used to be called "second-class", contain only some of these amino acids, and therefore should be eaten either with a small quantity of animal protein or in different combinations. If you are a vegetarian who eats no animal products, combine beans with a wheat product at the same meal – say, beans with wholegrain flour pastry, chickpeas with pasta or lentils with wholewheat bread.*

You will obtain adequate protein if every day you have one dish from each of the following categories: (a) one helping of meat or fish, two eggs, a cup of peanuts or cashew nuts; (b) 100 g (4 oz) of hard cheese, 200 g (8 oz) cottage cheese or 568 ml (1 pint) of milk (substitute soy or tofu); (c) four slices of wholewheat bread, a helping of brown rice or wholegrain pasta or one large potato that has been baked in its jacket. If you are a vegan and do not eat any animal products, you will obviously not want cheese and milk, and can have a good helping of pulses instead.

CARBOHYDRATES

You need carbohydrates for energy. They are found in foods you eat in bulk, such as bread, flour, cereals and root vegetables. Most foods containing carbohydrates have other valuable nutrients, too; potatoes – especially if you eat them in their jackets – can contribute protein and vitamin C as well as carbohydrates, and wholewheat bread provides B vitamins, iron and the fibre that helps to prevent constipation. If you eat small quantities of these foods daily, you need no other carbohydrates.

If you are already overweight before starting pregnancy, or if you are putting on a lot of superfluous fat during pregnancy (see above for a method of checking this), it is a good idea to try to cut out all white flour and sugar, as well as all the products containing them.

A balanced diet

Presenting food so that it looks attractive enhances the pleasure in eating and will help you digest it better, too. Even for a solo meal, arrange each plate of food so that it is a vibrant mixture of colours and textures. Below are suggestions for breakfast, lunch and supper dishes.

Bowl of muesli
A breakfast of cereal with fresh fruit and wholegrain toast.

Grapefruit snack
Citrus fruits such as grapefruit are a valuable source of vitamin C.

Fruit salad
Top a colourful, mixed fruit salad with a large spoonful of yoghurt.

Bean salad
Mixed beans and chick peas with vinaigrette and chopped herbs.

Carrot and artichoke soup
Serve this soup hot or cold, finished with a swirl of crème fraîche.

Salad sandwich
Use a mixture of young salad greens on wholegrain bread.

Fish dish
Serve with pilaf of rice, green vegetables and lemon.

Stir-fry
Arrange stir-fried baby vegetables in the centre of a decorative rice ring.

Pasta
Mix with tomatoes, red peppers, parmesan, olives and olive oil.

Cakes, desserts and biscuits do not do much to help your unborn baby's health. If you like sugar in tea and coffee, train yourself to enjoy both of these drinks without it.

FATS

Your body's need for fat is minimal. You can reduce your intake by trimming fat off meat, using less butter, drinking low-fat milk, boiling or steaming foods rather than frying or sautéing them, and cutting out rich sauces. You will find that fromage frais, ricotta cheese and yoghurt are useful ingredients of low-fat sauces, and that you can make fat-free sauces with puréed vegetables.

MILK AND DAIRY PRODUCTS

Milk is usually recommended for the pregnant woman, but unless your diet is grossly inadequate in protein you do not need more than 568 ml (1 pint) a day. Consumed in large quantities whole milk is fattening, and if you fill yourself up with drinks of milk you are likely to dampen your appetite for other foods you and your baby need. Some women do not like milk or are allergic to it. You can have fat-free milk or take cheese or yoghurt instead; if it is simply a matter of taste, disguise milk in sauces or dishes where you are not aware of it.

VITAMINS

It is important that most of your vitamin intake should come from food rather than supplements. Trying to get the right dosage of vitamins, and the right balance between different vitamins, from supplements is unwise. A well-balanced and varied diet including vitamin-rich foods such as vegetables, fruits and nuts will supply all the vitamins necessary for you and your developing baby.

FOLIC ACID

There is one exception to this. Folic acid supplementation in the first 12 weeks of pregnancy cuts down the risk of having a baby with spina bifida or other neural tube defects by up to 70 per cent, and also reduces the risk of cleft palate.

When women who had previously given birth to a baby with a neural tube defect (spina bifida or anencephaly) were given folic acid supplementation for one month before their conception and then up to the second missed period they were much less likely to have another handicapped baby.*

From the time of conception and through these crucial early stages the baby's spinal cord is being formed. If the spine does not close up then the baby has spina bifida, which can result in paralysis of the legs and incontinence. If the brain and skull do not develop properly the baby is anencephalic and is severely mentally handicapped.

A healthy diet does much to help to prevent neural tube defects. Even before you get pregnant, eat plenty of broccoli, spinach and other dark green, leafy vegetables.

MINERALS

Minerals and trace elements are a vital part of your diet, but if you are eating plenty of food that is rich in protein and vitamins you are unlikely to suffer from any mineral deficiency. Iron, calcium, magnesium and zinc are probably the only minerals about which you need be concerned during pregnancy.

Iron is necessary for the formation of red blood cells. Red blood cells contain a substance known as haemoglobin; if blood contains insufficient haemoglobin, not enough oxygen is carried to your baby and you become very tired. Vitamin C helps your body to absorb iron, whereas antacid medicines stop you from benefiting fully from it. Good sources of iron include dark molasses, egg yolk, whole grains, dried peas and beans, all dark green, leafy vegetables such as watercress and raisins, prunes, brewer's yeast and nuts.

Extra iron is often prescribed in pregnancy. If you eat foods rich in iron, you should have good reserves stored in your liver, and not need to take iron supplements. The fetus draws on these reserves, so that it can store enough in its liver to last several months after birth. If you are iron-deficient (anaemic) before embarking on pregnancy (and some women are without realizing it), a supplement may be advisable. Iron supplementation is not necessary for the normal drop in haemoglobin from mid-pregnancy. This reduced haemoglobin is a sign that plasma volume is rising and that the placenta is providing good nutrition for the baby (see page 70).

Calcium is necessary for the formation of strong bones and teeth. It enables blood to clot, muscles to work smoothly, and may protect against high blood pressure and pre-eclampsia. Oxalic acid in spinach and cocoa reduces absorption of calcium.

Your baby's teeth start to bud very early on in pregnancy, so your calcium intake in the first four months matters a great deal. Milk is a useful source, as are other dairy foods. Calcium is also present in leafy vegetables, sea vegetables, whole grains, pulses, nuts and carrot juice. You benefit from almost twice as much when you are pregnant.

Magnesium levels in pregnant women are often low. This may be one cause of muscle cramp. Good sources of magnesium are cereals, nuts, soya beans, milk, fish and meat.

Zinc deficiency may result in miscarriage, growth retardation in the uterus, stillbirth or congenital handicap.* There is also some evidence that zinc is necessary for muscles to contract well and, although it is difficult to measure accurately the concentration of zinc in human tissues, that shortage of zinc is one cause of long labour.* Taking an iron supplement can interfere with the absorption of zinc. High-fibre foods – especially bran – contain zinc, as do brazil nuts, Parmesan and other hard cheeses, seeds, herring and meat.

WOMEN AT RISK

Certain women are at "nutritional risk" and need to pay special attention to diet; for them vitamin and mineral supplements may be useful. The ones who may be at risk are those pregnant during adolescence (while they are still growing themselves), women who are underweight when they become pregnant, and women who are overweight because of excess consumption of carbohydrates and fats. Women living on a very restricted range of foods as with a macrobiotic diet, or who have lost a baby from miscarriage or stillbirth before, and women who have had three pregnancies within two years are also at risk. Included in this category are women suffering from some chronic diseases involving the regular use of drugs, smokers, heavy drinkers, and those with multiple pregnancies.

SALT AND FLUID RETENTION

It used to be thought that salt was dangerous in pregnancy and was one cause of pre-eclampsia (see page 139). It has now been established that salt is necessary for a normal pregnancy. When a group of expectant mothers were given no-salt diets they had *more* pre-eclampsia than a control group of women who had as much salt as they wished.* Cutting out salt can also cause cramp in hot weather. Since you tend to retain more fluid when you are pregnant, you will only maintain the usual level of saltiness in all your body fluids by having as much salt as your appetite dictates.*

Occasionally special diets are prescribed for pregnant women in order to reduce fluid retention, which used to be thought dangerous in itself. But these special diets can harm the unborn baby. Women with mild fluid retention (oedema) usually produce babies in just as good a condition as those who have no signs of it at all. Ankle, foot and leg swelling on very hot days, when you have been on an aircraft trip, or after you have been standing for a long time, is therefore nothing to worry about. If your skin is looking very puffy,

"My feet swelled uncomfortably in the heat while I was pregnant, so I showered my legs with cold water and rested with my feet up."

take more rest and look carefully at your diet to see if you should increase your protein intake (see page 95); if your fingers and face become swollen be sure to mention it to the doctor or midwife, as it is a sign that your kidneys are not coping well with the excretion of waste products from your body. This in turn may mean that your placenta is not working efficiently.

You cannot prevent oedema by cutting down on fluid intake, so drink as much liquid as you want. Four or five glasses of water a day help your kidneys to function well throughout your pregnancy.

EATING A BALANCED DIET

Bear in mind that you are providing nutrition for three distinct but interdependent biological entities: your own body, the developing baby and the placenta.* This triple nutritional task demands a good, diet rich in vitamins and minerals. A salad a day is a must, but remember that you can use finely chopped cabbage and other greens to make a change from lettuce. Experiment with salads and try mixing fruit and vegetables. Apples go with most savoury things. A baked potato with cheese and a cabbage-based salad are a good source of protein, vitamin C and calcium. If you can spare time to bake your own wholegrain bread, add extra wheat germ or soya flour and you have thereby added to your diet another valuable source of protein, iron, B vitamins and fibre.

Eating well does not have to mean eating expensively. Some women save money by avoiding unnecessary foods such as carbonated drinks, coffee, packaged desserts and soups, buns and confectionery and starchy, sugary puddings. Milk and cheese are relatively cheap, and a delicious main course can be made from a selection of vegetables in season covered with a white sauce and topped with a layer of grated cheese browned under the grill.

Drugs

Around 25 per cent of all the birth defects that occur are genetic in their origin. Around 65 per cent of birth defects have an unknown cause. Only 2 to 3 per cent are caused by drugs. This is partly because the total amount of water in a woman's body goes up by 8 litres (14 pints) in pregnancy, so drugs are more diluted.* On the other hand, the range of substances to which the embryo may be vulnerable is not yet known. For this reason it is wise to take the fewest possible medicines during pregnancy, especially in the first few weeks when the embryo is forming and when the placenta is only just starting to be active. (You should therefore take care during the second half of the menstrual cycle if there is any chance that you might be pregnant.) It used to be thought that the placenta acted as an effective barrier to all poisons that might be present in the maternal bloodstream. But it is now known that drugs can cross the placenta and may affect the baby.*

"At the restaurant I ordered a glass of wine. The waiter said, 'Have apple juice!' I felt so angry – I had no rights, no choices."

If you think of how the fertilized egg has to segment, travel along the fallopian tube, embed itself into the lining of the uterus and develop into a baby, you can imagine how such delicate and complex processes can be interfered with by chemicals that have been introduced into your bloodstream.

The liver and the kidneys are the organs of your body that deal with drugs and turn them into material that can be excreted in the urine. In an unborn – and even a newborn – baby these organs are still immature. The fetus is therefore not able to excrete many of the drugs that may reach it through the placenta. Instead, such drugs can accumulate in its body in toxic quantities. It is vital to remember, when taking any drug, that a dosage which may be right for you is far in excess of that which is suitable for your tiny baby. There was, for example, the thalidomide disaster,* when a sedative that was thought to be mild and safe was prescribed for women in early pregnancy. As a result more than five thousand babies were born with badly deformed limbs or none at all. Thalidomide is an extreme example of the effect that a drug can have on the development of an unborn baby. But all drugs, including prescribed drugs, medicines bought over the counter such as laxatives and painkillers and nicotine and alcohol, are potentially harmful if misused. Think carefully before taking any drug when pregnant, especially in the early weeks.

Drugs that are known to cause abnormalities of any kind are said to be "teratogenic". In the first few days of a pregnancy, any toxic or teratogenic drugs would probably prevent the egg from ever settling firmly in the uterus, so that you would not even realize that you were pregnant but would just have a delayed period; if you were to take the same drug slightly later, you would probably miscarry. At a later stage still, the pregnancy might continue, but there would then be a risk of the baby being damaged by the drug.

If the cell cluster is damaged sometime between conception and 17 days it either dies and there is a very early miscarriage, it is reabsorbed into the mother's tissues, or the embryo survives intact because cells multiply to replace those that have been lost. Organogenesis, the development of the different parts of the baby's body, takes place during the period 18 to 55 days from conception. After 56 days drugs do not cause major handicaps, although they may reduce growth and cause loss of function.

WEIGHING THE DIFFERENT RISKS

Some pregnant women need drugs and may be very ill without them. Illness in the mother can also affect the developing baby. For instance, running a very high temperature (see page 111) seems to be teratogenic at certain phases of pregnancy, so it may be safer to take aspirin to get your temperature down than to try and cope without taking any medicines. It is always a question of balancing the risks to the baby against your need and the stress that may be caused to you by not having drug treatment.

Since the thalidomide disaster there has been acute awareness of the need to screen all new drugs before they are prescribed to pregnant women, and doctors are being increasingly careful. However, drugs that have been in use a long time remain on the market without being tested. It is difficult to be certain about any drug, because animal experiments may produce damage in one species, yet not in another. This can work either way: rats may be affected, but not human babies, or babies may be affected when rats are not.

People are often ignorant about the chemical substances they introduce into their bodies. Antacids for the relief of indigestion, cough medicines, sleeping pills (barbiturates), antihistamines used in the treatment of hay fever, and antibiotics are just some commonly used drugs that alter the body's chemical balance. A great many pregnant women take over-the-counter as well as prescribed drugs of one kind or another in the first weeks of pregnancy, and no one has much idea of the possible risks. There are other substances that you may not think of as being drugs, including cigarettes and alcohol. Even tea and coffee have been researched for possible harmful effects, although normal use (up to half a dozen cups a day) seems to be fine.*

SMOKING

There are positive steps you can take to give your baby the best start in life and other things that you should avoid since they are known to be detrimental to your baby's health. First and foremost among the obvious dangers is smoking. Whether or not you inhale, nicotine passes into your bloodstream and from there into the baby's

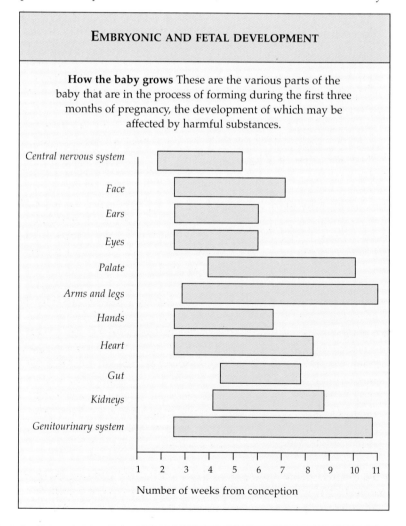

EMBRYONIC AND FETAL DEVELOPMENT

How the baby grows These are the various parts of the baby that are in the process of forming during the first three months of pregnancy, the development of which may be affected by harmful substances.

Central nervous system
Face
Ears
Eyes
Palate
Arms and legs
Hands
Heart
Gut
Kidneys
Genitourinary system

1 2 3 4 5 6 7 8 9 10 11

Number of weeks from conception

bloodstream. It makes the fetal heart speed up and into respiratory movements that are the baby's rehearsal for brea effect, the unborn baby coughs and splutters. Smoking interferes with the efficiency of the placenta and is the n. widespread and efficient way of pumping a powerful poison into a unborn baby's bloodstream. Nicotine makes the blood vessels in the mother's placenta constrict so that less oxygen and fewer nutritional substances can reach the baby.

Mothers who smoke bear babies who weigh less than babies of mothers who do not smoke and the baby's weight drops in relation to the number of cigarettes consumed.* This does not mean that some smokers do not have good-sized babies but that statistically babies of smokers are deprived of the best possible nutrition. It is not just that a woman who smokes tends to eat less food. Cigarettes have a direct effect on the growth and development of the baby.* It could be that some women make the mistake of thinking that labour will be easier if their babies are lighter in weight. Labour with a tiny, underweight baby is no easier or shorter than labour with a good-sized baby, and your baby is much more likely to be healthy and easy to care for if you have not smoked during your pregnancy. When a woman does not smoke herself, but her partner does, she and the baby are exposed to secondhand smoke, and fetal growth may well be affected as a result.*

Smoking after the fourth month of pregnancy is a major cause of prematurity and the birth of underweight babies who are stunted in development and may have to be cared for in a special care baby unit. Smoking also increases the chances of bleeding, miscarriage (women who smoke are twice as likely to miscarry as those who do not), premature rupture of the membranes, premature separation of the placenta, haemorrhage before or early in labour, haemorrhage after delivery, congenital abnormality, stillbirth and death of the baby in the week following delivery.* The more a woman smokes, the more likely these things are to happen.

How to give it up If you are a heavy smoker and dependent on cigarettes to get through the day it may be very difficult to give them up, even for the sake of your baby. Fortunately, the nausea of early pregnancy or just a sudden dislike of cigarettes prompts many women to cut them out. Even if this does not happen spontaneously you can use the techniques of aversion therapy to condition yourself to break the habit. Every time you feel queasy or vomit make yourself think "cigarette" and use the association between vividly picturing the act of smoking and the overwhelming sensations of nausea to train yourself to develop a dislike of cigarettes.

How to cut down If you are past the nauseous stage of pregnancy or feel perfectly fit throughout, as many women do, you can still try to reduce your cigarettes to at least half the usual number. Ask your partner to help by cutting down his consumption in the same way; if the two of you are making the same effort, your determination is strengthened. Also, cutting down on smoking is a concrete way in which your partner can contribute to your baby's health, by reducing the amount of passive smoking to which you are subjected. The more you can both cut down on your general consumption of cigarettes the better.

You may be feeling terribly guilty about smoking while still being unable to give it up. You may feel like a murderer, but the guiltier you become the more you want a cigarette in order to help you calm down. It is certain that guilt and emotional stress can also affect your metabolism adversely, including your heart rate, blood pressure, breathing, muscle tone and the adrenaline in your bloodstream. The question then arises as to how much stress you should tolerate in trying to give up smoking. If you know how to release tension you may be able to cope by smoking each cigarette only halfway down and still find that it helps you enough to be able to "unwind".

"Actually, it was very easy to give up smoking because I couldn't stand the taste or smell of cigarettes in the first couple of months. I cut out coffee for the same reason."

This is where your own judgment of the relative importance to you of smoking or not smoking in pregnancy is essential. Every pregnant woman has the right to be fully informed of the risks of smoking and to make her own decision on the subject of smoking during pregnancy. No one can *make* you stop smoking, however many dire warnings they give: you decide.

On the other hand, your baby cannot choose whether or not to smoke. A mother chooses for her child.

ALCOHOL

Because alcohol is socially accepted it is easy to forget that its use in pregnancy should be restricted. Fortunately, many women develop an aversion to it during pregnancy.

Alcohol crosses the placenta and the baby's blood levels are about the same as the mother's. The risk the baby incurs from alcohol depends on how often the mother drinks, how much she drinks, and the baby's stage of growth. Alcohol in early pregnancy is more likely to have a bad effect and even a single "binge" then can cause damage to the developing baby.

It depends on the mother's metabolism, too. Some women cannot break alcohol down into harmless substances, so alcohol passes through the placenta in its poisonous form. Heavy, chronic alcohol use can cause Fetal Alcohol Syndrome (FAS). The baby has distinctive facial features and may be mentally and developmentally retarded.

However, most women can drink in moderation during pregnancy and have a perfect baby. Limit your intake to 10 units of alcohol a week and spread them out over the week. One unit is a small glass of wine, a single measure of spirits or 300 ml (½ pint) of light beer.

BEING CAREFUL ABOUT DRUGS

Think about any drugs you may be taking when you intend to conceive and ask your doctor's advice. Do not wait until your first antenatal visit or even – if possible – until you are sure you are pregnant. If there is any chance that you might be pregnant, to be on the safe side it is best to avoid taking any drugs that are not essential to your health.

If a doctor other than your obstetrician is treating you, especially in the early months of pregnancy before it is obvious that you are having a baby, make sure that he or she realizes that you are pregnant before prescribing. This may be particularly relevant if you are ill when away from home and have to consult a different doctor.

Go through your medicine cabinet carefully when you stop using contraception. Make a list of the contents and ask your doctor whether there are any that are likely to be unsafe during pregnancy. Throw away, by flushing down the lavatory, any drugs that were not prescribed for you or that are out of date, in addition to those that your doctor advises you to get rid of.

MOOD-ALTERING DRUGS

Because so little is known about the effect of mood-altering drugs it is wise to limit their use or cut them out altogether. You may feel that cannabis or Valium helps you to relax on occasion when you cannot "switch off". But explore other ways of releasing tension. The effects of disciplined relaxation (see pages 185–195) are likely to help your unborn baby much more than anything you can take in through your mouth. They are some positive things you can do for yourself and your baby, ways of tuning in to your body rather than making an attempt to escape from it or deaden its sensations.

Cannabis Little is known of the effects of cannabis on the baby. Its strength varies widely, and its immediate effects on the user vary with expectation, the company in which it is taken, and previous experience of it. Claims have been made that it can be teratogenic, but this is still being investigated.

Cocaine Whether the drug is taken by inhaling a powder (snorting), smoking it (crack) or injecting it (shooting up), a woman using cocaine is very likely to have a baby who is small for dates or premature, and who is addicted to the drug. These babies tend to be irritable and jumpy and it is difficult to calm them down enough so that they will take a satisfying feed.*

Mild tranquillizers are often prescribed during pregnancy and do not seem to be harmful. Diazepam (Valium) is sometimes used in treating pre-eclampsia (see page 139) to bring blood pressure down. But it is best to stop taking even a mild tranquillizer as you approach the time when you expect to go into labour. Valium taken just before labour starts or during the course of labour can result in the baby having a low Apgar score (see pages 356–360) at birth as well as breathing difficulties. The baby may also take a long time to start feeding properly, as well as becoming chilled more easily than usual.*

Powerful tranquillizers such as chlorpromazine (Thorazine) and haloperidol (Haldol) should be avoided in pregnancy unless essential. If you think you might have conceived, talk it through with your psychiatrist and with a paediatrician. You could change to a milder tranquillizer and see if it is sufficient to control your anxiety and reduce tension. Strong tranquillizers taken in labour may make the baby lethargic or very stressed and trembling at birth.

SLEEPING PILLS

These include hypnotics, tranquillizers and antihistamines (see opposite). Hypnotics are of two different kinds. Some are barbiturates, which are highly addictive even over a short period and now almost never prescribed: phenobarbital (Luminal), amobarbital (Amytal), pentobarbital (Nembutal) and secobarbital (Seconal). Others are non-barbiturates: Chloral, Welldorm, Doriden and Mandrax (which also contains an antihistamine). Welldorm is often prescribed in pregnancy. Non-barbiturates also seem to be addictive if taken over a long period. Not enough is known about the effect of hypnotics on the unborn baby, but they are certainly cumulative. The drug concentrates in the mother's fatty tissues; the baby is doped along with the mother. Large doses of barbiturates can cause respiratory depression at birth and feeding difficulties. Over-the-counter sleeping pills have not been tested for safety in pregnancy. The best solution is to do without sleeping pills; try to overcome insomnia by making time for more conscious relaxation and exercise in the open air, and perhaps an aromatherapy bath at bedtime and lavender essential oil sprinkled on your pillow.

PAINKILLERS

Aspirin The most widely used painkiller is aspirin (salicylate) and its derivatives. If you have a headache or other pain, try to get rid of it by resting in a quiet, darkened room. If rest is not effective, a few aspirin are unlikely to be harmful. But never dose yourself repeatedly: a recurring headache should be discussed with your doctor. If taken regularly (say, every four to six hours) during the few days before you go into labour, aspirin can produce difficulties in blood clotting in both you and your newborn baby, and neonatal jaundice.

Codeine is used on occasion by many pregnant women as a mild pain reliever with no apparent ill effects, but it is addictive: the baby whose mother has been taking several pills daily throughout pregnancy may be born dependent, have severe withdrawal symptoms, and even die. Use it sparingly.

Paracetamol can cause liver and kidney damage in the person taking large doses. It should be used with caution in pregnancy, since the baby's liver and kidneys can suffer from relatively small doses.

Ibuprofen has not been shown to be safe. There is some evidence that it impedes the fetal and newborn circulation and may also cause cardiac malformations and delay the onset of labour.

Naproxen, like Ibuprofen, has not been found to be entirely safe for the developing fetus and has the same potential harmful effects.

Drugs to treat migraine can cause the uterus to contract during pregnancy, thus endangering the fetus. Discuss alternative ways of treating migraine with your doctor.

ANTI-SICKNESS DRUGS
Drugs for nausea and vomiting are of three different kinds: anti-cholinergic drugs, antihistamines and phenothiazines.* They can all have side effects. The first category treats nausea by acting on your nervous system; it reduces secretions, including stomach acid, and relieves muscle spasm. No one can be sure whether these drugs are completely safe for the fetus. Antihistamines, which include Cyclizine, Ancoloxine and Avomine, block the action of histamine (a substance to which some people are allergic) and may cause drowsiness. They are best avoided in pregnancy as high dosage may cause fetal abnormalities. The last category, the phenothiazines, are major tranquillizers, and are therefore inadvisable in pregnancy.

It seems then that drugs to control pregnancy sickness should not be used unless specifically prescribed by a doctor who knows you are pregnant, and then only when you have weighed together the advantages and disadvantages of taking the drug. Do not take any pills for travel sickness if you think you may be pregnant.

ANTIBIOTICS
Antibiotics may be prescribed in pregnancy; obviously their use is sometimes necessary and any disadvantages to the baby are out-weighed. Never use antibiotics left in a bottle that were prescribed for a previous infection, even if you have exactly the same kind of infection. Tell your doctor that you may be pregnant, or remind him or her that you are pregnant, when you ask for a prescription.

Penicillin appears to be a safe antibiotic that can be taken without risk at any time during pregnancy.

Sulphonamides (which are not really antibiotics but effective antibacterials) are used to treat urinary tract infections. If you need to have sulphonamide treatment you should stop a week or so before the baby is due to be born, to allow the drug to get thoroughly out of your system before you go into labour. Otherwise the newborn baby's kidneys may not be able to cope with excreting the drug and the baby may then develop jaundice, which can cause damage to its central nervous system.

Tetracycline, a wide-spectrum antibiotic, is deposited in the unborn baby's teeth and may then go on to cause an unsightly yellow mottling and staining. It can also stop the growth of the baby's bones while it is being taken, so it should not be used during pregnancy.

Streptomycin, another wide-spectrum antibiotic, should never be taken in pregnancy. One of the drugs used to treat tuberculosis, it can cause deafness in the baby.

DRUGS TO TREAT CONSTIPATION

Stool bulk producers, such as Normacol, do no harm provided that they are used in moderation.

Stimulant laxatives, which include senna-based laxatives such as Senokot, cascara and Dulco-Lax, seem to be safe for the fetus, but they may cause you to lose excessive amounts of fluid. Make sure that you drink plenty of liquids if you are taking any of these preparations.

Saline laxatives, including milk of magnesia and magnesium sulphate (Epsom salts and Andrew salts), can also cause dehydration if you do not drink plenty of fluids, but otherwise they do not appear to harm the fetus.

Various types of oil will lubricate the bowels. However, avoid liquid paraffin because it reduces the absorption of vitamins A, D and K. Lack of vitamin K may lead to disorders of blood clotting in the baby. Extra fluids alone may cure your constipation, especially if you adjust your diet to include a regular intake of bran. (See page 134 for more advice and information about constipation.)

DRUGS TO REDUCE FLUID RETENTION

Diuretics increase the excretion of salt and water from the body, and in so doing make your kidneys work very hard. They are used in the prevention and treatment of pre-eclampsia (see page 139). Since there is no proof that reducing fluid retention does prevent pre-eclampsia, it is almost certainly best to avoid taking diuretics altogether.* Discuss the matter with your doctor.

STEROIDS AND DRUGS TO TREAT ASTHMA

Steroids are used for the treatment of asthma and hay fever, eczema and other skin disorders, and rheumatism and arthritis. Severe and prolonged asthma attacks are more likely to harm the baby than the drugs that are used to control asthma.*

ANTI-DEPRESSANTS

There is very little known about the effects of anti-depressants on the development of a baby. But certainly the old tricyclate anti-depressants do not seem to be teratogenic; the risk of miscarriage or of congenital abnormalities does not appear to be greater than if a woman is not taking these drugs. Because drugs like Prozac – which are very long-acting – have been around for a much shorter period of time, psychiatrists usually err on the side of caution and do not prescribe them during pregnancy, even though there are no reports of their causing harm to the baby.

Women suffering from severe depression in pregnancy may need treating with drugs, especially if the woman is suicidal, and the possible risks of medication must always be carefully weighed against the risks of not having it. But doctors usually decide to take women off anti-depressants once they are known to be pregnant. If you do need anti-depressants during your pregnancy the sensible thing is to taper them off gradually so that you are no longer having them about four weeks before the baby is due. Then you can, if necessary, go back on them after the birth of your baby.

ANTI-PSYCHOTIC DRUGS

Clozapine should not be taken during pregnancy, as it affects bone marrow. It makes sense to avoid using anti-psychotic drugs that have only been on the market for a short time, and to stick to what has been tried and tested, and to those drugs the side-effects of which are already known. Anti-psychotic drugs affect the newborn baby's behaviour, and side effects in the mother will also appear in the baby after birth – if she is sedated, the baby will be too, for example – but these are reversible. However, in such

"I discussed taking the drug with my psychiatrist and she switched my medication to one least likely to affect the baby."

cases a paediatrician should be standing by at the birth to ensure that the baby is stabilized. Babies who have received anti-psychotic drugs are more likely to have convulsions and diazepam causes babies to get jittery as they come off it. So these drugs should be tailed off four weeks before the birth or reduced by half. To give the baby the best chance of dealing with the stress of being born, as little as possible of any drug should be taken.

DRUGS TO TREAT THYROID CONDITIONS

You may need to take drugs for an under- or over-active thyroid, but be aware that such drugs can have an effect on the baby's thyroid. Carbimazole should be used only in low doses during pregnancy. You should stop using it four or five weeks before the expected date of delivery, to allow the baby time to produce an adequate amount of its own thyroid hormones, which the drug destroys. Discuss the drugs you are taking with your doctor, if possible before embarking on a pregnancy.

ANTICOAGULANTS

These drugs are prescribed for deep-vein thrombosis or for a pulmonary embolism – both serious conditions that are caused by blood clots. Taken early in pregnancy, they may cause miscarriage. Anticoagulants can also cause haemorrhage in the baby and some, such as Warfarin, should not be taken in the last three months of pregnancy. If an anticoagulant needs to be given towards the end of the pregnancy, Heparin by injection is the safest one to use. Any adverse effects on the fetus can be reversed by small doses of vitamin K given to the baby after delivery.*

DRUGS TO TREAT DIABETES

Drugs that are taken by mouth in order to reduce blood sugar should not be used during pregnancy.* They can sometimes cause miscarriage or fetal abnormalities. Injections of insulin, however, are quite safe. If you are diabetic and you want to get pregnant, let your doctor know so that you can discuss in advance exactly how the pregnancy will be best managed (see page 141).

ANTICONVULSANTS

If you normally take anticonvulsants or antiepileptic drugs, discuss with your doctor the possibility of modifying your treatment before you conceive. These drugs may cause cleft palate and a range of other handicaps in the baby. Carbamazepine is probably the best anticonvulsant for pregnancy.

GENERAL ANAESTHETICS

There are times when a general anaesthetic may be necessary during pregnancy; but if possible such anaesthetics should be avoided because the baby becomes anaesthetized too. Make sure that your doctor or dentist knows that you are pregnant if he or she recommends general anaesthesia for anything.

Other risks

X-RAYS

In pregnancy it is wise to cut down the use of X-rays to the minimum, because there is no safe threshold for radiation, and hence no minimum level at which you can be assured that X-rays are safe for your unborn child. So avoid X-rays during pregnancy if possible, and in the second half of the menstrual cycle if there is a chance that you might be pregnant.

Radiation can partially destroy the genetic material that acts as the blueprint for the normal development of each cell of the body. A damaged cell is called a mutation. Radiation can have the strongest effects on an embryo in the initial stages of development, and a badly affected embryo is then likely to be aborted spontaneously. But X-rays taken in pregnancy can also have an effect after birth*: there is evidence that X-rays are associated with a higher than usual chance of developing diseases of the respiratory system, blood disorders and infectious illnesses in childhood.

There are some cases in which diagnostic X-rays are particularly important and the only means of discovering certain disorders during pregnancy. If a doctor or a dentist advises X-rays, take professional advice, but always check first to ensure that they really are essential. Your abdomen and thyroid should always be protected during the X-ray by a lead shield.

HIGH TEMPERATURE

If you find you are running a temperature, go to bed, drink plenty of fluids, and sponge yourself down with cold water, or take cool baths or showers to lower your body temperature. Do not just let your temperature rise since there is a slight chance that a very high temperature – say, over 39°C (102°F) – in the first four months of pregnancy can damage a baby.* The most crucial time is during the third and fourth weeks after conception. This is a horrifying thing to learn in late pregnancy if you know you had influenza earlier on, but most babies are born whole and healthy even when the mother has run a high temperature. Nevertheless, it is sensible to avoid becoming run-down, and so more susceptible to the risk of infection, if you think you may be pregnant. Keep up a high intake of vitamin C in your diet and have some protein each day to reduce the risk of contracting an infection. As far as we know, there is no longer any real risk of serious damage to the baby from a high temperature after the 16th week of pregnancy, but you could make the developing baby's heart race by getting over-heated yourself.

"It's like walking in a minefield – there are so many risks! In a way I think I'd actually be happier not knowing about any of them."

Saunas and long, very hot baths can also produce a temperature that is high enough to harm a developing baby, so always be sure to keep temperatures down. Your own comfort, however, usually acts as the best guide to your baby's safety.

FOOD POISONING

Listeriosis Soft and blue-veined cheeses and pre-cooked, chilled foods like ready-to-serve chicken and pâté are sometimes contaminated with listeria if they are not stored at sufficiently low temperatures. The symptoms of listeriosis are similar to those of influenza. If a pregnant woman suffers from this she may have a miscarriage, or her baby may be stillborn or have birth defects.

Salmonella Raw as well as partly cooked eggs are sometimes contaminated with salmonella, which causes food poisoning. It is wise for a pregnant woman to eat only eggs that have been thoroughly cooked, and to avoid eating mayonnaise and other dishes with raw egg as an ingredient.

Toxoplasmosis This is another disease that can harm the fetus. It is not usually thought of as a form of food poisoning because most people associate it with contaminated cat litter. It is true that it can come from handling cat litter or soil containing cat faeces, and if you have a cat you should always wear rubber gloves when emptying a dirty litter box and wash your hands afterwards. If you are a gardener be very careful to wash thoroughly after handling soil. But toxoplasmosis is also a food-borne infection. Eat only meat that has been completely cooked. Be particularly careful at barbecues, especially with kebabs. Meat should never be pink or bleeding, as it is with a rare steak. Do not eat raw, cured meat such as Parma ham. Wash your hands after handling raw meat and wash down kitchen surfaces and wooden utensils. Because toxoplasmosis may be present in soil, vegetables and fruit should also be well washed. Goat's milk and yoghurt made from it should be pasteurized. You can get further information from The Toxoplasmosis Trust, listed on page 414.

VACCINATION
Vaccinations are not recommended during the first four months of pregnancy, during which time there is a small risk of damage to the fetus. In the later months, most vaccinations (apart from rubella; see below) are considered harmless, although you should avoid smallpox vaccination throughout pregnancy, especially if you have never been vaccinated against smallpox before. If you are travelling to a country that still insists on smallpox vaccination you can obtain exemption with a certificate of pregnancy from your doctor.

Rubella (German measles) is such a mild disease that many people have it in childhood without knowing it. If you contract rubella when you are pregnant, the virus may cross the placenta and in the first 20 weeks it can have a serious effect on the baby. Even if you were vaccinated against rubella as a child, it is sensible to have a blood test before you become pregnant: if the test shows that you have never had rubella you can be vaccinated against it. Alternatively, if you are already pregnant and discover that you are not immune, you can be vaccinated immediately after the birth.

The protection afforded by rubella vaccination lasts at least seven years, and probably much longer. After vaccination, be very careful about contraception for the next three months, since you should not conceive until you have had time to build up immunity to the virus. Never have rubella vaccination if you think you might be pregnant.

If you were not vaccinated against rubella before pregnancy and have never had the disease, avoid all contact with children who might have it. If you think you have been in contact with rubella, get in touch with your doctor, who will offer an injection of gamma globulin. The risk of the baby being damaged by rubella in the first three months of pregnancy is high, especially in the first eight weeks; if you contract the disease you may want to consider a termination.

THE RHESUS NEGATIVE WOMAN

All blood is either Rhesus positive or Rhesus negative. By far the most common type of blood group is Rhesus positive. In fact, some 86 per cent of people are Rhesus positive, which means that their blood contains something known as the Rhesus factor. This factor is tested for early on in your pregnancy as part of your routine blood test. Its presence or absence is noted on your records, but is only important in one combination of circumstances: if you are Rhesus negative and the baby's father is Rhesus positive. There is no problem if the baby is Rhesus negative, however 40 per cent of all Rhesus positive babies of Rhesus negative mothers become anaemic, and if this condition goes untreated the baby may die before or after birth. If you are Rhesus negative with a Rhesus positive baby and some of the baby's red blood cells leak into your circulation, a risk can arise with the next pregnancy. This can happen after an

The Rhesus factor

A Rhesus negative woman rarely has problems with her first baby as the maternal and fetal bloodstreams never mix. However, at delivery, some of the baby's blood cells can enter the mother's bloodstream. If the baby is Rhesus positive the mother's blood develops antibodies. In a later pregnancy these antibodies may cross the placenta and attack another Rhesus positive baby's blood.

Each subsequent pregnancy

The first pregnancy

The Rhesus factor is only important when a Rhesus negative woman is carrying a Rhesus positive baby. At delivery some of the baby's blood may leak into the maternal blood. As a result the woman develops antibodies that destroy Rhesus positive blood cells.

In a second pregnancy, these antibodies may cross the placenta. If the new baby is also Rhesus positive its blood is damaged by the mother's antibodies.

The solution

Doctors inject a serum into Rhesus negative women within 48 hours of childbirth, or after a termination or miscarriage, to prevent creation of antibodies to Rhesus positive blood.

Key

| Rhesus negative blood |
| + | Rhesus positive blood |
| ▲ | Rhesus antibodies |

accidental haemorrhage in late pregnancy or at delivery, or if you have miscarried or had a termination. Your body then responds to the Rhesus factor present in the baby's cells as it would to an invader, and begins to manufacture antibodies against it. Then if some of these antibodies leak back from your circulation into the baby's circulation they proceed to destroy large numbers of the baby's own red blood cells.

The flow of red blood cells each way across the placenta is not usually substantial enough during a first pregnancy to cause your body to develop such antibodies. But when your first baby is born, some of its blood may flow from the placenta into your circulation. This triggers the creation of antibodies to the Rhesus factor in your blood. From then on you produce antibodies to the Rhesus factor, and the next time you are pregnant with a Rhesus positive baby your antibodies may attack the baby's blood vigorously. It may get jaundice, its brain may be damaged, severe anaemia may develop and, in the worst cases, it may not even survive.

There are several things that can be done about this. The first and simplest is an injection of anti-D immunoglobin at 28 weeks of pregnancy and another immediately after the birth of a Rhesus positive baby. It consists of a serum that stops the mother's biological defence mechanisms acting against foreign Rhesus substances. A fresh injection of this serum is then given during and after each subsequent pregnancy. The same routine is followed after a miscarriage or a termination of pregnancy, since it is possible that the fetus was Rhesus positive and that some of its blood will have entered into the mother's bloodstream.

It is no good giving this serum *after* a woman's body has already produced antibodies. If a high proportion of antibodies is detected in your blood during a second or subsequent pregnancy and your baby is known to be at risk, amniocentesis may be performed (see page 226) and the amniotic fluid analyzed for the presence of bilirubin (bile pigment). An anaemic fetus excretes into the fluid large amounts of bilirubin from destroyed red blood cells.

A woman who is Rhesus negative and whose partner is Rhesus positive is tested for Rhesus antibodies every two to three weeks. If there are antibodies present, a blood test is done on the baby inside the uterus, with ultrasound being used to guide the needle into the umbilical cord. If necessary, the baby can be given one or more blood transfusions before birth, again using ultrasound to guide the needle. If the baby is sufficiently mature to survive life outside the uterus, labour may well be induced early. If necessary, the baby can be treated immediately after delivery and given a complete blood transfusion which will thoroughly eradicate all the antibodies from its bloodstream.

Fortunately, as more and more Rhesus negative women are routinely immunized soon after the delivery of their babies, this situation is becomingly increasingly rare.

AN "INCOMPETENT" CERVIX

Occasionally a woman's cervix may be torn from a previous difficult labour or mid-pregnancy termination, or be damaged by a cone biopsy. She would not find this out until her next pregnancy, when she might lose her baby after the fourth month as a result of "cervical incompetence" (see page 374). The term "incompetent" is an unfortunate one and makes women feel as if they have failed to reach some standard of reproductive ability.

An obstetrician may recommend cervical cerclage – sewing the cervix closed for the duration of any subsequent pregnancy. This is a relatively simple procedure: once the pregnancy is established, a suture is inserted under anaesthesia and is threaded through and around the cervix like the drawstring of a purse. The suture is removed at about the 36th week of pregnancy or later. Some obstetricians like to induce labour at this point because they say it is simpler, since contractions often start shortly after the removal of the suture anyway. You are not compelled to have labour induced, however, and should decide whether this is what you want in such circumstances. There is wide variation in the degree to which obstetricians in different countries use cervical cerclage. It is fashionable in France, for example, whereas in Britain it is used more by private obstetricians than those working in the National Health Service. A random trial of cervical cerclage, conducted on women at high risk of giving birth prematurely, produced no evidence of its benefit.* Since twins and triplets are often born a few weeks early, some obstetricians perform cervical cerclage to try to prolong a multiple pregnancy. This does not work.*

PRE-TERM LABOUR

If you pass blood (which could be coming from the cervix), feel a sudden rush of warm liquid from your vagina (which could be the membranes rupturing), or have regular contractions like menstrual pains that get longer, stronger and closer together over several hours, chances are that you are going into labour. If this happens before you have reached the last month of your pregnancy the baby may need special care at birth. So call your doctor or midwife, or go straight into hospital. It is best for the baby to be born in a centre that has intensive care facilities, with a neonatologist standing by in case the baby needs help with breathing.

If the baby is very premature you will be given corticosteroids to mature the fetal lungs, and this gives the baby a much better chance. There is evidence that administering ethanol, diazoxide or progestogens in an attempt to stop labour is likely to be harmful.*

Your physical wellbeing

To make the most of the experience of being pregnant, you will probably want to get your body in good condition. Healthy activity can be pleasurable in itself as well as being an excellent preparation for labour. Sometimes books on pregnancy and even childbirth educators give the impression that childbirth is an athletic event for which you have to train like a marathon runner, a kind of examination for which you must study assiduously, or even an ordeal with which you are unlikely to cope but which will be quickly forgotten afterwards. No wonder expectant mothers become anxious! No mention is made of the excitement, joy and sheer pleasure that many women experience in childbirth.

Most women look forward to childbirth with excited anticipation. They know that there is a slight chance of something going wrong but that the better they have prepared themselves with body-toning movements and exercises, the more likely they are to be able to handle any problems that occur during pregnancy.

Getting to know your body

Before beginning exercises, it is useful to gain an awareness early in pregnancy of how your body works and what is taking place in your reproductive organs. One way of doing this is to have a closer look at your genitals. To get a clear view, you can kneel or squat over a mirror. A torch might help you to see the area better.

YOUR PERINEUM
The perineum is the tissue around your vagina and over the area between your vagina and anus. Just before delivery the perineum begins to bulge and its tissues fan out and open up as the ball of the baby's head begins to press through it.

YOUR VAGINA
The vagina is the soft, cushioned canal that holds the penis during sexual intercourse; it is also the passage through which the baby is delivered. The outer part of the vagina is the vulva, consisting of layers of outer and inner lips (labia) constructed like the overlapping petals of a rose. During pregnancy they change in colour from red to violet as the blood supply to them is increased. Pregnancy hormones also darken your nipples, and you may notice dark patches on your face and on other parts of your skin.

Insert one or two fingers gently into your vagina and feel around the stretchy folds inside. Although the sides of the vagina are normally touching each other and there is no hollow space, notice how readily they spread apart. They open like an accordion when the baby is pressing down through them to be born, and the action of hormones that are released into your bloodstream will make them become even more flexible during the last few weeks of pregnancy.

YOUR CLITORIS

The clitoris is like a bud rising from the inner lips at the upper (front) end of your vagina. The base of the clitoris and the inner lips around it are very sensitive, and pressure on or stroking of these parts produces sexual excitement. As you touch its root, you may notice that it swells up. You will feel that there is a hood or fold of skin surrounding the clitoris and that this connects up with the inner lips. So anything in your vagina that stretches the inner lips apart will also pull on this hood and will stimulate the clitoris, too.

A woman's genitals vary as much as a man's. Just as penises are different sizes, for example, the clitoris may be the size and shape of a small pea or more like the curved centre of an orchid. Women's labia vary, too. Some are firm, some soft, some large and fleshy, others smaller. A woman may worry that masturbation might have changed the shape of her labia or clitoris, but these organs are so flexible that pulling, pressing or rubbing them does not produce permanent structural changes. Doctors and midwives cannot tell anything about your sexual habits by examining your vulva, although many women harbour a secret fear that they can, especially if they have suffered sexual abuse.

At delivery the baby presses against this whole area that you are examining, easing forwards the tissues so that they open up like elastic, and then slides out with a rush of liquid. After the baby is born these flexible tissues spring back again; at first they will not be as firm as they were before, but they will gradually gain in tone.

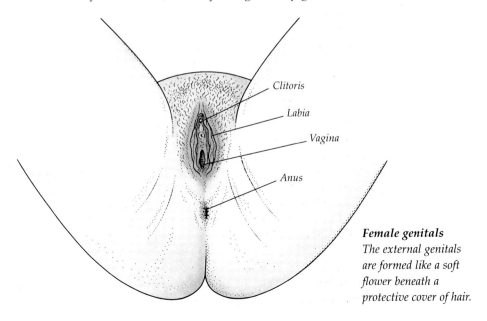

Clitoris

Labia

Vagina

Anus

Female genitals
The external genitals are formed like a soft flower beneath a protective cover of hair.

117

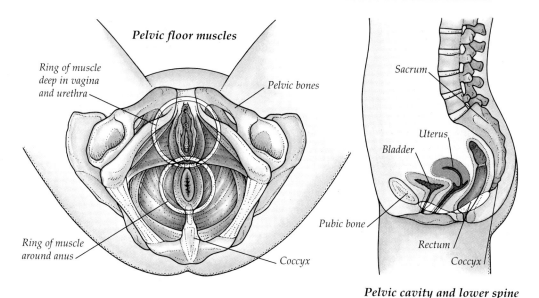

Pelvic floor muscles

Ring of muscle
deep in vagina
and urethra

Pelvic bones

Sacrum

Uterus

Bladder

Ring of muscle
around anus

Coccyx

Pubic bone

Rectum

Coccyx

Pelvic cavity and lower spine

Pelvic floor

The muscles of the pelvic floor form a springy support for your uterus, bladder and rectum.

YOUR CERVIX

Now introduce your longest finger deep inside your vagina and you meet the rounded, firm cervix (the neck of the womb), the part of the uterus that will open (dilate) when you are in labour. Early in pregnancy it will feel like the tip of your nose. You may notice a little dip in the middle, like the dimple in the centre of a buttoned cushion. This is where the mucous plug is situated, and this plug, like the cork in a bottle, seals off the uterus from the outside. At the end of pregnancy the cervix will have softened and, when you touch it with your finger, it will feel more like your mouth when it is soft and relaxed than like your nose. This is one of the signs that you are ready to go into labour. The cervix is "ripe", and ready to open up.

YOUR PELVIC FLOOR

The muscles that support everything inside the pelvic cavity (including the uterus, the bladder and the rectum) form the pelvic floor. They have special significance for your health, whatever age you are and whether or not you are pregnant. The upright position that humans have adopted in preference to the all-fours stance puts an extra stress on these muscle layers in pregnancy.

Although these muscles form a co-ordinated working structure, they are not really a "floor" at all. They are slanted at different angles and levels and can be held with varying degrees of firmness. The easiest way to find these muscles, of which some women are unaware, is to interrupt a stream of urine, since you bring all of the pelvic floor muscles into play when you do this. Or you can think of them as forming a figure eight around the vagina and anus. In the middle of the eight is a horizontal bar, the transverse perineal muscle. When the muscles of the pelvic floor are contracted, the circular shapes of the figure eight change to almond shapes and the transverse perineal muscle is pulled towards the pubic bone (the firm ridge of bone just above the clitoris) like the opening lid of an old-fashioned roll-top desk. You can feel this from both inside and outside if you put one finger inside the vagina and a thumb over the pubis.

Your pelvic floor muscles contract spontaneously during love-making, increasing your sensations of pleasure and those of your partner. Awareness and control of these muscles are important in labour, too, when you will need to be able to release them as you press the baby down the birth canal to be born.

Some people can hold their pelvic muscles contracted for much longer periods than others, and you may notice, when you first try to contract these muscles, that they tire and tremble. To exercise your pelvic floor muscles gradually, you can pretend that this area is a lift that you are taking up to the first floor. You hold it there, then move on to the second floor, and so on until the muscles are fully contracted. Then release them gradually to the ground floor. Finally end with a toning movement by drawing the muscles up to the first floor again. If you do this 10 or 12 times a day you will be able to hold them firm for longer periods, building up to a count of eight or nine without holding your breath or tightening up your shoulders. But always remember to alternate tightening movements with resting spaces to allow the muscles to be reoxygenated in the intervals between activity.

Caring for your spine

The spine is a flexible column of vertebrae that acts as the central scaffolding of the body and which, because it is sinuous and lithe, enables all the parts that are attached to it to move freely. Your spine is not rigid like a lamp post. It is both strong and elastic. Caring for it properly depends on using it well. When it is used like a crane, you run the risk of backache and back injury.

The section of the spine situated at the rear of the pelvis is the sacrum. It is the central pillar to which the pelvis is fixed. The large, flaring ilia, the bones that look rather like elephant's ears, are fixed to the sacrum by the sacroiliac joints.

The spinal vertebrae are cushioned by discs, like a dynamic hydro-elastic pillow.* When you bend, these cushions soften the movement. When the vertebrae are pulled apart the discs open up like segments of garden trellis. The discs contain fluid that is gradually lost during the day if you have been in an upright position, especially when you have been sitting a lot. For this reason, a person is nearly 2.5 cm (1 in) shorter at the end of the day than at breakfast-time. Lying down enables the discs to fill up again, but they depend on *movement* to suck in fluid. In pregnancy the sheer weight of your body, and the extra weight of the baby and all its luggage, also sits heavily on the discs in your lower spine. The result is that all this extra weight squashes the discs even more. So to have

Posture and balance

Good posture is essential to your physical wellbeing during pregnancy. This means not only learning to stand and walk in the best way so that your baby is cradled in the pelvis in a position that is comfortable for both of you, but also performing other everyday movements, such as getting out of bed, in a way calculated to avoid unnecessary strain. These exercises will help you to achieve good posture, to improve the tone of your muscles, and to learn how to use only those muscles necessary for whatever you are doing. If you are looking good and walking with a spring in your step, you will probably also feel much better.

Standing well

Stand with your feet evenly planted, as wide apart as your hips, and parallel to each other. Keep your knees loose. Release any tension across your buttocks. Listen to your breathing. As you breathe out, feel the weight of your seat bones and sacrum pressing down through your heels, and imagine a thread attached to the crown of your head, drawing you upwards through your spine and neck. Let your shoulder blades drop apart and relax, and your arms hang loosely by your sides. Visualize your baby nestling towards the inside of your spine. Be aware of your breathing.

Relax shoulders

Keep knees loose

Standing badly
If the weight of your uterus makes you stand back on your heels, with your bottom stuck out and your shoulders back, your spine hollows and you get low backache.

Tailor sitting

This is an ideal way to release tension in the lower back. It can be one of the most comfortable sitting positions during pregnancy, as long as you make sure you do not slouch.

Drop knees towards the floor

Avoid slouching shoulders

Sit on your seat bones, cross-legged, and let your knees drop naturally towards the floor. Allow your spine to lengthen upwards as in standing well. Sometimes you could try sitting with your back against a wall for support.

a heal
know
and h
period
on to
the be
so tha
pregna
spine

Beca
weigh
small
wrong

Four-l
abdon
back l
well-to
these a
on too
verteb
the dis
may s
Girdle
health
own tu
provid
abdon
know

The
abdon
late pr
centre
your p
navel
wome
of a po
caving
pulled
muscl
somet

You
rectus
rest yo
shoulc
area th

The rocking-chair exercise

This encourages good posture during pregnancy by allowing you to press out the small of your back, while keeping the rest of your body aligned. For the exercise, you become like a rocking chair that rocks to and fro, and you need a partner to set you in motion. Avoid hollowing your back at any time as you do this.

1 *Stand well, as described opposite. Your partner should face you, with her hands resting firmly on your hips.*

Rest hands on hips

2 *Bend your knees very slightly and breathe easily as you rock your pelvis gently backwards and forwards between her hands several times.*

Rock pelvis backwards and forwards

Rest hand under lower tummy

3 *Your partner should stand at your side and put one hand firmly on the small of your back and the other over your lower tummy.*

Rock pelvis backwards and forwards

4 *Continue rocking, pressing against her hand with the small of your back, then releasing away from it.*

Keeping fit during pregnancy

While you are pregnant it is easy to allow muscles that were previously firm and elastic to sag. You are putting on weight, your figure is changing, and you may assume that sagging muscles are an inevitable accompaniment to these changes. However, gentle toning exercises, aimed at firming up your abdominal muscles and avoiding back strain, can do you and your body nothing but good. Through all the movements it is important to be aware of your breathing, and never to hold your breath.

Pelvic rocking

For this exercise you should lie on a flat surface with your head and shoulders supported by pillows, and your knees bent with the feet flat. Experiment by pressing the small of your back against the floor or the bed, and then releasing it so that you produce a gentle, rocking movement. Then roll your hips around in a slow, circular, hula-hoop movement.

Rock up and down gently

1 *Keeping your heels firmly down, neck and shoulders relaxed, raise your hips and buttocks as you breathe out and rock them gently to and fro, breathing freely.*

Roll your pelvis in a circular motion

2 *Relax and breathe easily as you roll your pelvis around—as if you were doing a slow, languorous belly dance while lying down.*

Keep your feet flat on the floor throughout the exercise

Exercises to avoid

Although double-leg raising and sit-ups are exercises often recommended for pregnant women, they do not in fact strengthen the abdominal muscles. These muscles do not work to lift the legs but to stabilize the lower back. If they are not strong enough to start with, they cannot cope with the effort involved when the legs or trunk are raised, and the result is back strain or torn abdominal muscles.

Double-leg raising
This exercise is rarely effective in toning abdominal muscles, and should never be done in pregnancy or the four weeks following birth.

Sit-ups
These can cause harm, and should not be done with straight knees or back if you are pregnant or in the first six weeks after childbirth.

Leg sliding

Leg sliding is a gentle exercise that allows you to tone up your tummy muscles both ante- and postnatally. Do it five or six times at first, and gradually build up until you can do it comfortably 10 or 15 times. If you feel your back aching, stop. Leg sliding is best done lying on your back on a firm surface with a pillow under your head. Keep your neck, shoulders and arms relaxed. Follow your breathing rhythm, moving on an out-breath, allowing your breath to flow in between movements.

1 *Keeping the small of your back pressed down, bend your knees so that your feet are flat on the floor.*

2 *Slowly extend both legs until they are straight. Keep the rest of your body relaxed as you extend.*

Draw up each knee alternately

3 *Draw one knee back up, then the other, without lifting the small of the back off the floor.*

Testing for separation of the rectus muscle

If you are starting exercises in the last months of pregnancy, find out whether you have already damaged your rectus muscle. You will need to be careful when doing exercises for toning your abdomen if this muscle has separated (see page 123).

Stretch your arms to your knees

1 *Lying on your back with knees bent, keep breathing as you tuck your chin down, and slowly raise your head and shoulders about 20 cm (8 in), stretching your arms towards your knees.*

Keep your legs bent and knees up

Feel below your navel

2 *Place your hands on your tummy. A small, soft bulge like a marshmallow in the middle below your navel indicates that the rectus muscle has probably separated.*

125

case you can rehabilitate it with postnatal exercises after the baby is born (see pages 398–401). Meanwhile concentrate on leg sliding (see page 125). Some exercises that are intended to strengthen the abdominal muscles can cause the rectus muscle to separate. You should not try double-leg-raising exercises while you are pregnant, or even single-leg raising unless the muscles are already in very good condition. Nor should you do exercises that entail putting your feet under heavy furniture and then raising the upper body or try any sit-ups without using your hands. Not only can these exercises damage the abdominal muscles, they can also strain the back.

EXPLORING PELVIC MOVEMENT

The bones that form the pelvis are like a cradle for the baby growing inside you, a cradle that can rock in all directions. Feel your pelvic bones with your fingers. Start with your hip bones. Press in over their upper ridges and then walk your fingers around and down into the small of your back where your hip girdle joins your spine. The point at which it does so is the sacrum, the bone that forms the back of the pelvis and the outlet through which the baby descends. Now walk the fingers around again to the big bones at the side, then down into the groin and around the front till they meet at your pubic bone. This forms the front of the pelvis and the baby dips down under this bridge of bone just before delivery. Notice that your pubis is much lower than your sacrum. The human pelvis is tilted. Once you have found exactly where these bones are and have a clear picture of them, get your partner to feel them, too. Guide his hands so that he is able to track your pelvis accurately.

Sacrum

Pubis

Female pelvis
The female pelvis forms a kind of cradle for the developing baby.

PELVIC ROCKING

Lie on any flat surface (it can be a firm bed) with head and shoulders supported by two pillows and your knees bent with the feet flat. Explore the capacity for movement in your pelvis. Experiment with gentle, rhythmic rocking. Then try rolling the cradle around as if you were doing a very slow hula-hoop movement. This is a kind of belly dancing while lying down, in which you tighten your tummy muscles while pressing your buttocks together. As you do so, notice how the different sets of muscles are alternately tightened and released and the way in which tummy and buttock muscles work together in a co-ordinated fashion.

Now combine this movement with controlled breathing. Each time you pull your tummy muscles *in* and press your buttocks together, give a long breath *out* through your mouth. Then, as you release the muscles and rock your pelvis gently forwards (it is a very slight movement), allow your lungs to fill up with air, breathing in through your nose. Do it at your own pace, emphasizing the breath out and letting the breath in take care of itself. This movement done in early pregnancy is a good way of toning abdominal muscles in preparation for the work they must do later.

Now rest your fingers on the big bones at the front of the pelvis on either side. Continue the movement with the breathing and notice the swing up and down of these bones. This is the distance the bony cradle rocks as you walk and move around in pregnancy. The baby is thoroughly accustomed to these movements during its intrauterine existence, and it is therefore not surprising that rocking a newborn baby quiets and soothes it. Research shows that a baby who is being rocked is most likely to be comforted by a swinging movement of 7.5 cm (3 in) to either side of the central position.* This corresponds exactly with the arc of the pelvic rock.

A position with firm support for your spine is best for practising this pelvic rocking. Other positions may hollow your back, which can be harmful, especially in advanced pregnancy, because it puts stress on the sacroiliac joint situated at the top of your buttocks. Such strain is particularly bad for you when you are pregnant because your ligaments are already softened by hormones released into the blood to make the vagina and cervix more flexible in preparation for the birth. Once these ligaments have softened, any form of pelvic rocking which involves back *hollowing* can cause more backache.

Exercise in pregnancy

Exercises to help you cope with the stresses of pregnancy should be matched by others designed to help your adjustment after childbirth, since this is the time when the speediest and most dramatic physical changes are happening to you. Postnatal exercises are simply a modification of the ones you learn in pregnancy, so there is no need for you to learn completely new ones after the birth. In this book postnatal exercises are described on pages 398–401.

POSTURE AND BALANCE
Good posture maintained every day is much more important than pregnancy gymnastics. As the load you are carrying changes during pregnancy you should give conscious thought to balance and body mechanics, something that is usually taken for granted. It is not just a matter of "standing straight, head up" like a Victorian young lady walking with a book on her head, but of understanding how to economize on muscle work and use only those muscles of the body that are needed for any particular task. This results in graceful and comfortable movement without strain and effort.

Standing To achieve good posture, stand with your back to a wall, heels far enough away from it for your seat and shoulders just to touch it. Release your chest, press the small of your back towards the

Aches and pains

In late pregnancy you are carrying extra weight that, instead of being evenly distributed, is centred in one area and so affects your balance. This extra weight alone can cause aches and pains by straining muscles and causing you to adopt an unnatural stance, leading to further strain. The way the baby is lying can also cause discomfort and occasionally a sharp shooting pain when the baby is pressing against a nerve. These exercises will help you ease such aches and pains.

Foot exercises

Foot exercises discourage varicose veins in the legs by stimulating the blood flow back to the heart. When you are sitting down or having a rest, practise drawing the alphabet with your feet, one foot at a time, keeping your legs still. You will find that you can easily read or do some work at the same time.

Draw letters, or even whole words, moving only your feet and ankles

The shoulder roll

Upper backache, which is caused by poor posture or heavy breasts, can be relieved by doing the shoulder roll exercise.

Put your fingers on your shoulders and rotate your elbows back

The angry cat

However many exercises you do with your back supported, it feels good to get the weight of the baby off your spine occasionally. You can do this by going on to all fours and rocking your pelvis, an exercise sometimes known as "the angry cat". This is a kind of pelvic rocking.

Spread your shoulders wide

1 *Get on to all fours, keeping the small of your back flat, not hollowed and your neck aligned with your spine. Your palms should be placed flat on the floor.*

Incorrect posture

Never, under any circumstances, allow the lower back to cave in while doing this exercise.

Keep your elbows still

2 *Without moving your elbows or knees, keep breathing as you tighten your tummy muscles and hump up your lower back. Relax back to the flat position after holding for several seconds.*

128

Wall stretching

A good way to lift your ribs off your expanding uterus is simply to stretch up your arms. First raise one arm up in the air and then the other, until you are comfortable. A similar result may be achieved if you do the exercise while sitting with your back pressed firmly against a wall to help alignment.

1 *Sit with the base of your spine pressed against a wall and lengthen up as in standing. Keep your shoulders soft and wide as you extend your legs in front of you and breathe easily.*

2 *Keep your seat and legs grounded and your back flat against the wall as you swing your arms out to shoulder height. With your palms pressed against the wall, walk your fingers up it.*

3 *When you have reached as high as you can, turn your palms outwards and spread your shoulders wide. With each out-breath let your seat bones drop and your spine lengthen up the surface of the wall.*

The wheelbarrow

Towards the end of pregnancy many women have pain in the groin. This usually occurs as a result of pressure from the baby on the joints of the pelvis. To relieve the discomfort, try this exercise, your partner kneeling very close to you.

1 *Lie on your back with your knees bent. Your partner should hold your hips at either side.*

2 *Your partner should slowly lift your hips. She should hold them up for a moment, then lower them.*

wall, and feel your seat tucking under and your tummy muscles working to straighten your spine. Make sure not to tighten your shoulders. Keep them dropped. Now imagine that a string is pulling your head up from the centre at the top and notice the back of your neck lengthening. Relax your jaw. (Your jaw muscles cannot force your head up!) Walk a few paces away from the wall. You will find that you are now standing in a stiff, exaggerated stance like a soldier on duty. Let the muscles settle into a more comfortable state. The rocking-chair exercise (see page 121) encourages good posture, too, and can be done with the help of your partner.

"I've always been very active physically and was determined I wasn't going to give up because I was pregnant. So I've cycled everywhere and gone on with my yoga and swum every day."

Walking Whenever possible, walk rather than stand. The healthiest, most rhythmic, and natural all-round exercise is walking. If you have to stand around, exercise your feet while you do so, even if only by screwing up and extending your toes, going up on to the ball of the foot and down again, and shifting weight from one foot to the other. Muscles in the feet and legs pump blood back to the heart, so movement is important to maintain good circulation in the legs.

You can also increase the tone of your buttock muscles and help the circulation in your legs by bridging (see page 122).*

Sitting Sit back on your chair and make sure that your spine is well supported. If necessary, put a small cushion in the small of the back to provide support while you are sitting down. In the last few weeks of your pregnancy you may need more support than this; try sitting well back against a large bean bag or a firm floor cushion. If you have to write or type at a desk or table for any length of time, remember to rest your head down on it occasionally and gently stretch the back of your neck. Use a low footstool (so that your knees are level with or slightly higher than your hips) to rest your back when you have to sit for a long time.

Bending and lifting Use your legs, not your back, when you reach down for anything. This means that, whenever possible, you should bend your knees and get right down in order to grasp the load. Kneel or squat when you are working low down, cleaning the bath or making a low bed, for example. Avoid misusing your spine as if it were a crane. For some household jobs, such as wiping or polishing a floor, it is most comfortable to get on to all fours. This takes the weight of the baby off your spine and is surprisingly comfortable, especially if you do have backache.

Lying down and getting up The front-lateral or "three-quarters-over" position is often the most comfortable when you are lying in bed. It may help to put a pillow under your upper knee. Allow a good amount of space between your legs. Avoid hollowing your back when you are lying down, too. If necessary, put a small pillow under your hips so that your back does not cave in.

Whenever you get up from lying on your back, roll over on to one side first, swinging your shoulders around, and push with your upper arm, drawing up your knees at the same time till you are in a kneeling position; tighten your buttocks and then rise from that position. This movement will avoid unnecessary strain on your abdominal muscles. It may sound complicated but it can come to be a beautifully smooth, co-ordinated movement, making you feel like Cleopatra rising from her barge.

Aches and pains

Although bad posture is often responsible for aches and pains during pregnancy, you may have other aches and pains that are just the result of being pregnant. If this is the case all you can do to relieve them is concentrate on relaxation and experiment with different positions in which you feel more comfortable.

If you have backache a chiropractor may be able to put it right and show you how to use your muscles more effectively and avoid strain. Chiropractors use a special couch that can easily be adjusted to leave room for your bump, and they can make spinal adjustments right through pregnancy without harming the baby.

Low backache In late pregnancy, if the baby is facing towards your front and engages as a posterior (see page 263) with the back of its head pressing against your sacrum, you may develop backache. Rest in positions in which the weight of the baby is tilted off the spine, and take every opportunity to get on to all fours. Washing a kitchen floor can provide extraordinary relief from backache. The angry cat (see page 128) is an exercise that combines this position with pelvic rocking to relieve your spine of the baby's weight.

Upper backache This occurs when you try to compensate for the weight of your pregnancy dragging you forwards by flinging your shoulders back and tightening the muscles in the upper back. To relieve it, roll your shoulders backwards whenever you have the opportunity and do the shoulder roll exercise (see page 128).

Pubic pain The cartilage of the joint in the front of the bony pelvic girdle is softened and stretched by hormones in your bloodstream during pregnancy. This makes more room for the baby to come down during birth. Sometimes from around the middle of pregnancy this stretching starts to cause pain. Your pubic symphysis may be tender to touch and you may have low back pain as well as pain along your inside thighs. A pelvic support belt can help, so ask your doctor or midwife about this. A bag of frozen peas or corn wrapped in a cloth placed over the painful area may give some relief when you are resting. When you roll over or get up out of bed be careful to keep your knees together.

Tingling and numbness You may sometimes feel tingling and numbness in your hand. This is known as carpal tunnel syndrome. It results from pressure on the nerves and tendons caused by swelling of the hand and wrist. You will be most aware of it in the morning, after your wrists have accumulated fluid during the night. To relieve the discomfort, try the shoulder roll exercise or hold your hand above your head for a few minutes and flex and gradually extend the fingers upwards.

Pain under the ribs You may experience pain below the ribs on either side when the top of the uterus (the fundus) is high after 30 weeks of pregnancy (see page 73). This pain normally tends to come on whichever side the baby is lying.

You will discover that you are only comfortable when sitting straight on a rather high chair and will not want to slump down on to your uterus. In spite of folklore about the dangers of an expectant mother lifting her arms above her head, you will find that it helps to stretch upwards so that your whole rib cage is lifted off the uterus. You can also do stretching exercises while sitting with your back against a wall for support (see page 129).

Pain in the groin In late pregnancy this is the consequence of the stretching of the round ligaments that go from either side of the uterus into each groin. Avoid rapid movements such as standing up too quickly. Also avoid standing for long periods, and even when sitting change position frequently. Symptoms can be relieved by doing the wheelbarrow exercise (see page 129). Some women get stitch in the side because the broad ligament on either side of the uterus is stretched. If you are lying down on your side, you may find it helpful to place a small pillow beneath your uterus to prevent this from happening.

Cramp in the leg Occasionally, pregnant women get recurring cramp, especially if they are trying to maintain a salt-free diet. Eating something salty before you go to bed may make the cramp disappear. A magnesium supplement can reduce cramp in the leg. Sometimes calcium tablets are prescribed for cramp on the grounds that your body must be short of calcium, but research shows that this is actually useless as a treatment for cramp.*

"I always wake him up to massage my leg cramps. At least he'll be well prepared for seeing to the baby in the night!"

Avoid curling your toes while you are sleeping. It is best to use a duvet or make up the bed loosely so that your toes are not pressed down by the weight of the bed linen during the night.

132

Lifting your feet above the level of your heart will also help circulation and relieve cramp. However, in advanced pregnancy this position may give you indigestion, so you are left with a choice between two discomforts. While you are lying with your feet up, roll them around in circles from the ankles to help stretch the calf muscles, or practise drawing the letters of the alphabet, one foot at a time, keeping your legs still. If you do get cramp, ask your partner to grip your heel and, using his or her forearm, push your foot up while holding your knee straight with the other hand. It is a useful precaution against getting cramp to do this regularly about ten times before you settle down for the night.

Common problems during pregnancy

Although your baby can grow inside you without your having to think consciously or do anything about it, the baby's development affects your whole body and every system in it. You may worry about disconcerting changes taking place if you do not understand what they are and why they have occurred.

VARICOSE VEINS
The valves that help direct the blood through the veins back to the heart may soften in pregnancy and become unable to propel the increased amount of blood through the legs. This causes pooling of blood and swelling of your veins, especially when standing.

Avoid all positions that allow pooling of blood in the legs: prolonged standing, sitting with your legs crossed or with your thighs pressing against the edge of your chair, for example. Foot exercises will help keep the blood moving. If you are advised to wear elastic stockings, choose semi- or full-support styles and put them on *before* you get up in the morning. Bend a knee, put one leg on and wriggle it up; then do the same with the other.

Vaginal varicose veins Sometimes a woman develops varicose veins in her vagina and labia. The discomfort may be eased by wrapping some ice cubes in a handkerchief, knotting it and packing it against the sore areas. Obviously you cannot walk around like this, but it is a good excuse to lie down for a while, thus offering a position in which the whole weight of your uterus is not pressing down on the swollen veins. Sometimes vitamin B6 (pyridoxine) can help, and you might take pregnancy vitamins that contain B6.

Haemorrhoids (also known as piles) are varicose veins of the rectum and can be caused by constipation. If you have piles avoid any straining on the lavatory. This condition should be treated quickly because haemorrhoids can become prolapsed (protrude through the anus), causing extreme pain. Your doctor may give you a prescription for a relieving cream, or a lint pad soaked in witch-hazel will help.

CONSTIPATION

You are more likely than usual to be constipated during pregnancy because extra hormones produced while you are pregnant cause the intestine to relax and become less efficient. First of all, ensure that you are eating the right kinds of food (see page 96). Eat plenty of fruit, vegetables, fibre and whole grains, and drink as much water as you can. When you are on the lavatory, allow your pelvic floor to be fully released and bulging down. Take your time over emptying the bowels, and have a brisk walk every day if possible. If you are still constipated, ask your doctor to prescribe a bulking agent.

BLADDER CONTROL AND INFECTIONS

In the first three months or so of your pregnancy the developing baby and enlarging uterus are pressing against your bladder, while extra progesterone flowing through your bloodstream softens the tissues. So it is quite normal for a pregnant woman to have to urinate very often. This may be even more noticeable at the very end of pregnancy when the baby has gone down into your pelvis.

Cystitis Pressure and engorgement of blood vessels in the pelvic area mean that a pregnant woman is more exposed to the risk of urinary infection. If you notice a stinging, burning feeling when you urinate, this usually indicates that you have developed cystitis. If left untreated, cystitis rapidly becomes very uncomfortable.

If you suspect that you have cystitis, go to your doctor, who will probably prescribe a course of antibiotics. It is sensible to seek help when you first notice the symptoms since delay can allow the infection to take hold more firmly.

As a general treatment for cystitis, drink plenty of liquid. Drink a glass of water every time you have used the lavatory. Drinking cranberry, orange, lemon or grapefruit juice may help, an alkaline-based drink such as a mixture of sodium bicarbonate and sodium citrate can be beneficial. One natural remedy that is effective is marshmallow tea. Wear cotton pants and avoid any clothing that is tight on the crotch. Wear tights that have a cotton panel or air holes between the legs. Spend time on the toilet to empty your bladder as completely as possible. When the baby is pressing against your bladder in late pregnancy, you will be able to shift position so that the baby moves a little, allowing you to void some more.

Pyelitis If you have a temperature and low back pain, and if it hurts when you apply pressure over your kidneys on one or both sides, you may have pyelitis (a kidney infection). Sometimes the infection also causes nausea and vomiting. Seek treatment immediately, since this is not only painful for you but can affect the functioning of the placenta. Antibiotics are effective, but all the measures suggested for coping with cystitis are also helpful and you will probably appreciate a hot-water bottle placed against the painful area. Women with pyelitis are often admitted to hospital to allow a proper diagnosis of the problem. The right drugs will usually clear it up completely within two weeks.

YEAST GROWTHS

It is normal to have an increased vaginal discharge in pregnancy, but if your vulva becomes itchy and your vagina is red, sore and burning, you probably have thrush ("candida" or "monilia"). Pessaries of a group of drugs called imidazoles are the most effective treatment for thrush. If you get repeated infections, try cutting out sugar and white flour and basing your diet on whole grains, fruit, vegetables and protein. Painting gentian violet (which you can get from a chemist without a prescription) over the affected area works well but is a messy process; wear a sanitary pad to prevent staining.

BREAST TENDERNESS

The normal breast tenderness of the early weeks of pregnancy can be acutely painful for some women, and they walk about with stiff arms to protect themselves in case anyone brushes against them. A good supporting bra is important even if you do not normally wear one, since if the breasts are increasing in size, as they usually are at this stage, their own weight can be uncomfortable. If your breasts become extra-sensitive like this, you will not enjoy your partner's most gentle touch until about the middle of pregnancy.

INVERTED NIPPLES

Some women have one or both nipples shaped like dimples. These are called "inverted" nipples. If you have a nipple like this but can press it out, or if it projects when you are sexually excited, the baby will be able to get hold of the nipple well and draw it out further. Otherwise you may find it more difficult to fix the baby on to the breast with a good mouthful. However, if you do manage to start the baby off, he or she will soon suck the nipple into a good projecting shape. It is a fallacy to think that you have to have prominent nipples in order to be able to nurse successfully, and there is no point in wearing nipple shells in pregnancy or trying to pull and squeeze your nipples in order to encourage them to project.*

Women with inverted nipples (also called dimpled nipples) can still breastfeed.

VOMITING

For some women the nausea and vomiting that are very common in the first three months of pregnancy (see page 24) go on much longer, and this prolonged sickness is known by the medical term of hyperemesis. A woman with hyperemesis is really ill because she cannot take any food by mouth. Surprisingly, the cure may simply be admission to hospital and often no further treatment is necessary. This is why some psychiatrists and obstetricians have suggested that hyperemesis is a symptom of disturbed relationships and that if the woman has a chance to get away from the relentless day-to-day

135

contact with a partner, mother, mother-in-law or anyone who is part of the stress to which she is reacting, the vomiting will ease. Part of the cure may simply be that she does not have to do any cooking or smell kitchen odours, however.

If you find that you are vomiting consistently at all hours of the day, cannot be sure of keeping any meal down, and are feeling really wretched, it is worth trying to get right away from your normal daily routine and surroundings. Try and spend time with people you know only slightly or not at all, and who will therefore not fuss over you too much. If this gives you the opportunity to do something that you have never done before (not hang-gliding!) or see something you have never had the chance of seeing before, so much the better. There is a phrase that is sometimes used about a person who is "run down": "she needs to be taken out of herself". A woman who is vomiting almost without interruption may need to be taken "out" of herself and her usual relationships until she can cope emotionally, and then, when her pregnancy has settled down, she can come back "into" herself with new strength.

NASAL CONGESTION

Sinusitis The mucous membrane inside the nostrils and sinuses often swells up during pregnancy because of the action of hormones liberated in the bloodstream that are also, fortunately, softening up your vagina and cervix. Some women seem to have a permanent cold in late pregnancy for this reason. Sinusitis does not interfere with your breathing during labour, so there is no need to worry about this, although you may be more comfortable breathing through your mouth rather than through your nose. This means that you will feel better if you take frequent sips of water or

"I seem to have had a stopped-up nose for months. It'll be good to be able to breathe easily again."

have a small spray bottle filled with ice water to spray into your mouth between contractions. A lip salve to smooth on your lips will help prevent any soreness. The symptoms of sinusitis will go away completely after you have given birth.

Nosebleeds are very common in pregnancy. These, too, are associated with higher hormone levels and congestion. A tiny blob of Vaseline in the nostril will usually stop a nosebleed, and you should avoid blowing your nose hard.

VAGINAL BLEEDING IN EARLY PREGNANCY

Bleeding from the vagina at any stage of pregnancy is always worrying. In early pregnancy it may be that the level of your pregnancy hormones is not sufficiently high to avoid breakthrough spotting. There is no way you can stop this without possibly affecting the developing baby. Cut out unnecessary exertion and, if the bleeding started at a time when your period would have been due, take life gently then and see if you can manage a few days in bed. Practise deep relaxation every day. There is further information about how to deal with a threatened miscarriage on page 372.

VAGINAL BLEEDING IN LATE PREGNANCY

If you notice any bleeding in late pregnancy it may be a sign that labour is about to start. It is usually blood from around the cervix and, except in those cases where there is a polyp in the cervix that has started to bleed, shows that thinning out and some dilation is now taking place. If your baby is due within a month and the bleeding looks like the beginning of a period, a blood-stained mucous discharge (a "show", see page 242), do not worry but accept it as a normal sign that your body is in good working order for labour and that you may start within a week or two.

Bright red bleeding, which flows as if you were at the height of a period, is another matter entirely. It is known as antepartum haemorrhage (APH) and, although quite rare, is serious. If you start to haemorrhage, you should telephone your doctor or go to hospital immediately. You should actually avoid both vaginal and rectal examination because they can make things worse. Ultrasound is the best way of finding out what is happening.

Placenta previa Sometimes blood flows from the placental site when it is too low-lying and partly in front of the baby's head. Intermittent APH from 27 weeks onwards is a typical symptom of this condition, known as placenta previa. Placenta previa occurs in about one in every 200 births and it almost certainly means that the delivery will be by Caesarean section. During a vaginal birth, as the lower segment of the uterus thinned out, the placenta would be torn away from its roots, thereby depriving the baby of both nourishment and oxygen. If you start to bleed when you are as much as 37 weeks pregnant, or thereabouts, you will be admitted to hospital and, if bleeding continues, will be advised to continue to stay there until the baby is mature enough to be born.

In fact, ultrasound at 16 weeks often reveals that the placenta is lying in the lower part of the uterus. Although this tends to be taken by some obstetricians as an indication of the need for Caesarean section, it is absolutely normal in early pregnancy and, by the end of pregnancy, when the wall of the uterus has stretched and enlarged, the placenta is usually in the right place in the upper part of the uterus. Only 6 per cent of low-lying placentas detected by ultrasound in early pregnancy turn out to be lying over the cervix.*

Abruptio placenta APH can also mean that a part of the placenta, situated in the upper part of the uterus as it should be, has peeled away. This is called accidental haemorrhage (accidental in that the haemorrhage has occurred by chance) or abruptio placenta. Sometimes there is constant pain in the abdomen and the uterus

becomes and remains firm. The severity of accidental haemorrhage depends on how large a portion of the placenta has separated from the uterine lining, but it is a potentially serious problem, and the doctor should be informed immediately. You will be advised to go to hospital for bed rest and, if the bleeding stops and all is well with the baby, will be discharged after four to five days. It is probably wise to avoid intercourse and orgasm until after the baby is born.

HIGH BLOOD PRESSURE

Every time you go for an antenatal visit your blood pressure is checked (see pages 44–45). This is because, although slight fluctuations are normal during pregnancy, any significant rise may be an indication of pre-eclampsia. If the diastolic figure (the second number) in your blood pressure reading rises by as much as 15, you are considered to have hypertension – high blood pressure.

Low-dose aspirin is sometimes used prophylactically by women who already have high blood pressure at the beginning of pregnancy so that they are less likely to develop pre-eclampsia. Unfortunately it also increases the risk of abruptio placenta (that is, the placenta starts to separate from the wall of the uterus before the baby is born) and does not reduce risks to the baby.*

Hypertension can be an early signal of pre-eclampsia. When a woman has pre-eclampsia the placenta does not continue to work as well as it should. So if you have high blood pressure, bed rest may be prescribed, the idea being that the placenta functions more efficiently if you stay in bed. But hypertension is over-diagnosed. For every woman who has sustained high blood pressure, another is diagnosed as having high blood pressure because it happened to shoot up at an antenatal visit. This may be because she had to rush to get there, was sitting around for ages worrying about her older child, was made anxious by information she heard in the waiting room, or simply because having her blood pressure checked by a doctor or nurse resulted in "white coat hypertension". If you can, refuse to be hassled and stay as relaxed as possible about your blood pressure. The more checks that are made for hypertension and the presence of protein in the urine in pregnancy, the more often they are found. Frequently they are chance findings.

PRE-ECLAMPSIA

The full name of this condition is *pre-eclamptic toxaemia*, but it is also known as pre-eclampsia, or *toxaemia*. The Australian name for it is *hypertensive disease of pregnancy* or *HDP*, and it is also called pregnancy-induced *hypertension* or *PIH*, and even gestosis. All these names reflect the uncertainty as to its cause. A 19th-century doctor called it "the disease of theories" and this still remains true today. Pre-eclampsia affects between 5 and 10 per cent of all pregnant women, but rarely occurs in the early part of pregnancy, unless a woman has been malnourished for years.

Take some time to really relax each day, breathing deeply and concentrating on the new life within you (opposite).

Symptoms Your blood pressure rises, the level of uric acid in your blood goes up, and you retain a lot of fluid. A rise in blood pressure alone does not mean that you have pre-eclampsia, and neither does an increase in fluid retention. The two symptoms in combination, however, indicate the need for some form of treatment.

If mild pre-eclampsia is left untreated, eventually protein appears in the urine. Blood tests may show that the liver and kidneys are not functioning normally. Babies of mothers with a high proportion of protein in their urine may be born prematurely; once a woman is excreting a lot of protein, or her blood values are seriously abnormal, pregnancy is unlikely to continue for longer than two more weeks.*

The danger of pre-eclampsia is not so much to you as to the unborn baby. If the condition is allowed to progress, clots and fatty acids build up in the placenta, blocking the arteries and causing the placenta to fail. This means that labour occurs prematurely, before the baby is necessarily mature enough to be able to survive. In its most severe form pre-eclampsia becomes eclampsia, and it can seriously affect you as well as the baby, causing convulsions and possibly even a state of coma. The following symptoms can all be signs of eclampsia: headache, flashing lights, nausea, vomiting and pain in the abdomen. Do not make the mistake of thinking that you have gastric flu if this happens to you in late pregnancy. Get in touch with your doctor immediately.

Causes No one is certain what causes the disorder, but research indicates that it may be due to thinner than usual blood vessels in the placenta. The problem starts between the 6th and 18th week of pregnancy, when placental cells do not infiltrate arteries in the uterus deeply enough to make the blood vessels expand so that they can nourish the baby (see page 70). There is another element in pre-eclampsia, too; it seems to be a process similar to graft rejection. It is as if the baby is a transplant in the mother's body, and her immune system recognizes it and produces cells in order to expel the intruder.

The risk of pre-eclampsia is highest in the first pregnancy. But it also has something to do with the man; if the woman has a new partner for a subsequent pregnancy, the chances of her developing pre-eclampsia are about the same as if it were her first baby.

Poor nutrition may play an important part in pre-eclampsia. You may be able to avoid the disorder by eating well, ensuring you have adequate protein throughout pregnancy (see page 95). If you have had pre-eclampsia in a previous pregnancy, start out on a programme of good nutrition *before* you conceive again. Dietary restriction to try to prevent pre-eclampsia is definitely harmful.*

You are more likely to get pre-eclampsia if any of the following apply: you have diabetes or kidney disease; you normally have high blood pressure (140/90 or higher); you are having twins or more; family members have high blood pressure or have had pre-eclampsia; you are in your teens or are over 40; you are under 1.6 m (5' 3"); you have had pre-eclampsia before (in which case there is a one in ten chance of its recurring); you suffer from migraine.

Treatment Many doctors think that staying in bed at the first signs may avoid further developments. Certainly bed rest coupled with relaxation of body and mind will reduce your blood pressure and improve the blood flow to the baby. Do not lie flat on your back in bed, but on your side or well propped up. Left-sided bed rest is most favourable for blood supply to the placenta.

If you have high blood pressure with protein in your urine, or high blood pressure alone, above 170/110, your doctor will probably admit you to hospital on the same day. You will be kept in bed and your blood pressure and urine checked every four hours. Sedatives are sometimes prescribed. After a couple of days you will be allowed up for short periods: if your blood pressure falls below 90 and stays there, and if there is no longer any protein in your urine, you will probably be allowed to go home after three or four days.

Many women feel trapped in hospital when they have pre-eclampsia, because they may not feel ill. In these circumstances, knowing what is happening to you and why helps you to care for yourself rather than just put up with having things done to you. Ask questions: find out about your condition and its progress, and understand the reasons for the treatment you are receiving.

Eclampsia If your pre-eclampsia has developed into eclampsia an intravenous drip will be set up through which a drug will be introduced into your blood to prevent convulsions; injections will be given to lower your blood pressure. Your baby may then be delivered by Caesarean section.

DIABETES

For young diabetic women with tightly controlled insulin, childbearing is as safe as for others. Every woman of childbearing age should know that it is important to control the condition carefully, particularly before conception and during the very early stages of pregnancy, since otherwise there is an increased risk of fetal abnormalities. The alphafetoprotein test, or the antenatal risk profile, which is the first screening procedure in a series that can reveal the risk of handicap, is more likely to yield an inaccurate result than in non-diabetic women, so this should be anticipated. It does not mean that anything is wrong. The

"The diabetes came as a complete surprise, because I'd felt so well right through pregnancy till then."

accumulation of glucose in a diabetic woman who is pregnant is absorbed by the baby, who then grows very fast. It is now possible for a woman to monitor her blood-sugar levels at home using a glucose meter; when linked to a computer at hospital, the meter provides details of the levels of blood sugar in the average day, so that she can adjust her sugar intake as necessary. A single ultrasound scan is an inaccurate way of trying to find out what the baby's size is likely to be at birth, so the obstetrician may recommend a series of scans during the latter months of pregnancy. If it is thought that the baby is growing too big to pass easily through your pelvic outlet, early induction of labour may be recommended. If labour is induced, although the baby may be large, it may not actually be mature, and may need special care after birth (see page 366). Some babies of diabetic mothers are delivered by Caesarean section because induction is performed before the mother's cervix is soft and ready to open. There is absolutely no good reason why a diabetic woman should not breastfeed her baby, and many women do so very successfully. In fact, breastfeeding reduces the chances of the child becoming diabetic later on in life.

Gestational diabetes This has been called "a diagnosis looking for a disease". It is much better to consider it more simply as the discovery of sugar in the urine and blood.

SUGAR IN THE URINE

Your urine is tested for sugar whenever you see the doctor or midwife (see pages 44–45). Nearly all women at some time during pregnancy produce sugar in their urine, indicating that they may have raised blood-sugar levels, which contribute to a baby's growth. Very occasionally the presence of sugar in the urine can be a sign of diabetes but most of these women *are not diabetics*. It is merely a biochemical variation, not an illness. When you are pregnant, you have more blood circulating in your system than normally, and there is therefore more blood sugar that must be dealt with by your kidneys. You are more likely to have high blood sugar if you are an older mother, if you are overweight, have had any repeated infections of the urinary tract, or if you smoke.

"I've found that I get sugar in my urine if I eat bananas and sweet things and don't get daily exercise. I also try to eat little and often rather than have a few large meals."

You can reduce the sugar level in your blood by modifying your diet: cutting out sugary foods, bananas and caffeinated drinks and by having small, frequent meals instead of a few large ones. If you go for a long time without food, body fat may be burned up and ketones start to appear in your urine. This is definitely not a good idea. It means that you are starving yourself. By all means restrict your weight gain if it makes you feel better, but ensure that you have good nutrition. Sugar levels can also be reduced by making sure that you get some exercise each day.

If sugar is found in your urine your doctor or midwife will probably want to take a blood sample for a *random blood glucose test*. If the glucose content of this blood sample is high you will be asked to take a *glucose-tolerance test*. Some obstetricians expect their patients to take the glucose-tolerance test as a matter of routine at approximately 28 weeks. It is up to you whether you accept this offer. You are given a sugary beverage to drink (or you may be asked to eat a specially prescribed meal with measured amounts of carbohydrates) and then have a blood sample taken one hour later. If the glucose content of this blood sample is high it does not mean that you have "gestational diabetes". If fact, there is an 85 per cent chance that you do not but you will be asked to take a longer, more complex and more sensitive glucose-tolerance test. If this indicates "gestational diabetes", you will be asked to monitor your own blood-sugar levels and modify your diet. It may also be recommended that you take insulin, on the grounds that this will keep the baby smaller, although there is no evidence that taking insulin reduces the size of the baby in women who are overweight.

Being labelled "gestationally diabetic" and treated as if you were diabetic during pregnancy can be extremely stressful and intrusive: strict dietary advice, frequent blood tests, insulin administration, multiple ultrasound scans, and the likelihood of induction and operative delivery. Most research suggests that this kind of surveillance is unnecessary and even harmful, and it certainly does nothing to help the baby. In the majority of cases a woman's blood-sugar level soon falls back to normal once the baby is born.*

ANAEMIA
It is normal for your haemoglobin level to fall during pregnancy. Iron used to be prescribed automatically in pregnancy, but now we know that it can be harmful, and that when a woman's haemoglobin level does not fall in pregnancy she is more likely to give birth pre-term. Laboratory tests of haemoglobin concentration and ferritin levels (for which the normal range is 125–150) are not useful.*

If you are genuinely anaemic, you can tell because you tend to feel very tired, become exhausted when you do anything vigorous, have dizzy spells and are frequently short of breath. Women who suffer from anaemia in pregnancy are less able to cope with any heavy bleeding at the time of the birth and are more likely to have an infection. Adjust your diet so that you get more iron-rich foods, protein, B vitamins (especially B12) and vitamin C, and take the folic acid supplement which your doctor will prescribe (see page 97). All are necessary to ensure that your blood can carry enough oxygen to all the tissues of your body. Your doctor will also prescribe iron tablets. If they make you constipated, ask for another kind. If you have a very low haemoglobin level (see page 40) after 30 weeks, injections of iron may be prescribed.*

HEADACHE
There is no reason why you should have more headaches when you are pregnant than when you are not pregnant. In fact, some women who usually suffer from migraine find that it disappears throughout

pregnancy. You can have tension headaches while you pregnant just as at any other time. If your pregnancy is fraught with anxiety, or you are taking on more than you can handle, you will probably be prone to headaches. Decode the messages from your body, modify your lifestyle and, if you are worried about labour, find out how you can help yourself (see page 149). A sharp, blinding headache in late pregnancy that affects your eyesight should always be reported to your doctor as it could possibly be associated with pre-eclampsia.

DIGESTIVE DISTURBANCES

Indigestion and heartburn are problems of the last three or four months of pregnancy. There seems to be so little room in your abdomen and it feels as if all your organs are being crushed.

It is better to have many small snacks than several larger meals a day, and it is sensible to avoid fried, rich or spicy foods. Some people find that they cannot digest bread or products containing yeast and that, by cutting out these foods, they can eliminate heartburn. Many women discover that they cannot drink during a meal and that meals have to be taken dry. You need to experiment with different combinations of food and liquid to find the kind of diet that suits you personally. There is no perfect diet that is right for everyone. Since heartburn results from acid present in your stomach flowing back into the oesophagus, try to find positions for sitting and sleeping in which the upper part of your uterus is not pressing against your stomach. You will probably prefer upright chairs and at night will feel better if you sleep well propped up with pillows. Make sure jeans, trousers and skirts are comfortably loose at the waist if you want to avoid indigestion.

"When I stopped trying to fight the pregnancy and let myself slow down I began to enjoy it."

SHORTNESS OF BREATH

When the baby is high, after about 34 weeks, and before it drops into your pelvis, you will probably find that you are short of breath whenever you exert yourself or even just climb the stairs. Your uterus is putting pressure on your lungs, and your diaphragm may be shifted out of place by as much as 2.5 cm (1 in). Again, sitting straight and sleeping propped up can help and you will probably discover that you have to take life rather more slowly in order not to become breathless. There is a rhythm to everything in nature, and this is a phase of pregnancy when your body is telling you to slow down.

Daily care and comfort

When you are pregnant you find that you carry around your own efficient central heating system. You do not need to dress as warmly as usual and in hot weather you will probably feel more comfortable in cotton dresses and skirts, and should avoid synthetic materials. Many pregnant women suffer from varicose veins in the legs, rectum or vagina (see page 133). Boots should not grip so tightly that circulation is impeded. Make sure that jeans or trousers do not interfere with the circulation in the groin.

SHOES

Shoes should allow the feet to keep their normal shape and should not be so high that your weight is thrown forwards on to the balls of your feet. In late pregnancy you may find that your feet are wider than usual and so need a wider-fitting shoe or a half-size larger. Although lace-ups give good support to the arches, you may not be able to tie them easily in late pregnancy. For the same reason slip-on sandals are better than shoes that have elaborate buckles.

BRAS

Since breast changes and enlargement occur from the first days of pregnancy, you will need to acquire a bra that gives good support and, if you are heavy-breasted, one with straps that are sufficiently wide not to dig into your shoulders.

Heavy breasts, allowed to hang without support, may develop stretch marks (see page 146), which will leave you with silvery streaks after the pregnancy. A woman with large breasts may prefer to wear a lightweight bra at night, too, during pregnancy.

TEETH

Although the baby needs calcium in order to grow strong teeth, your own teeth are no more likely to fall out in pregnancy than at any other time. However, as your gums soften and become spongier along with other tissues in the body as the result of the action of pregnancy hormones in your bloodstream, you may be liable to get a gum infection. Good nutrition (see pages 93–100) is the first line of defence against this. Mouth hygiene is also important, with regular tooth brushing, especially after breakfast and before you go to bed at night. Arrange a dental examination and cleaning – but not X-rays – once you know you are pregnant. Have another dental check-up when the baby is about five months old.

SKIN PIGMENTATION

For many women pregnancy is better than a beauty treatment: skin improves, eyes shine and hair is in better condition. But some women develop patches of darkened (pigmented) skin on the face, and this can be distressing. The technical term is "chloasma", but it is also called "the mask of pregnancy". It is a result of the high level of hormones, and also occurs in some women taking oral contraceptives. It is made worse by exposure to sunlight. The kind of cosmetic cream sold for minimizing birthmarks often disguises it effectively. The mask usually disappears once the baby is born.

145

You will notice that other parts of the body already pigmented become darker, for example the circles around your nipples and the skin of your labia. You may also develop a dark line down the middle of your tummy from your navel, where the rectus muscle is stretched. It is particularly obvious in dark-haired women. All these colourations should disappear once the baby is born.

STRETCH MARKS

Stretch marks (striae) may appear over your tummy, buttocks and breasts. They are dark streaks and are a sign that the skin has been stretched from underneath. They never disappear completely but, after the birth, they change from brown or deep violet to a silvery shade, rather like the marks on some fine, gauze-like fabric that has not been properly ironed. Many women use a rich cream or oil to "feed" the skin, and there are some on the market especially for stretch marks. However, these are expensive and any readily absorbed cream, or even vegetable oil, will do. If your skin is very stretched, and especially if you are having twins, it is marked like this because of pressure on the layers underneath which cannot be reached by anything applied from outside. Still, it can be relaxing for you to stroke your tummy; even though you may still have stretch marks, there is nothing to be lost and some pleasure to be gained from gentle massage with a rich, slippery cream.

ITCHING

A pregnant woman may get very itchy and uncomfortable in hot weather. It is important to wear cotton rather than synthetic clothing and underwear that is as loose as possible. Calamine lotion or an equal mixture of a few drops each of camomile, lavender and bergamot essential oils in some (about 50 ml (2 fl oz)) witch hazel or rosewater is soothing when stroked into the skin.

If itching is really bothering you, consult your doctor or midwife. Rarely, it is a symptom of liver malfunction – obstetric cholestasis – which puts the unborn baby at risk, and for which the only treatment is the induction of early labour.

SPORTS

Any sport you already do well is probably fine to continue with during your pregnancy: if you are really good at something, you do not waste muscular energy and your movements are smoothly co-ordinated. As pregnancy advances, you will notice your balance changing as the centre of gravity is becoming more concentrated in your tummy. This will almost certainly limit your sporting activities, although I heard of

"I've continued with horseback-riding – it's wonderfully relaxing – but I don't do jumps anymore."

a tightrope walker who practised daily on the high wire until she went into labour – an exceptional woman! Swimming is splendid exercise during pregnancy, and dancing, too, provided that you are not in a stuffy room. Although strolling through the shopping centre does not provide good exercise, brisk walking in fresh air, wearing comfortable shoes, with arms swinging and breathing deeply, is an excellent means of exercise.

Cycling is also beneficial, although if you can avoid heavy traffic and its inevitable fumes it is much kinder to both you and your baby. It is sensible in pregnancy to avoid all competitive sports that might make you overexert yourself.

TRAVEL

Travel in pregnancy is usually quite safe, but the exhaustion that may easily result from it is not. For this reason it is important to divide up long journeys into short, manageable sections if you can possibly do so; rest in between. Do not sit immobilized in a car, train or aircraft for longer than two hours at the most without getting up and walking around for five minutes. Sitting for long periods reduces the circulation of blood in the pelvic area. Also remember to empty your bladder regularly, since you are more likely to get a bladder infection during pregnancy (see page 134).

Travel in loose, comfortable clothing and shoes that allow for a little expansion. Soft slipper-socks are usually the most comfortable. Take any opportunity of dropping off to sleep. Pack an eye shade made of soft material to block out light.

Flying On an aircraft drink water or fruit juice; avoid alcoholic drinks, as air travel is dehydrating, and alcohol will dehydrate you even further. If you are more than 36 weeks pregnant, some airlines will require a letter from your doctor saying that it is all right for you to travel. Your doctor will probably agree to write such a letter as long as the risk of your going into labour on board an aircraft is only slight. It would be quite reasonable of your doctor to refuse consent if, for instance, your blood pressure is high, or if you suffered a threatened miscarriage in the early part of the pregnancy. In such cases a change in altitude could bring on premature labour. Similarly, it is unwise to fly in a small, unpressurized aircraft, as the supply of oxygen to the fetus can sometimes be drastically diminished. Some airlines, however, place no special restrictions on travel for pregnant women. You might also bear in mind, if you are thinking of flying a long distance, the strain caused to you by jet lag.

Driving is perfectly safe if you do not find it exhausting, and if you are not subject to dizzy spells. It is a good idea to try and avoid the rush hour and breathing in exhaust fumes. If you have a heavy standard shift, the sheer hard work of changing gears can cause discomfort in the later months. Automatic transmission makes lighter work of driving. Make sure your seat belt is strapped under your tummy and the shoulder harness is used properly, not so tight as to interfere with breathing or digestion.

REST AND SLEEP

During the first and last three months of pregnancy you will probably feel much more tired than usual, and it is advisable to rest as much as possible, rather than trying to fight off the tiredness. It is much better to rest *before* you become completely exhausted and feel you cannot go on any longer. Towards the end of your pregnancy there may be several reasons why you cannot sleep as much as you would like. Nearly every pregnant woman goes through a period when she either cannot drop off to sleep or wakes in the night because the baby is kicking her, she needs to empty her bladder, or she has had a violent and disturbing dream and cannot get back to sleep. Sometimes the insomnia occurs because she is lying in bed worrying and in the darkness her fears gain the upper hand.

If you have recently given up work, you may feel that your pregnancy has become a time of passive waiting and is stretching out longer and longer, so that you cannot see an end to it. You probably cannot sleep because you need action, and sometimes vigorous exercise during the day can be a remedy for this problem. You could also try the traditional remedies for sleeplessness, such as hot milk after a luxurious warm bath at bedtime. The problem with this, though, is that you are more likely to have to get up to empty your bladder.

The stillness of the middle of the night provides a marvellous opportunity for practising your relaxation and breathing techniques and for getting in touch with your baby. Use the time to centre down into your body and become more aware of the developing life inside you. Find a comfortable position to relax in, well supported by pillows wherever you need them, and let the pillows take the weight of your body, your limbs and your head. Concentrate on your breathing and allow it to flow right down through your body to where the baby nestles deep inside you. Cup your hands over the lower curve of your abdomen and breathe deeply so that the wave of the inhaled breath presses your hands up, and as you give a long breath out, your hands sink on the receding wave. Listen to the rhythmic sound of your breathing and think of it as being like waves flowing over shingle.

Relax and enjoy lying there with your baby. Once you have begun to lose yourself in these feelings, you will find that your breathing has relaxed and you are drifting off to sleep. Talk and sing and have private conversations with your baby. In the later months of pregnancy the baby can hear you, and when the baby is jumping around you may find that it soothes you both.

Emotional challenges in pregnancy

Many expectant mothers look and feel radiant. A healthy woman who is looking forwards to a much-wanted baby, who has a loving and secure relationship with a considerate partner, and some knowledge about childbirth and what she can do to help herself at that time, often revels in her pregnancy. Many women say "I feel fitter than I have ever felt before" or "I'm really enjoying being pregnant" and are surprised at the vitality and sense of inner fulfilment that they experience. Yet probably all of us are assailed by darker thoughts at times when we are overtired or under some special stress. Some of the negative feelings that women experience in early pregnancy have been discussed on pages 24–25. But as your pregnancy advances, more specific anxieties may preoccupy you at times. Anxiety may grip you in the middle of the night when the baby has kicked you awake or when you have had to get up to empty your bladder and cannot get back to sleep again. Every fear is magnified in the darkness as you lie trying to sleep and unable to relax.

WORRIES ABOUT THE BIRTH

Labour can be an intensely pleasurable, all-absorbing and deeply satisfying activity, which it is really possible to enjoy. But just as some people do not like climbing a mountain, even though the view at the summit is magnificent, and just as some people feel that sex is overrated, whereas others think it is one of the best experiences that life can offer, different women have very different attitudes towards childbirth.

This attitude is not simply a matter of what happens to you physiologically or how you are treated in hospital, but also depends on what kind of person you are. Anxiety can cast a shadow over childbirth and produce the speeded-up heart rate, high blood pressure, muscle tension and other physical results of stress that actually make birth more difficult. It is important to think through it and to understand why you are anxious.

Anxiety about labour is probably best dealt with first of all by finding out more about it – not just its mechanics, but the physical and emotional sensations each phase brings – and learning the relaxation, breathing and focused concentration that can help you to work with your body instead of against it. The simple process of sharing fears also often results in feeling much more lighthearted, so that women begin to enjoy their pregnancies. A good childbirth education class where discussion is encouraged and you can talk freely about your apprehensions, as well as your hopes, is often

effective in developing self-confidence and helping you to look forwards to labour as a peak experience that brings delight and fulfilment, not just an ordeal to be endured.

Pain A woman having her first baby often thinks "I have never had anything really painful. How will I stand up to the pain of labour?" and since she has no idea what that pain is like or what contractions feel like, the thought can bring terror. Learning about labour, about how contractions work and how they may feel at different stages of labour, is the most effective way of coming face to face with this anxiety and doing something about it. There is a whole chapter in this book about pain and pain relief (see pages 295–313), but the important thing to understand is that for most women the pain of labour is quite different from the pain of injury. Some women describe it as "positive pain" or "pain with a purpose".

Loss of control For many women anxieties about labour are linked with a dread of losing control. For your whole life you have been taught to control physical processes and your own behaviour, and suddenly something is about to happen that clearly cannot be controlled and that will take over your body. You are told that you may cry out or groan, for example, that you may lose inhibitions, be impatient or irritable with your partner or whoever is helping you in labour, and swear and say things you never meant to, and are horrified to hear that during labour you may involuntarily empty your bowels or your bladder.

You also learn that the waters may break suddenly. In any group of women discussing the events of labour, first-time mothers nearly always ask those who have already had babies when their waters broke, whether it was sudden, and if so where it was; they express keen anxiety that they may break in the supermarket or on a bus or in another public place. What these women are saying is that they are fearful of letting their bodies function freely because of the embarrassment and social stigma attached. It is as if degrading physical processes, above all dirty ones that involve getting rid of waste products from the body, are taking place in public.

Think through why you find the thought of your waters breaking in public so upsetting. You are having a baby and it is perfectly obvious that you are going to give birth soon. If your waters do break in public, is it really so very terrible? You will attract interest and sympathy, but not disgust. You may see it as a kind of sexual act in front of other people. You are quite right, and understanding this can help you in labour. Birth, just like lovemaking, is a sexual process. If you can go *with* your labour instead of fighting it the experience can be fulfilling in a strangely pleasurable way. Prepare the way to this through body awareness and relaxation. Touch relaxation (see pages 186–194) is a special kind of release that teaches you to flow towards sensations of pressure and heat. It will help a lot in labour.

During a second pregnancy (opposite) you may worry that you will not have enough love to share between two children. You will.

Loss of dignity and failure An anxiety closely connected with loss of control is the fear of making a fool of yourself. Some women think doctors and nurses will laugh at them if they find themselves making uncontrollable noises, for instance. You may feel that you are on public display in labour and approach it as a test of endurance. You may also be anxious about "letting down" a partner who puts great faith in your ability to cope, or even of "failing" a keen childbirth teacher. Some men who participate in classes and the other preparations for the birth become so enthusiastic and obsessional that they are in effect "trainers", rather like athletic coaches. The woman then feels that she is expected to put on a performance and must excel in it. Childbirth classes that are geared exclusively to techniques used in labour, rather than focusing on wider aspects of the total experience, can reinforce this feeling.

Just as the elaborate techniques performed to "ensure" satisfaction in lovemaking can sometimes disturb the spontaneous rhythm of sex and interfere with the intense feeling and play of emotion between the couple, so breathing exercises and "distraction" techniques can sometimes intrude on the experience of labour.

"I was always awkward in my overweight body. But in labour I swam through contractions like a seal or a dolphin. I felt triumphant!"

Exercises need to become "second nature" and be made a part of yourself. It is like learning to play the piano: there is a vast difference between laborious scales and playing a sonata. The exercises are important because they prepare you for playing music. But the eventual aim is to let the music flow through you, rather than to superimpose tricks and techniques. Such a physical and emotional surrender is simple in labour because of its intensity. Birth involves mind and body working together in a completely absorbing, exciting and passionate way. There is no success or failure in labour. You cannot make a fool of yourself, let anyone down or fail an examination in birth.

Fear of managing alone Some women approach labour as a medical incident like having an appendectomy, an unwelcome interruption of normal life rather than an experience that can be satisfying in itself. They feel totally dependent on the technology provided by the hospital and worry about whether they will get there on time, or whether the right people will be present to deliver the baby. Such dependence is reinforced by contemporary obstetrics and by every programme on television which illustrates the latest marvel of science applied to childbearing. The impression is readily given that women must depend on lifesaving machines, and that without them it is not safe to have a baby. The fact is, however, that although these machines can be extremely useful in diagnosing difficulties when a baby is at risk or when special problems arise in pregnancy or labour, the majority of women can give birth perfectly well without them. It is not advances in medicine but improved conditions, better food and better general health that have made childbirth much safer for mothers and babies today than it was 100 years ago. The rate of stillbirths and deaths in the first week of life is directly related to a country's gross national product and to the position of the mother in the social class structure.

It is a disturbing thought that it is twice as safe for a professional woman to bear a child than it is for a poor, unsupported mother. The challenge is to find out which mothers and babies are at risk, and to offer them everything that can make birth safer, and to enable all women to give birth naturally if they can.

Loss of autonomy Another frequent anxiety is that of being denied the right to function as an adult and being under the control of doctors, nurses and even machines. Many pregnant women resent the feeling that they cannot make their own decisions. Increasing numbers feel that they do not want to hand their bodies over to professional caregivers in pregnancy and childbirth, and are seeking maternity care in which they can take an active part, sharing the decision-making with their advisers.

If you are not sure whether your doctor is being quite open with you, or whether the hospital will really let you do the things in labour which you have asked to do, the uncertainty can produce a sick fear in the pit of the stomach. Too often pregnant women are treated very much like children or as patients in categories, such as "high risk", "low risk", "primigravida", "multigravida" and so on, who have to be processed through the hospital system, passive receivers of care rather than active birthgivers.

Fear of hospitals For many women hospitals are threatening places. People usually go to hospital when they are ill. This may be the first time that you have been a patient in hospital and the sights, sounds and even smells of hospitals may alarm you. Society has given little thought so far to designing and decorating maternity units so that they are intimate and look more like home, or at least a good hotel. Hospitals are sometimes still places with long, green-painted corridors and white tiles and instrument trolleys. Delivery rooms in otherwise splendid modern hospitals can be windowless boxes and antenatal clinics, your first introduction to the hospital, are often forbidding places without pictures and with back-ache-inducing chairs set in rows. Even more important than the surroundings are the attitudes of members of hospital staff and the ways in which they interact with patients. If you meet cool indifference, rigid authoritarianism or patronizing behaviour you may dread going for your antenatal appointments, and this anxiety may colour your whole approach to labour and childbirth.

There is a certain kind of emotional climate in which anxieties flourish and unfortunately it is one that our society often provides for many pregnant women. If there is no one readily available of whom you can ask questions and who will answer in clear terms that you can readily understand, the seeds of anxiety are often sown. Then they are nourished by the insecurity of seeing different members of the antenatal staff at each visit.

Women often feel apologetic about being anxious, about not being "sensible", as if they were revealing some shameful lack of emotional stamina. They are sometimes regarded as having something psychologically wrong with them if they show anxiety. But many of the fears you have during your pregnancy are not the result of inadequacy but a response to stresses caused by an environment that is alien and unfriendly, and by care that is impersonal. In such a situation anxiety is *realistic*.

Although you may not be able to eradicate anxiety about the birth itself, it is sensible to tackle it directly. Take a tour of the maternity ward. You can call the hospital to learn when tours are scheduled. Ask to see around the birth rooms (see page 183), including the machinery that may be used. Although you might prefer childbirth classes that are run independently of the hospital, attend at least some of those at the hospital, too, so that you can get to know some of the staff, and talk with your doctor or midwife about the style of childbirth that you would like if possible; ask him or her to note down any particular requests on your chart. Read the section on talking to doctors (pages 45–53) before you go to see your doctor.

Loss of attractiveness Some pregnant women are deeply concerned that their sexual attractiveness may be completely destroyed by childbearing. They are frightened of losing their figures; they may also be anxious that the vagina will be slack and changed in shape, and that they will not be able to make love with their partners in a mutually satisfying way. Fear of a tear or a cut (see page 320), often discussed in childbirth education classes, is not so much about pain resulting from stitches. It is really anxiety about genital mutilation.

Episiotomy In many hospitals episiotomy is more or less routine for all women having their first babies and for a large percentage of those having second and subsequent babies. Now this is changing fast. Women are questioning the need for what amounts to surgical intervention in normal birth and the creation of an artificial and painful wound. Obstetricians are asking why this has become so widely used without any proper evaluation. In fact, recent scientific trials have shown that this procedure, except in cases of fetal distress or other rare situations, has no advantage and causes unnecessary damage to the perineum. Women are often more anxious about the practice of episiotomy than any other invasive procedure during childbirth. The thought of being cut or injured, in such a sensitive place is horrifying, and some women feel as though they are being punished for enjoying sex. Many women are concerned that giving birth will damage them so they will never be the same again.

There are various ways in which you can prepare the tissues of your perineum – the area between your vagina and your anus – to become soft and supple during pregnancy, so that you enter labour fully confident that you can give birth without injury. Pelvic floor movements (see pages 118–119) can contribute to the sensitive awareness, co-ordination and control that help you in the second stage of labour, allowing you to open your body for the baby to be born and reducing stress on the pelvic muscles and perineal tissues. Many women find that massaging the tissues with vegetable oil can also help. Certainly getting in touch, literally, with this part of your body and feeling how flexible the tissues are will give you the confidence to know that your vagina and perineum are able to fan out and open wide like a great peony or a rose spreading thick, fleshy petals. Since in late pregnancy it can be quite difficult to reach your perineum and exert firm pressure, you may want to ask your partner to help you with this gentle massage. It feels especially good if the oil is warmed first and your partner's hands move slowly.

"'I can't, I can't' I wailed. 'You can' she said, 'I know you feel you're splitting in two, but trust me, you won't.'"

If you are concerned to avoid an episiotomy, discuss the subject with your midwife or doctor in advance. Say that you would like help at the delivery so that you can breathe the baby out rather than push it out, and ask for this to be noted on your chart. It is wrong to think that a woman who is anxious about episiotomy is in any way "neurotic", although doctors sometimes assume this.

You are better able to understand the healing process after an episiotomy if you know what has happened, and where. Exploring the vagina with your fingers during pregnancy (see page 116) and after giving birth, and looking at it in a mirror, helps you to feel that it belongs to you; you can gradually rehabilitate the muscles through practising gentle pelvic floor movements (see pages 118–119).

WORRIES ABOUT THE BABY

Almost every woman wonders at some stage during her pregnancy whether her baby is normal. Fear of producing a handicapped child is often connected with anxiety about not being able to live up to standards set by somebody else, usually either or both of the woman's own parents. It may seem almost impossible that you could produce from the dark interior of your body anything that is completely perfect. This is probably the most persistent, gnawing fear of all, and the only way of coming to terms with it is to develop self-confidence, a process that, not surprisingly, takes time. This is where regular attendance at childbirth education classes, which encourage you to have trust in your body and in your ability to give birth, rather than depending on others, can help enormously.

One woman who had disappointed her parents academically became pregnant outside marriage, in a desperate effort to show them that at least there was *something* she could do. She then lay awake wondering if her baby was deformed. Talking about this fear in a childbirth discussion group led her to reveal that she was having awful dreams. It then emerged that five out of the twelve women in the group were having very vivid dreams, and that even some of those who had not admitted to any worry about whether the baby would be "all right" were having dreams. In these dreams the baby was disposed of because it was not "good enough", or was taken away and looked after by other people because they, the mothers, were not good enough. She felt relieved and reassured that she was not alone. Dreams often reveal emotional tangles that cause distress in pregnancy until they are brought out into the open.

Most women who fear bearing an abnormal baby have little reason to expect that the baby will not be perfect. The minority who know of inherited diseases or handicaps in their or their partners' families, or who are pregnant after the age of 40, can seek genetic counselling and have alphafetoprotein (AFP) or other screening tests (see pages 220–229).

WORRIES ABOUT THE FUTURE

Change When a woman expresses anxiety about "things never being the same again", it helps to think through what exactly this means for her. One couple who had a deeply satisfying relationship saw the pregnancy and the birth as an "interruption": "We don't want to change our lives for a child," the woman said, "to be swamped by it. How long will it take before we get back to normal again? Sometimes I'm frightened we'll *never* get back to normal." She said that she did not want to become the same kind of woman as her mother. Most of all she was afraid her partner would not love her any more and that she would be desexed by maternity.

"We were happy and didn't want things to change. But now we're falling in love with the idea of each other as a mother and father. We're falling in love again."

Loneliness Some women having their first babies move during pregnancy, to a larger flat or house, and find themselves in an area where they know nobody at all. They stop work in late pregnancy and no longer even have the daily contacts with friends and colleagues at work. At home and alone for the first time, they are initially delighted, but quickly become bored and depressed.

If you find yourself in this position make plans to take up an activity which brings social contacts: learn something new; join a club of some kind; attend childbirth classes; track down interesting places in the locality to which you have moved, and invite people to your home. Your doctor or midwife may be able to tell you about other pregnant women or mothers with new babies who live near you and whom you can meet. It is worth investigating the possibilities while you are still pregnant. When you are busy with a baby it may be difficult to make new friends, especially during the winter months, so take the opportunity of making them now.

Social expectations A woman told me that her pregnancy made her feel that at last she was fulfilling a socially acceptable role and her own mother was proud of her for the first time in her life. She resented this. Doctors expected her to be a "good patient" and be processed through the busy antenatal clinic like all the others with their swelling bumps. She suddenly felt miles away from her former colleagues and others with whom she had worked, separated by the inescapable fact of her pregnancy. But by the end she felt guilty that she had resented the baby at the beginning of her pregnancy. At night as it moved inside her she lay wondering whether she would ever be a good mother. She said, "I sometimes feel so sorry for the little thing in there that I end up crying". In an antenatal discussion group where women had the chance to talk about their feelings it emerged that several of the women in the group were also lying awake at night worrying. What had seemed personal handicaps proved to be an experience shared by a number of women.

If you realize that you are not alone with your fears, and are not being "odd" or neurotic, anxieties usually become much less disturbing. Thinking about inevitable change may worry you in different ways: you may be afraid that the relationship with your partner will deteriorate; that you have no maternal instincts; that the loss of a job and the money and sense of freedom associated with getting out of the house and earning your own living may bring a real deprivation. You may wonder if you will be able to tolerate being at home all day with a "screaming brat", and whether you will miss all the interesting people at work.

Although such anxiety is realistic in the sense that these changes are dramatic and demanding for many women, most expectant mothers worry more about labour and the baby than about how they will cope after the birth. Many take the unknown "afterwards" more or less for granted. It is as if they can see only as far as the birth, which dominates the horizon. The postpartum experience may then come as a shock. So some anxiety about life after the baby arrives is a healthy sign, and indicates that the emotional work is taking place that prepares a couple not only for birth but also for parenthood.

Many anxieties during pregnancy, for both the woman and the man, offer clues to the challenges confronting them. It is a waste of emotional energy to try to "forget" them or put them to the back of your mind. They are there to be worked with. It is often the man and woman who are determined to take it all in their stride and carry on as usual, and who do not acknowledge feelings of apprehension, who face the most shattering crises when they finally have the baby. The discomfort produced by anxiety can force you to think through the meaning for you of the coming of a child into your life. Without stress and challenge of this kind, emotional preparation for birth and parenthood may be overlooked. Anxieties are a vital element in the emotional changes necessary if you are to face up to the reality of birth and then to the astonishing reality of the new baby.

Becoming a father

Becoming a father is a major step in a man's life. It can also be a daunting one. Yet it is an experience usually treated as insignificant in comparison with that of becoming a mother. As a result, the emotional upheavals and stresses of the future father are little understood, and men are not prepared for the impact of pregnancy. If people do notice that a man is finding the going difficult they tend to laugh rather than sympathize. In fact the nervousness and anxiety of the father-to-be are favourite subjects of jokes and anecdotes, ranging from the picture-postcard variety – showing a man wide-eyed and desperate in the hospital corridor as his wife produces triplets – to those amused tales about male ignorance and incompetence shared between women over coffee.

In childbirth classes and hospital lectures for parents-to-be a man is often discussed only in terms of how he can help his partner, and his own emotional needs are neglected. One result of this is to make him feel isolated and resentful, finding it difficult to reach out and give his partner the support she needs. She is the princess going to the ball and he feels a bit like the back legs of a pantomime horse.

An expectant father may feel jealous of all the attention given to the future mother, absurdly envious of her reproductive powers and sometimes even jealous of the coming baby. Then he feels guilty about succumbing to these emotions and decides to concentrate on his work – because that at least is one thing he can do properly. And the more he immerses himself in his own preoccupations, the more isolated and left out of the pregnancy he feels.

Some men become depressed during pregnancy or experience violent mood swings similar to those that a pregnant woman may go through. A few even walk out of the relationship because the stress is too great for them to handle. So it is important to remember that usually there are *two* people having a baby and that the man also goes through a transitional period of stress when deep emotions may be stirred and his behaviour may be difficult to understand.

REACTING TO FATHERHOOD

The sheer responsibility of having a baby can be frightening. The woman may be planning to give up work for a time, or even for good, and the man is expected to support the family. The financial burden may be too great for some men to shoulder without anxiety. For many men money problems constitute a rationalization, a socially acceptable explanation for anxiety, without getting to the root of what they really find disturbing. In fact, some men find that the prospect of becoming a father brings with it a crisis of identity. Although it is a common occurrence and one which in due course brings about creative change, it is nevertheless still a crisis.

A father discovers new depths of love and compassion, and life becomes more precious (opposite).

The changing relationship One element in this crisis involves grieving over a relationship that is bound to change. The easy ways, the lack of routine, the spontaneity of the early stage of the relationship, all have to give way to an existence centred around a baby. Some men see their partners as their mothers. When the woman becomes pregnant it is as if the man is losing a mother and is being replaced in her affections by a new baby. As his partner becomes more involved in the pregnancy and the baby to whom she is giving birth, he feels increasingly rejected and finds this inevitable shift of focus very threatening.

The changing woman Some men acquire a woman as a kind of showpiece, proof of their success in hunting down and possessing a desirable sexual object, or evidence of their social success, a demonstration and a symbol of a lifestyle that embodies achievement. Delighted as such a man may be to be fathering a child, he may find it quite difficult to cope with his partner's new concentration on the pregnancy rather than on him. He feels that the physical changes in his partner's body are upsetting as conventional attractiveness is replaced by a very different body – no longer the outline of a neat figure but a melon-shaped abdomen and heavy, swelling breasts covered with a network of tiny blue veins. A man who has valued a woman as a status or sex symbol may feel that he is being cheated.

The developing baby It is sometimes difficult for a man, who does not have the baby growing inside his body, to acknowledge its reality. He often begins to become more aware of the child at about the time he feels it bump and kick at night. Some men find this sensation not only astonishing and exciting but rather eerie, and they take a while to adjust to the idea of another being living and growing inside the body of the woman they know so well.

The future grandparents When a couple have a first baby they may have to work through a painful transitional period in which they must forge a new adult relationship with their own parents, which allows for the responsibility and commitment they have to the child they are bearing. This may produce stresses with the future grandparents, and a man may get caught up in a difficult relationship with his own mother just as a woman may with hers. When a man's mother is fearful that she is losing her son she becomes demanding. He may feel the pull of her possessive love drawing attention away from the needs of his wife and baby. Sometimes a woman sees this, whereas the man is completely unaware of it. It is important to understand that the older women, the ex-mothers, are being replaced, and they may feel hurt and unwanted. If there is a problem of this kind, the couple should talk about it together and be honest about their feelings.

THE FATHER'S NEW ROLE

Having a baby used to be solely the concern of the woman, with her mother standing in the background giving advice. Nowadays it is much more something for a woman and a man to share.

There are still some men who say they do not want to get involved in "women's things" and who feel that their manliness is being threatened. They have the uneasy suspicion that learning about childbirth means that they will no longer be potent, virile males. Some imagine that it is expected that they will be able to hand the woman over to the experts and retire from the scene. They believe that the professional must know so much more than they do that they are bound to be in the way during the birth and have no function in the delivery room.

Thirty years ago some midwives and obstetricians looked askance at men who became involved in the process of childbirth, as if they were slightly odd. Go back fifty years or so and men kept well away from anything to do with birth; pregnancy was a "certain condition" which a man pretended he knew nothing about.

My mother told me that my father felt embarrassed to go out with her in advanced pregnancy, so that walks they took had to be after dark, with her enveloped in a wraparound coat. And as for a father wheeling a stroller, or changing a nappy – it was unheard of; even a man who might have liked to try his hand at such things rarely got the chance. This was partly because in those days there used to be what one perceptive psychoanalyst called a male "taboo on tenderness". Men were frightened that to be seen to be involved with women's activities would humiliate them in the eyes of other men. And childbirth was the epitome of all feminine mysteries. Both women and men were prevented by these rules from discovering their full potential.

"He found it really hard to believe there was a baby there till it kicked him one night. He got very excited."

Many modern men are determined to share as much as they possibly can in pregnancy and birth. They enjoy the woman's changing shape and the reality of the baby's kicking against their hand. But a man often still feels he will be a novice at fatherhood. He wonders just how much he can do, since the baby is growing in his partner's body, not his. In a way, the partnership between the mother and her unborn child is already complete. And pregnancy often seems to be so carefully managed by the obstetric team that a man can sometimes feel like an intruder.

But a woman depends on her partner's support and needs the special relationship with him, which is quite different from any others that she has. She may not realize just how much he is sharing in the pregnancy emotionally and the heights and depths of his own feelings about it. There is no longer any need for a man to square his shoulders and pretend he is not stirred by what is happening. Take the opportunity to talk together about your feelings.

FEELINGS ABOUT BEING PRESENT AT THE BIRTH

Most expectant fathers today approach childbirth with curiosity and interest and in a very different spirit from that thought suitable by their fathers and grandfathers. Although they may wonder whether they are going to make fools of themselves while playing an unfamiliar part, and may be nervous about unpleasant procedures involved in labour, they want to understand what is going on and to help and support their partners. They realize that hospital staff are usually extremely busy and working with more than one patient at a time. It is therefore impossible for other people to give the constant companionship and loving care that a woman craves as she is swept through the intensely powerful physical and emotional experiences of labour, and the very unfamiliarity of the surroundings can make the most courageous woman apprehensive.

"I wouldn't have missed it for the world. I wasn't sure that I wanted to be there, but it turned out to be an incredible experience."

She needs her partner or someone else who loves her. She needs someone who is there not simply as an onlooker but as a companion, who understands what happens in childbirth, who knows what her antenatal preparation has been like, and who is able to help her in labour. (For more about the father's role at the birth, see page 277.)

The man who fully involves himself in the birth shares in an experience that is exciting, challenging, intensely moving and deeply satisfying. It is a question not only of helping his partner have their baby but of an often surprising encounter with his own emotions and the discovery of a peak experience that is bigger than anything he anticipated. There may be an astonishing, incredible joy and wonder at being so close to the beating centre of life. In a very direct way, love is made flesh.

Being supportive about antenatal care

Pregnancy can be a time of great emotional upheaval as a woman adapts to the extraordinary things happening inside her body. She has to go through all sorts of physical examinations that are not always conducted in a warm, sympathetic way. It is clear that many women are made anxious by the kind of antenatal care they receive.

THE CLINIC

Some men find a woman's anxiety difficult to understand. They say that they find the sophisticated technology that is used today reassuring and fascinating. But if the man imagines something happening inside his own testicles or penis, he may find it easier to comprehend. How would he feel if his testicles started to swell up and change shape dramatically, forcing him to visit a doctor regularly and be prodded, poked and examined by strangers who seemed concerned only with the lower end of his body? He might find it impossible to get information about what was happening to him, knowing only that he faced an ordeal at the end of nine months when whatever was occurring must be terminated and the thing inside him somehow got out. How would he like lying flat on a high table, sometimes with his legs up high and wide apart in metal stirrups, while various women in white coats peered at him with little lights and probed his body with special machines? Out of the corner of his eye he could see them writing up case notes full of technical terms and abbreviations apparently suggesting a disease.

A man has to go to an antenatal clinic only once to discover how intimidating it can be. In the atmosphere of a hospital clinic women often feel that they have become part of a factory process. Questions about treatment or requests for advice go out of their heads, or else seem to interrupt the smooth running of the institution and mean that other women waiting their turn have still longer to wait. Often a woman returns depressed and anxious. If her partner can attend occasionally and meet the doctor, he can give her moral support and build the foundation for a good working relationship with those who will be present during labour.

If this is not possible, he can still help his partner by providing comfort and security if this is what she needs, and by talking to her about the things that ought to be discussed with her caregivers. It is helpful to write questions down and keep a notebook for this purpose, together with information that you want to consider.

CHILDBIRTH EDUCATION CLASSES

By attending classes in preparation for the birth with his partner, a man can learn a good deal about the physiological processes and emotional changes of labour, can understand his own part in it, and often has the chance to see films of birth where men are giving support to their partners using skills learned in class.

EVERYDAY HELP

In the last three months a man can help by seeing that his partner takes more rest and lies down every afternoon or evening. Extra labour-saving equipment or additional help in the house can ensure that she does not get worn out. She should not be doing heavy shopping, so he may take over supermarket duty, or go with her to load the bags of groceries into the car. If there are jobs in the house like moving furniture, these are his now. And if she cannot get down to bath the toddler or strip the bed, the man can make these his responsibility now while she does some of the easier tasks. On the other hand the woman does not need to be treated like an invalid, and the couple can enjoy going out together, especially at the end of pregnancy when time may seem to pass very slowly and she feels she has been pregnant forever. A man can also protect his partner from all the well-meaning and often confusing advice that comes from other people both before and after the birth. He can support her in doing things the way they have both decided.

Your changing relationship

Pregnant women are not only obstetrical patients or even just future mothers. They are also usually in a loving relationship with a man. Pregnancy can be a time of great opportunity for both partners in the relationship to discover things about themselves and each other. However two people feel about each other, the emotional changes of pregnancy are bound to affect them. If they do not communicate easily it can be a time when small irritants turn into major crises.

THE COUPLE UNDER STRESS

There are some couples who find the transition period of pregnancy an especially difficult time. It can put stress on the couple who have an informal, even casual, relationship and who have not attached particular importance to getting married, but who perhaps marry when a baby is on the way. It can put equal stress on a couple who both enjoy their careers and have never seen themselves as parents, but who nonetheless decide to continue with the pregnancy when the woman conceives by mistake. It can bristle with challenges, too, when a woman has been on the pill, stops taking it because the couple think it might be a good idea to have a baby, and then immediately becomes pregnant before she has had time to switch her mind to the actual possibility of motherhood. In these situations rapid adjustment is necessary, and either or both parents may feel trapped at the same time as they are feeling delighted.

As soon as they tell other people about the pregnancy they may feel that a social machine has swung into action. Some couples say that they felt strong disapproval from relatives, especially their parents, when they put off having a baby because they were both busy with their careers. Then when the woman eventually did become pregnant they were overwhelmed by the relief and pleasure these people expressed, as if at last they were doing the socially acceptable thing. Even positive reactions may feel like a public intrusion on their intimate and personal relationship with each other.

SHARING THE PROBLEMS

When a pregnancy starts, a man and a woman often begin inhabiting different worlds. He may think that she has become psychologically unpredictable and vulnerable. She may see him as unsympathetic, unloving and crude. He may feel he can no longer talk to her about "rational" matters, and that she has lost interest in everything except the baby. He may even feel pushed out into the cold, as if he were living with a different woman. Because they are often isolated from other couples facing similar difficulties, they may be under the impression that such problems are unique to them. Talking to others expecting babies can help them to detect the social pressures on prospective parents and the cultural style of childbirth in modern Western societies, which often creates emotional stress. Attending classes together can provide a bridge between the different socially assigned gender roles of man and woman, and can help draw them closer.

TALKING IN A GROUP

At one antenatal group couples discussed together the effect of pregnancy on their relationship. One woman, who was feeling that she had lost her individuality in the universal category of expectant motherhood, remarked that she was frightened of what this was doing to her relationship with her husband. Would they, she worried, become just "Mum and Dad" and cease being lovers? Her concern about this was even making her resent the baby at times.

In discussion the members of the group found that other couples, too, were experiencing these pressures and the same kinds of anxiety. Some of them felt strongly that they wanted to be different kinds of parents from their own parents and to have a happier marriage than their parents had. It was agreed that it was important for a couple to share these thoughts with each other and to discuss not just the practical arrangements to be made for the baby, but their ideas about the kind of parents they hoped to be, and what they thought about their partners as prospective parents as well. Becoming a mother involves emotional "growing pains" that can be as disturbing as those of adolescence. A similar psychological process often occurs in a man, too, but he usually feels he has even less justification to talk about it because *he* is not physically pregnant. Yet to be able to nurture their young, both the man and the woman have to change and become different kinds of people.

Another couple who had been through this process with an earlier pregnancy said that talking about it had helped them to understand each other better and that they came to like their changed roles. At first they were merely play-acting the parts of "Mummy" and "Daddy", but then they found they were good at them. As they grew to become confident parents they became aware of qualities they had never imagined the other possessed.

DEVELOPING CONFIDENCE

Many couples have a funny name for the unborn child, and talk about it as a friend. When doctors prod and poke at the antenatal clinic or when the woman goes into labour, a couple can feel as if an intimate relationship between the three of them has been invaded. "Our" baby has become "the" baby, or even "the hospital's" baby. A woman needs to feel that the baby belongs to her.

Other couples have problems in family relationships (especially with their in-laws), which they imagine to be peculiarly their own and that they do not realize are shared by many others. Each partner

USING SEX TO INDUCE LABOUR

If you are "due", especially if induction of labour has been suggested by your doctor, lovemaking is one of the ways in which you might be able to start things off naturally. Some women are thought to be especially sensitive to prostaglandins in semen. (Prostaglandins cause the uterus to contract, and semen has a higher proportion of them than any other body substance.) It is best to choose a position in which the woman lies on her back with her legs raised on the man's hips. But since such a position may be very uncomfortable at this late stage of pregnancy, it should be done gently.

Breast stimulation in late pregnancy also sometimes produces a strongly contracting uterus. This worries some people, but unless you have reason to think that the baby may come too early it is

Lovemaking in pregnancy

Some women find that pregnancy makes lovemaking more exciting. Others want nothing to do with sex. Both reactions are normal. Sex in pregnancy should always be gentle and tender. For many couples it presents an opportunity to find new ways of making love.

Whatever position you choose . . .

. . . your partner on top, but with his weight off your abdomen . . .

. . . you on top . . .

harmless, and may be a good thing, because the contractions that result help to prepare the way for labour, softening and drawing up the cervix and dilating it a little even before labour begins.

NIPPLE STIMULATION DURING LABOUR

Stimulation of the nipples can restart a labour that has come to a halt. Some doctors have tried it in place of the oxytocin drip. But it does not always work. It may depend on how the stimulation is provided: perhaps someone you love may be more effective than a breast pump. The midwife or doctor may agree to go out and leave you. It makes sense to try the natural way of stimulating the uterus first. The emotions you have as lovers are not in conflict with the feelings of compassion and tenderness you have about a baby.

. . . relaxed and languorous side by side . . .

. . . almost on all fours . . .

. . . or even if you decide that you do not feel like full intercourse, the important thing is that you feel able to give each other physical pleasure without fear of harming your unborn child.

Pregnant again

Pregnancy the second, third or more, time around is quite a new experience. It is never exactly like the first time. It holds different challenges. Coping with these changes involves flexibility and resourcefulness on the part of both parents. In some ways things are much easier: you know what to expect and have probably developed self-confidence in your role as a childbearer. You may sail through the pregnancy with style. But there may be difficulties that come as a surprise because you thought it would be simple this time.

REACTIONS TO ANOTHER PREGNANCY

Other people's reactions The first problem you may encounter is the reaction of other people to a new pregnancy. Whereas your first was greeted with delight, friends and relatives are usually far less interested in the next pregnancy and may even raise their eyebrows and criticize you if you already have several children or if you are pregnant again after a very short interval. They can make you feel that what you are doing is not very public-spirited and even socially harmful. Some women say they were asked "Do you want it?" or "Don't you think you've had enough?"; others cite sympathy offered by well-meaning friends: "How ever will you manage?"

Your partner's reaction You may find that your partner is not so excited about the next pregnancy. He may be busy and preoccupied and even seem totally uninvolved. Many men feel an extra burden of responsibility and financial anxiety when a second or subsequent baby is on the way. One baby was fun but now he feels "trapped" into having to provide for a growing family for years to come. Some women are desperately disappointed at their partners' reactions to later pregnancies and feel that they are missing out on all the joy of the first baby and the companionship that drew them close together the first time. Talk about your feelings together so that you can come to appreciate what the experience means to each of you.

FINDING TIME TO RELAX

When you already have a lively two- or three-year-old or a group of energetic youngsters to look after, pregnancy can be very tiring. The first time around you were able to look after yourself and even occasionally luxuriate in afternoon rests, with time for thinking, planning and dreaming. Caught up in the hustle and bustle of family life, doing the school run, coping with the enormous meals children can consume and facing the everyday battle with tricycles in the hall and crumbs on the carpet, you may have to relegate pregnancy to the back of your mind. You simply do not have time to think about it. This may result in your neglecting yourself, your nutrition and your relaxation, and also missing out on time when you can just focus your thoughts on your baby and yourself. When you realize this, in the short and infrequent intervals between your commitments as wife, mother, nurse, psychotherapist, teacher, hostess, chauffeur, house cleaner, chief cook and bottle washer, the chances are that you will feel guilty. You begin to feel apologetic to the little baby who is growing inside you, and perhaps also fearful that you cannot give him or her the time or even the love that you have devoted to the others.

This feeling may be intensified after the birth, when to some extent the new baby has to be fitted into family life rather than your own activities being modified to the baby's needs. If you are sitting a two-year-old on the potty, or calming down three children in the bath having a very splashy game that threatens to submerge the toddler, it is difficult at the same moment to fix the new baby comfortably on the breast and to enjoy the release of milk.

Talk about these feelings of inadequacy with other women who are facing the same problems. If you do feel guilty, the only solution is to try to organize your life so that every day you have at least some time to think about and plan for the coming baby or, once the new baby has been born, to give him or her your whole concentration. It is certainly difficult to find even a short space of time for such attention; but you may be able to enlist someone who is willing to take your other children for a walk some afternoons, or your partner might bath them and put them to bed every evening, giving you time to concentrate on yourself and your new baby.

TAKING CARE OF YOURSELF

A new pregnancy may produce aches and discomforts that you have not experienced before. Lifting bigger children and the inevitable clearing and cleaning may contribute to backache associated with bad posture. This is accentuated by fatigue and doing things in a rush. If your child still wakes in the night, does not *ever* like the idea of an afternoon nap or wakes very early in the morning and comes jumping into your bed during the hours after dawn, a restless bundle, you may be running short of sleep and long for a solid uninterrupted 10 or 12 hours. Perhaps it is possible to arrange this when your partner is at home at the weekend.

Chances are that you look and feel more pregnant with this baby, too, partly as a result of poor posture and tiredness, but also because of the stretching your uterus has already withstood during the previous pregnancy or pregnancies. This may mean that you do not feel at all happy about your body; a lack of pleasure in yourself is then expressed automatically in the way you stand, walk and sit. It is a vicious circle only too easy to get into.

Ask your childbirth educator to help you firm up your abdominal muscles. Use your buttock and leg muscles to help support your spine and tummy and do a few rhythmic exercises daily (see pages 124–125).

171

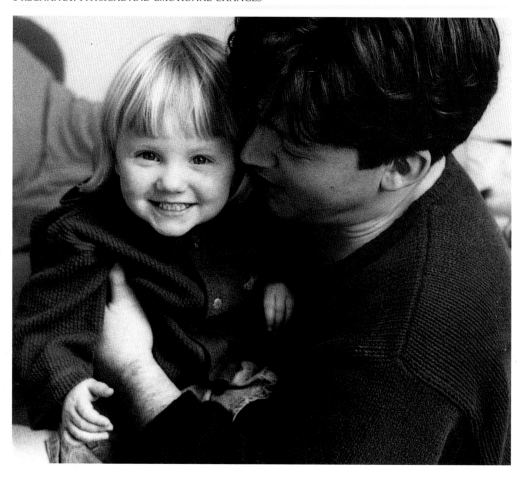

Birth provides an opportunity for an older child to learn about and share in a major life transition, and to develop new social skills and awareness.

Your older child may enjoy doing them with you. Then make an opportunity to cherish yourself a bit. Ask your partner for a massage. Think about what would cheer you up.

Preparing an older child

Some parents worry a great deal about how to prepare an older child for the new baby. This problem can seem almost insurmountable if the older one is clinging and very dependent. Childbirth educators* have come up with the idea of making a book for such a child, with photographs of himself, and starting with a simple description of how a baby grows inside its mother, complete with line drawings and a photograph of the mother when she was pregnant. You could show preparations for the birth, and then your child as a newborn baby, being suckled or bathed. These pictures could be followed by a series of photographs of the older child eating, drinking, playing, helping in the house and garden. Perhaps the last page could be left blank for a photograph of the new baby. All this helps an older child to prepare for the new baby and to realize that he was once just as small and incapable as it will be. If possible borrow a baby for a few hours or have a mother and her small baby in the house for half a day or so. This will help your child to confront the reality of a baby and also observe how a mother cares for it. Many older children expect a new baby to be either a passive bundle that can be handled like a doll or a playmate who can join in their games immediately.

If you are moving an older child from a cot to a bed, do so several months before the birth, so that it does not seem a consequence of the baby's arrival. And if you are going to have extra help after the birth, encourage the helper to become friends with the older child well before the advent of the new baby.

When another baby is on the way, the relationship between the father and the older child is of great importance. It is a time when the two can draw closer together and enjoy each other's company for longer periods, something that will help you a great deal after the birth when you are busy with the new baby.

SIBLINGS AT THE BIRTH

If you are thinking about having your older child or children present at the birth of this baby you will need to involve them in your antenatal care and prepare the child for the experience of birth by giving simple but vivid descriptions of how the baby is born, what happens in labour and how you may behave. Children are fascinated by how the baby grows in the uterus, and there is a book of mine which may help with this. It tells the story of how the baby grows inside the mother through photographs and text describing what the baby can do at each stage of pregnancy.* But remember that children need not only see pictures of giving birth but can also get familiar with the breathing and other sounds you may make. Only you can know if this experience will be right for a child. It can be a great education.

At the birth children should have an adult companion whom they like who is responsible solely for that child. Labour is often long and children get bored. They want to play, to run around outside, to eat, drink and sleep. They also need explanations of what they see and hear at the time: "She is grunting because she wants to push"; "That creamy white stuff kept the baby's skin soft, smooth and watertight so it did not get all wrinkly inside". The child's companion should be well informed as well as comfortable with being at the birth. An anxious adult conveys this to a child. Whenever a child expresses the wish to leave the room or do something else the companion should respond instantly. Your midwife or doctor should be involved in planning ahead for a child's presence at birth, and have a chance to get to know the child and build a friendly relationship. By the time a child is around four years old you can help him or her to construct and write a birth plan: "I would like to cut the cord . . . hold the baby after mummy has cuddled it . . . cut the cake at the birthday party after the baby has come out". It is best to arrange for your other children to be present if you are having a home birth, and for some women this is a reason for choosing not to have a hospital birth.

PREGNANCY

Anticipating the birth

In tune with your body for labour **176**

Windows into the uterus **220**

The last few weeks **231**

In tune with your body for labour

Part of preparation for birth consists of exercises, but it is even more important to *think* about labour in a constructive way. Give yourself time to imagine what is going to happen in your body and what you may feel, and so build up a picture that has meaning for you. This picture will be quite different from illustrations in obstetric textbooks: it is vital that it relates to *feelings* and is not just composed of intellectual information. Only then can the subjective sensations you experience in labour fit into a pattern that makes sense to you and that can help you adjust to each challenge as it comes.

So during pregnancy take time to imagine the birth of your baby. Think of different kinds of birth (see pages 262–276) and how to cope with them. Avoid restricting your fantasies to only one kind of labour when it may turn out that the labour you have is very different.

CHILDBIRTH EDUCATION

If you are having a baby without having been to childbirth education classes, your body will probably respond naturally to the situation. However, education for birth helps you to know more about your body and so feel happy with it during pregnancy. You learn how to prepare yourself so that when you are in labour it is possible for you to work *with* your body instead of fighting it, so that you understand the activity of the uterus, and so that, through relaxation, breathing and focused concentration, you can gradually come to achieve harmony with the birth process. This is important not only for the hours that you are actually in labour, but also for how you feel about the whole experience, yourself and the baby afterwards. Birth is not "just another day in a woman's life". Women remember their births and the intense emotions that were stimulated with extraordinary clarity years later, often into old age. They remember vividly how they felt when labour started, when the bag of waters popped, how it was when they got to hospital, what doctors, nurses, midwives and their partners did, interventions that occurred in the birth and, of course, their first meeting with the baby. Positive experiences remain as good memories. Negative experiences, far from being forgotten, intensify over time.*

Choosing an antenatal class

Once you have begun your antenatal care, it is time to think about arranging childbirth classes, so that you and your partner can learn about the physiological changes of pregnancy and labour and the possible emotional impact of the stresses likely to be involved.

It pays to shop around for classes and discover different ones available in your area. You would not dream of walking into a hairdresser's and asking them to cut and style your hair without finding out what sort of work they did. Learning about childbirth is even more important, so you should approach childbirth education classes with the same discrimination. For the quality of teaching to improve, critical, informed consumers are needed. Any antenatal teacher worth her salt learns from her students, and continues to modify her teaching on the basis of the feedback she receives from them and the ideas they share with her.

FINDING OUT ABOUT CLASSES

When you inquire about classes, do not assume that they are successful only if those who have attended them have had easy labours and births. If you have to have a forceps delivery or a Caesarean section it does not mean that you have "failed" in applying what you have learned. Having a baby is not like passing an exam or winning a race. You are not expected to come out "on top" with a two-hour labour, or to take no pain-relieving drugs. It is much more a question of learning how to adapt your responses – mainly those of breathing and relaxation – to the particular challenges of your own labour. So it can be useful to talk also to women who have had labours that were not straightforward, and to find out from them if attending classes helped them at all.

"I was working hard in the office through most of my pregnancy and the classes gave me special time that was just for myself."

Even though women all the world over have babies in much the same way, birth can be a vastly different experience for different women. Just as sexual intercourse involves certain mechanical and physiological processes that are the same everywhere, what people feel about birth, exactly what they do, and the meaning the total experience has for them varies with the individual and the occasion. Childbirth is not primarily a medical process, but a psychosexual experience. It is not surprising that adapting your responses to the stimuli it presents should involve a subtle and delicate working together of mind and body.

When looking into classes, ask a woman who has attended them whether she found the skills that she learned in class helpful when she was actually in labour, and whether she felt confident and understood what was going on. If she says "Nothing helped", it implies that the classes did not relate in any way to the reality of labour; if she says that she was absolutely terrified from beginning to end, it sounds as if the classes did not help her either, although she may have enjoyed getting to know the other expectant mothers.

Your local hospital may offer antenatal classes, although frequently they focus on the routines and procedures you may expect to have done in that hospital rather than on the choices, and on baby care rather than on what you can do to help yourself during labour. Your doctor or midwife may know of other classes. Write to the National Childbirth Trust and the Active Birth Centre (addresses for these are given on pages 413–414) and ask them to let you know where antenatal classes are held by their teachers.

WHAT MAKES A GOOD ANTENATAL CLASS?

Good classes are progressive in the sense that you learn a little more each time; you should not feel at the third or fourth lesson that you have sat through it all before. There should be opportunities for you to ask questions, discuss freely, and practise the exercises rather than simply listen to a formal lecture. Breathing and relaxation exercises that can be of practical use in labour should be included. Their relevance to labour should be specifically described, together with why and how they are used.

Relaxation is not as simple as it might sound. It is not just a question of flopping in front of the television screen or lying down with a bar of chocolate and a good book, but of learning complete awareness and control of muscle groups all over the body so that they can be contracted or relaxed at will, including muscles you may not even know you possess. Relaxation also means learning how to relax *under stress*, not just lying in a deck chair on a sunny day or in a classroom while a cool voice tells you that a contraction is beginning, continuing and then fading away.

It helps to learn different patterns and rhythms of breathing for the different phases of labour (see pages 201–208). So when you are asking about classes, try and find out from any woman who has been to them whether she learned breathing in detail.

An effective teacher helps her students realize something of what labour feels like, and the reality and power of its challenge. She also explains things fully, without fear that she is burdening her students' minds, and does so honestly and clearly. Unfortunately, in some classes there is far too much talking down to pregnant women.

"I didn't want just reassurance and talk about 'discomfort'. I wanted complete honesty so that I could make rational choices for myself."

You have a right to understand what is happening to your own body and what people are proposing to do to you. A good teacher does not answer a query with "Oh, you don't have to bother about that", or imply that everyone will do what is best for you and your baby, and that all you need to do is to have complete trust in your birth attendants. Discussion should always be a real exchange of ideas between you, not simply a few questions to which answers are fired back without any recognition of the apprehension and the sometimes nightmarish fears that can lie behind them.

You can see from this that a good deal depends on the personality of the teacher. It is not so much "the method" that is good or inadequate as the quality of the teaching itself, and perhaps most of all the relationship that the teacher has with her students. I have seen teaching that seemed woefully inadequate or mechanized, or that involved learning a number of rather irrelevant physical exercises, and yet, because of the personality and attitude of the teacher, the women participated joyfully in their labours.

THE READ METHOD

There are different approaches to childbirth education and the names associated with them can be confusing for expectant mothers. The Read method is named after Dr Grantly Dick-Read;* it is the oldest method and is usually associated with "relaxation classes". The philosophy behind this approach is that ignorance produces fear, which leads to tension, which in turn quickly produces pain. So teachers concentrate on overcoming fear by teaching deep relaxation and the breathing that accompanies it, along with providing full and accurate information about the childbearing process, exercises to keep you supple and poised, and discussion of breastfeeding. Today, there are few Read method teachers, but most childbirth educators incorporate his concepts into their classes.

PSYCHOPROPHYLAXIS

Psychoprophylaxis is a highly systematized training centred on techniques of breathing rather than relaxation. This method originated in the former Soviet Union, was developed in Paris, and was then introduced to Great Britain.* Psychoprophylaxis classes begin by deconditioning the women from their fear and doubts about childbirth, and then proceed to recondition them to respond to labour contractions as helpful stimuli and not as pains. Exercises are taught both for limbering up and for use in labour. Full information is given about the anatomy and physiology of pregnancy and labour. In the 1970s many National Childbirth Trust teachers taught psychoprophylaxis with a lot of "huffing and puffing", distraction techniques and strenuous exercises for pushing the baby out. They now have a much more broad-ranging and flexible approach.

In the United States, women know psychoprophylaxis by the name of its French originator, Lamaze, whereas in France itself it is often called *accouchement sans douleur* (birth without pain) or *asd*. This name is thoroughly misleading and might make any woman having pain in labour feel that something is going wrong. For most women who have been to antenatal classes the pain of labour is not the most salient thing about the experience but is a side effect with which many of them, helped by techniques of adjustment and by emotional support and guidance at the time, can cope very well without any pharmacological aids. Other women may want some additional pain relief in labour, and should certainly have it.

In North America and Britain, psychoprophylaxis methods have changed radically since they were first introduced. Dogma has disappeared, breathing is no longer regimented, and the whole approach has become more relaxed. Many teachers have learned to be skilled in group dynamics and psychological counselling, and different educators have evolved their own approaches to childbirth.

THE BRADLEY METHOD

In the United States an obstetrician, Robert Bradley, has created "husband-coached" childbirth, in which the man acts as the woman's teacher and supporter in pregnancy and labour, breathing is slow and full, obstetric intervention is kept to the minimum, and pain-relieving drugs are not used. Many Bradley enthusiasts opt for home birth. The Bradley organization is known as The American Academy of Husband-Coached Childbirth.

THE AUTOGENIC METHOD

On the continent of Europe a system of training for labour based on the Schulz methods of relaxation and breathing is taught in many antenatal hospital classes. A woman is taught to relax by conceptualizing warmth and weight in different parts of the body; her breathing should be slow and relaxed.

ACTIVE BIRTH

Janet Balaskas has developed an active method of preparing for birth based on hatha yoga, with the focus on moving around and changing position throughout labour, and giving birth squatting, kneeling or on all fours. To be able to do this freely and with comfort, it is very important to practise "stretching" exercises beforehand, and a woman learns how to adopt "open" positions with help from her partner.* Some methods of preparation for active birth are now often incorporated into other classes, and Janet Balaskas's great achievement is that in many hospitals all over the world she has succeeded in getting women off the labour bed and the delivery table and on to the floor.

THE ODENT APPROACH

Although a surgeon, Dr Michel Odent perceives that childbirth is very different from surgery. For him, it is important to provide an environment that facilitates a spontaneous psychophysiological process in which the woman who is left undisturbed will feel as if she is "on another planet".

Instead of holding childbirth classes, Odent organizes singing get-togethers in which new parents, pregnant women, and their partners, midwives, doctors and little children all join. He has rediscovered the use of water in birth, offering the woman a deep bath of warm water in which she can float in a peaceful, darkened room. For delivery, he favours the standing squat, with the woman supported from behind by her partner or another helper. Michel Odent's ideas have been incorporated into many classes run by midwives or other childbirth educators.

The Kitzinger psychosexual approach

My own "psychosexual approach" originally grew out of both the Read and psychoprophylaxis systems and now incorporates many active birth positions and movements. The approach is based on the idea that the woman is an active birthgiver rather than a passive patient. It focuses on birth as an experience rather than as a series of exercises in breathing and relaxation.

Psychology and social anthropology have contributed much to my own approach, and especially my observations of how women behave in and feel about labour in many different cultures. I have learned most from women themselves. Labour often involves barely glimpsed feelings about ourselves that have developed through the formative years of childhood: attitudes to and fantasies about our bodies, feelings about the relative size and positions of organs and orifices, and concepts of cleanliness and pollution, beauty and ugliness. All of these are partly social in origin, products of our upbringing and family relationships.

Labour is a social situation, not just a physiological or even a private emotional experience. Because it involves human relationships at a sometimes tense and demanding time, it helps to know how to talk with the different people assisting at the birth and how to understand what may be in doctors' and midwives' minds. All antenatal teachers agree that students need plenty of information about how their bodies work and what goes on in hospitals. Most classes make a visit to hospital and a tour of the delivery room. Yet it is not just a matter of knowing what will happen to you, but also of learning how to negotiate to get the kind of birth you want.

"The role play helped a lot, exploring ways of engaging with doctors and nurses, and how to handle resistance."

The aims of antenatal classes

So you will see that there is wide variation in exactly what is taught and how, although there is general agreement that six sessions of one and a half or two hours each are the minimum required. The aim is not to retreat from contractions but to adjust to them and respond actively. There is more and more emphasis on a woman being in the kind of setting and having the loving emotional support that enables her to be confident in her own powers and to behave spontaneously, without having to do "exercises" or wondering whether her performance is good enough. In the classes partners can learn how to help in pregnancy and labour and understand something about the feelings involved in becoming a parent. It is important that a woman be allowed to bring a woman partner if she wishes, and classes should not be restricted to heterosexual couples.

Your partner in childbirth classes may be male or female, a lover, husband, friend or relative. If you are offered less than these options in the classes you attend, you may feel the need to supplement them with other classes, reading or extra private tuition.

WHEN TO START CLASSES

Whatever method you finally opt for, do not leave booking classes or your reading till the last moment. Start finding out what is available and begin your course of reading four or five months before the baby is due, even though classes may not be offered till the last nine weeks or so. Where teachers run classes only for those in the last two or three months of pregnancy there is often an opportunity to meet the teacher earlier. This is an excellent idea, although some teachers of psychoprophylaxis believe that students get bored if they start too soon. Even if you do not start to practise any breathing techniques till the last weeks, it can only be beneficial to learn good posture in early pregnancy, and something about how the baby develops inside you and how to cope with any minor discomforts of pregnancy. It is also an advantage at any time, whether or not you are pregnant (and for men as well as women), to know how deep relaxation can help you get to sleep.

Whatever approach you select, provided you are happy with your teacher and develop confidence in yourself through the instruction, the teaching will be right for you, and you will find that you have a variety of tools which you can use to help you cope with contractions in labour. Labour need not be a fearful ordeal, but a positive, rewarding experience and a really *happy birthday*.

MAKING YOUR OWN SPACE

Some women want to be absolutely alone during labour. Most women, however, welcome understanding support from someone else in whom they have confidence and with whom they can "be themselves" and do what comes spontaneously.

Labour should not have to be a public performance. Unless there are especially urgent and demanding reasons why total strangers – nurses, doctors, students, medical auxiliaries, hospital porters and cleaners – should be there, you have the right to ask for privacy and have only those people with you whom *you* have chosen. You could make this absolutely clear in the birth plan that you hand over to be inserted in your chart (see page 50).

When women talk about their birth experiences in hospitals, especially large ones, they often talk about all the people who wandered in and out, anonymous faces looking through the porthole window in the door, and conversations about them, not *with* them, conducted over their supine bodies. Can you imagine the effect of having strangers and other observers around you when you took a bath, sat on the lavatory, tried to sleep, or were making love? Birth is a psychosexual activity that involves revealing that which is usually physically and emotionally private. It is patterned by rhythms similar to those in other physiological functions that entail letting your body open up. It involves strong emotions like those of intense sexual arousal. The tides and waves of labour culminate in the birth passion. To be watched by someone with whom you have

A typical birth room

If you plan to have your baby in a hospital it is a good idea to look at a birth room. Some equipment seems daunting until it is explained to you. Many hospitals arrange tours of their maternity departments for expectant mothers.

1 The clock is used to record the length of each stage of labour and for noting the time of the baby's birth.
2 The resuscitation trolley for the baby is equipped with oxygen and suction apparatus to extract any mucus from the baby's lungs.
3 Curtains screen harsh daylight so that it does not disturb the mother. They are intended to provide a reassuring element in the birth room and you can ask to darken the room for your first meeting with the baby.
4 Some hospitals have a chair bed, a comfortable seat for the birth partner that can be folded out as a bed.
5 The birth bed has three sections: head, middle, and foot, which are adjustable. The head can be raised or lowered. The entire bed can be raised or lowered. The foot can be lowered or removed as shown here.
6 A squatting bar gives a firm support to hold on to if you want to adopt a squatting position.
7 The adjustable stool is for the doctor or midwife.

8 A plastic container catches fluids and waste products.
9 A low stool is usually provided and is useful for helping you get on to the bed.
10 An electronic fetal monitor with sensing devices that are attached to your abdomen can be used intermittently or continuously during labour, or not at all. It detects and records the fetal heart rate and your uterine contractions.
11 Near the bed is a gas-and-oxygen machine for you to use if you need to relieve pain.
12 Behind the bed is the apparatus for measuring blood pressure. There is also a supply of oxygen available should the mother need it and spare electric sockets for other purposes.
13 A pole will hold the fluid if a doctor decides to set up an intravenous drip.
14 Adjustable footrests are on either side of the bed. When the mattress at the foot of the bed is removed, the mother may place her feet here.

no intimate and trusting closeness, to be inspected, criticized, applauded and urged to do better, can interrupt and prove an obstacle to psychophysical co-ordination. This is why it is important to create your own space for birth, and to arrange to have one or more companions with you with whom you feel not just comfortable, but completely at ease. If you are going to be giving birth in a large hospital with people whom you have never met before it is all the more vital to choose a birth companion who can be like an anchor in a stormy sea.

CHOOSING A WOMAN BIRTH COMPANION

Research carried out in various countries shows that if a woman has another woman with her during labour and birth she has less need for pain-relieving drugs and her labour is shorter. There are fewer operative deliveries (forceps, vacuum extractor and Caesarean sections) and fewer episiotomies; babies are in better condition at birth, and mothers are much more likely to look back on the birth as a positive experience. Some studies have also revealed that such women have fewer perineal lacerations, are more likely to be breastfeeding at six weeks and are less likely to be depressed.* Ten randomized controlled trials involving 3,000 women in childbirth who did not even know their companions before they went into labour have confirmed the benefits of having a support person through labour and birth.* The evidence is that the constant presence of a birth companion who is focused on your needs is one of the most effective forms of childbirth care introduced in the last 25 years. It is the rediscovery of a practice that was elemental to birth in many different cultures all over the world, including Europe and North America, until professionals took over. Women have always had other women with them. In medieval Europe women birth companions were known as "God sibs" – literally, "sisters in God".

"My sister was marvellous during my labour – really supportive – and it was lovely having her there and sharing the miracle of the birth with her."

In the United States today, and increasingly in Britain, the term "doula", which is a Greek word meaning "a female birth companion", is used. A doula can be present at the birth either instead of the baby's father or to support the couple who want to be together.

Doulas are women who are especially interested in birth and in helping women through birth. They have had training and experience in providing emotional and physical support and information. If you are thinking of who this person should be, consider your childbirth teacher, a student teacher, a close friend, or anyone in your family whom you feel has the right personality and experience and who will give you loving emotional support. A "doula" is often described as someone who will "mother the mother". In fact, this may not be exactly what you want. Many women do not look for mothering, but welcome woman-to-woman understanding and practical help from someone more like a sister.

Hospitals used to lay down strict rules stating that only one other person could be with a woman in childbirth. This has now changed. More and more hospitals recognize that having not only your partner but also a friend or family member whom you know and trust, and whom you have selected, helps you relax and increases self-confidence, with the result that labour is more likely to go well.

Relaxation and massage

Relaxation is the art of letting go and allowing peace to flow through you. The skill is in being able to release your muscles at will and not only when you are in a special mood to relax. It is not just an exercise, but as necessary a partner to – and interlude in – strenuous activity as is the breath out to the breath in.

THE IMPORTANCE OF RELAXATION

Relaxation is vital for labour. If you cannot relax you are likely to become exhausted as a result of muscles tightening up all over your body in reaction to the challenging stress of contractions. By tensing muscles unnecessarily you are wasting energy, and if you are exhausted any pain will be felt more keenly and your ability to control it is bound to be diminished.

Generalized tension and anxiety can sometimes affect the way the uterus contracts, producing inco-ordinate uterine action, which causes painful contractions that are not very effective in pulling open the cervix. Because it alters your whole body chemistry, marked tension lasting a long time can also reduce the oxygen supply to the baby. Just as the smooth co-ordination of your digestive system, the beating of your heart and your breathing are all affected by acute tension, so stress and anxiety can slow down the unfolding process of childbirth and make it more difficult.

When you know how to relax you can adjust to your labour with special breathing and positions, and other techniques. Relaxation helps keep your mind clear so that you are able to understand what is happening and can respond to it purposefully and creatively.

CENTRING DOWN

To explore and enjoy the skills of relaxation, you need to be able to "centre down", to use an old Quaker term, and be still and enjoy peace of body and mind. Lie down on your side, well supported with plenty of pillows, back rounded, head and shoulders forwards, legs and arms bent. Or sit in a comfortable chair with cushions supporting all of your back, including the back of your neck. You may also like a cushion under each arm or underneath your thighs. Before starting any exercises spend time thinking of the journey the baby makes to be born. Read pages 252–253 and then focus your thoughts on that part of your body. Concentrate on feeling your muscles and flesh heavy, all tension released.

Touch relaxation

Tension makes childbirth unnecessarily painful. Learn how to relax to your partner's touch so that this is a spontaneous reaction in labour. To practise touch relaxation, first sit on the floor, well propped with cushions and with legs and arms bent and spread a little. Give a long breath out through a relaxed mouth. Now you are going to contract different sets of muscles – especially those you tend to tighten under stress – noticing how you feel when they are tight. Your partner rests one or both hands over the area you have tightened. As you feel the touch, relax as if you were flowing out towards the touch.

Relaxing your abdomen

Under stress, the abdominal muscles tense up and this can lead to a more painful labour than need be the case. Tense abdominal muscles also cause shallow breathing. Massaging your lower tummy can relieve your tension and contribute to an easier labour. During labour the pull of the dilating cervix often feels painful and then light massage over the area just above your pubic bone can also be helpful in easing pain and tension. Practising how to relax abdominal muscles allows you to learn how to respond to your partner's touch in advance of labour.

Pull in your abdominal muscles

1 *Tense up by tightening your abdominal muscles and pulling them in towards your spine. As you do this, notice how the tension feels. You will find that you have also tightened the muscles at the bottom of your back and that your breathing is affected too.*

2 *Sitting or kneeling by your side, your partner can massage with both hands in a continuous, flowing movement, one hand following the other, stroking slowly and evenly over the lower curve of your tummy in a half circle. Light massage just above your pubic bone usually helps too.*

Relaxing your shoulders

Most people tighten their shoulders when under stress. Tight shoulders result in strained breathing and, because the tension is in the back of the neck too, can cause a headache. In labour, tension in the shoulders very soon results in heavy, panicky breathing, which in turn leads you to hyperventilate. A side effect of this is a reduction in the amount of oxygen reaching the baby. If you know how to release your shoulders, you will not hyperventilate. A woman may tense her shoulders when she is finding it difficult to cope with strong contractions in the first stage of labour. She presses her shoulders and her head back into the pillows. Try doing this while lying down and notice how you feel. Is it affecting your breathing?

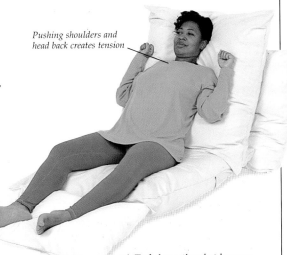

Pushing shoulders and head back creates tension

1 *To feel exactly what happens when your shoulder muscles become very tense, concentrate on pressing your shoulder blades back towards each other as if they were angel's wings and you could make them meet at the back.*

2 *Your partner should rest one hand firmly over each shoulder, applying pressure with the heels of the palms at the front of your shoulders. You should release immediately, flowing out to the touch. The hands should be slowly removed.*

3 *When tension is building up in labour, firm pressure on your shoulders, or the shoulder on the side nearest your partner, enables you to release this tension.*

Relaxing your head

This exercise helps to release tension in the muscles of the scalp. We often forget about the scalp muscles because they are under our hair, but tension here can lead to a frozen, strained facial expression, as well as giving you both head- and neckache.

Release tension in response to pressure on temples

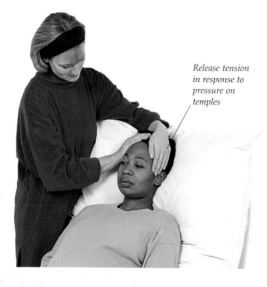

1 *Push your eyebrows up towards the top of your head. Notice how you feel when you do this. The scalp muscles can become this tense during labour.*

2 *Your partner should form her hands into a cap, which is rested against the top of your head. As you feel the pressure, release. Let your eyes close slowly. As your partner becomes aware of your tension easing, she reduces the pressure slowly. As this happens you visualize any residual tension flowing out of your head.*

Relaxing the face

If a woman in labour is concentrating hard, or feels anxious about what her body is doing, the muscles around her eyes become tense and her brow furrows. Her jaw stiffens, her mouth gets tight, and it becomes difficult to release the vagina and perineum too.

1 *Frown as if you had a headache and were in a very bright light. Notice how you feel when you screw up your eyes and forehead. This is how you may feel while concentrating hard in labour.*

2 *Using two fingers placed on each side of your head, your partner presses gently on the bone of the temples. Release muscular tension as soon as you feel this touch. Then very gradually your partner reduces the pressure, as you visualize any residual tension flowing out and away.*

Relaxing your arms

When you are experiencing a very strong contraction, it is tempting to grip someone or something with your hand and to contract muscles in your arms. This makes pain worse and, along with tension in the shoulders, interferes with breathing, so that you start to gasp.

Hold tension in arm

1 *Tighten the muscles in the arm that is nearest to your partner. Notice how your arm feels. Your partner watches to judge when the muscles look tight and then applies gentle pressure on the arm.*

2 *Your partner places one hand firmly on the front of your shoulder, with the other hand over the inside of your upper arm, cradled around the big muscle there, the biceps. The hands are held as if they are moulded to your body. As soon as you feel the warmth and pressure of the touch, release your arm muscles completely.*

3 *The hand on the inside arm moves slowly and firmly, stroking right down to your wrist. The other hand stays firm on your shoulder. As the hand moves, focus on the feeling of any residual tension flowing down your arm, out and away. Movements like this, from the centre of the body towards the periphery, are helpful because tension always flows from the centre, out and away. This slow, firm stroking down the inside arm can feel very good in labour. Try it at the start of each contraction.*

Relaxing your legs

When a woman feels her baby pressing down to be born she often tightens the muscles of her inner thighs in direct response to the pressing sensation. A vital part of opening up in order to allow the baby to be born is the complete release of any tension in your inner thighs.

1 *Press your knees very firmly together. As you do so, notice how tense the muscles of your inner thighs feel.*

2 *Your partner rests one hand on the outside of each leg and you relax towards the touch, letting your knees roll outwards naturally.*

Easing cramps

Sometimes in labour the inner thigh muscles get so tight that the woman's leg becomes stiff and her foot drawn up so that she gets a painful cramp. This can be released with massage.

1 *Stretch one leg out straight, so it feels stiff and taut, then flex your foot. Concentrate on feeling the muscular tension that results.*

2 *To help release the tension in the muscles, your partner places one hand on the inside of your thigh, moulding the hand to the leg, then strokes slowly and firmly down to your ankle. You release to the warmth of the touch.*

Releasing tension

This massage is particularly useful as you
reach the end of the first stage of labour, when
contractions are coming about two minutes
apart, and last a minute or more. At this time
a woman often feels that her legs are cold and
tense. She may begin to shiver and shake,
until her whole body is trembling. If this is
your experience, you will find that massage
of the inner thigh muscles warms your legs so
that you feel they belong to you again and you
can consciously release tension in them.

*1 See what happens when you press
both your knees outwards so that
your inner legs are uppermost.
Concentrate on feeling the tension in
your inner thighs as you do so.*

*Inner thighs become
tense as knees are
pressed out*

*2 Your partner rests both hands on the inside
of your upper thighs, and you relax
towards the touch. With hands shaped around
your inner thighs, your partner strokes slowly
from the top of your legs down to your knees.
She should use a very firm stroke as the hands
slide down the inside of your thighs and a
gentle stroke coming up over the outside of
the legs in a continuous flowing movement,
helping tension flow out from the centre of the
body, down and away. It is as if the hands are
giving the message to your body "Open up,
open up, the baby's coming out".*

Releasing your pelvic floor muscles

This type of massage reminds you to release
your pelvic floor muscles so that you can
help the baby's head bulge forwards in your
vagina. Each downward movement of the
hands has the effect of releasing the muscles
through which the baby is coming to birth.

*To focus on this feeling, first contract your pelvic floor
muscles as if they were a lift going up to the second,
third and then fourth floor of a building. Pull them
up and hold them. Then your partner rests both
hands on your inside thighs, and you release the
pelvic floor muscles down to them, as if the lift
were going down to the basement. As your partner
slides her hands towards your knees, release still
more, bulging your perineum forwards.*

191

Relaxing your back and shoulders

For the next set of exercises, lie on your side, making yourself comfortable with pillows. Your back should be rounded, your head and shoulders well forwards and your underneath arm behind your back. If a woman is lying on her side during childbirth and she becomes tense, she often adopts a fetal position. Having someone hold your shoulders in this position is helpful if you tend to overbreathe during contractions. A thumb massage over your upper back and shoulders or each side of the spine may help too.

1 *Curl up into a fetal position and hunch your shoulders. Notice how you feel when you do this. Your shoulders will have tightened up so that they are now near the level of your ears. Your breathing will probably be affected too.*

2 *Your partner rests her fingers on your shoulders and applies firm pressure with the palms. You release, flowing out towards the touch.*

Cushion gives extra support

Locating tension in the small of your back

Many women experience backache in labour, usually around the sacrum – the bone in the small of the back where the pelvis joins the spine. The tension that results from such backache means that you suffer more pain from your own stiff muscles.

1 *To find out exactly where the sacrum is, ask your partner to place her fingers over the large bones at the side of the pelvic cradle and then trace the shape of the pelvis around to where it dips downwards at the back to meet your spine.*

Tension is created when the small of the back is pulled in

2 *Still lying on your side, imagine that you have a bad pain around your sacrum. Pull in the small of your back to tense up muscles all down your back. You will find you are sticking your bottom out and throwing your shoulders back. This is what happens when a woman has back pain in labour.*

Relieving backache

The tension that results from backache can be greatly relieved if your partner applies firm pressure over this area. Relax your muscles and let go of tension while your partner presses along each part of your lower back.

To help you release, your partner presses firmly and steadily over the sacrum, using the heel of the palm (not the fingers). As soon as you feel the warmth and pressure, you relax, letting go and flowing out towards the hands. Muscles right down your back soften and loosen immediately.

Relaxing your back with massage

In childbirth, firm counterpressure, as above, may feel good, or you may prefer to be massaged. Massage is usually best done by moving the flesh – both skin and muscle – on the bone, rather than by merely creating friction.

Your partner can use either a firm, circular motion with hands more or less stationary, or slide the hands across the top of one buttock to the top of the other and back again.

Relaxing your partner's back

Partners using counterpressure or doing back massage often develop backache too, because they are relying on muscle strength in the arms rather than allowing their own body weight to flow down *through* their arms. Your partner may want to rest one hand on your hip, but should be careful not to exert pressure there or lean on you, since that will cause you discomfort.

The exertion of giving a massage can give your partner backache too. She may want to relax by resting one hand on your hip.

193

Relaxing your buttocks

A woman in labour may tense her buttocks because the baby is pressing against her rectum and anus as it comes around the curve of the birth canal, and she feels as if it is coming out of the wrong hole. She is often convinced that she wants to go to the lavatory. She resists the sensation by tightening up her muscles. When she tightens her buttocks she also tightens her pelvic floor muscles against the baby's head, as if shutting the door on it. Contracting these muscles can hold up the descent of the baby's head and cause unnecessary pain.

1 To tense up the muscles, press your buttocks tightly together as if you have a piece of paper between them and somebody is trying to take it away from you. As you hold on to it, notice exactly how you feel. This is how tense you may become during labour. Your partner watches for the tension, then rests one hand on each buttock, on the lower inside curve, and as you feel the warmth and pressure you release. Your partner will feel the tension slide away.

2 Your partner can help you relax by firmly massaging your buttocks as if kneading bread dough. It is important for him to get down into the fat and muscle, very slowly kneading both buttocks at once. As soon as you feel the firm, reassuring touch, you will relax.

Relaxing your "tail" muscles

Firm pressure, or rhythmic "rocking" massage, at the very base of the spine relaxes the "tail" muscles. These muscles form part of the pelvic floor.

Imagine that you have a tail like a kangaroo. You can lift it off the ground and then drop it down again. Now kneel in front of a chair with your forearms on the seat, and lift your "kangaroo muscle" up. Your partner firmly rests a curved hand at the very bottom of your spine, just around the curve where your anus is. You release towards the touch.

Touch relaxation

With touch relaxation, a partner gives you a message of touch to say, in effect, "release here". You respond to the pressure and warmth of the hands with immediate relaxation. If you learn to respond to your partner's touch in this way during pregnancy, it will be a spontaneous reaction when you are in labour. In effect, it will amount to your partner being able to draw the tension out of you.

To practise the technique, you contract different sets of muscles one set at a time. Your partner then rests his or her hands over the area that feels tight, and as soon as you feel the touch, you release, as if you are flowing towards it. Sometimes it helps if the touch develops into a gentle massage over the part of the body that is tense. This massage should always be very slow; a partner who is worried or excited may massage in fast, jerky movements and this has the effect of communicating tension rather than relieving it. Whenever massage is performed on bare skin, it is a good idea to use a little powder or warm oil, so that the hands glide smoothly and you do not feel itchy.

Between each exercise it is important to discuss whether it feels right for you – whether you want the touch firmer, lighter or in a slightly different place. During labour, too, you can talk together between contractions so that your helper understands exactly what you want. Some examples of touch relaxation for different parts of the body are given on pages 186–194. In childbirth, touch can be enormously comforting. It helps you to release all the muscles you do not need to use in order to have the baby. It relieves psychological stress, too, because you feel secure and nurtured.

On the other hand, some women find that the experience of giving birth is so total, so overwhelming, that touch would be superfluous. While touch relaxation can be an important part of preparing for the birth, when you are in actual labour you may come to a phase when you do not want to be touched at all. If so, simply tell your partner this. It is vital that you have the kind of support *you* want and that your partner be willing to stand back and let you do things your way.

Release of tension By practising relaxation techniques like this with you, your partner becomes aware of any tensions you are feeling and, when you are in labour, will be able to notice if there is a build-up of tension in your body long before anyone who does not know you well realizes what is happening. Then, all that is needed is to reach out a hand with the message: relax! If your shoulders are getting tense, for example, a firm hand rests on your shoulder. If your legs are knotting up, loving hands stroke your legs firmly.

One great advantage of this is that it does not involve giving directions and "coaching" in labour. There may be times – especially at the very end of the first stage – when positive guidance is invaluable, but there is no place at all for bullying a woman in childbirth. Through learning touch relaxation, your partner will have the self-assurance to give you just the kind of help you need.

Responding to the doctor or midwife Experiencing touch relaxation together also prepares you to respond to the touch you receive when the doctor or midwife examines you. Instead of feeling threatened, tensing up and pulling away like a snail drawing in its horns, you will be able to relax. This makes having your tummy palpated and pelvic examination much easier and more comfortable.

Pressure from the uterus During childbirth the stimulus coming from the uterus feels remarkably like a strong, intense kind of touch radiating from inside. As the uterus contracts it squeezes tightly. A powerful pressure builds up and there is a sensation of heat. When the cervix is being opened and pulled wider, still more pressure is exerted. Then, as the baby moves down through the cervix, pressure is produced by the ball of its head. It feels as if a grapefruit were being pressed down first against the anus and then through the vagina. To all these stimuli a woman may respond either by tightening up or by releasing her muscles.

"I hadn't realized that I clenched my jaw when I tensed up around my eyes or how often I curled my toes when I concentrated."

Learning to flow with a contraction Now imagine that you are in labour and that the pressure of the uterus is increasing with each contraction. Visualize the pressure of the baby's head, too. Then release and flow towards these sensations. Some women experience each contraction as warmth building up to heat and then dying down again. One woman told me that every contraction was like an oven door swinging wide open; at its peak she received the full blast of the heat and then the oven door closed again.

When the baby's head is on your perineum and coming through the vagina, all the tissues fan out like the petals of a flower. As they open you may feel a warm, tingling sensation, as if the whole area is being flooded with heat. If you have learned always to relax in response to the pressure and warmth from your partner's hands, you will be able to respond to these physical messages from *inside* your body too, not by pulling back, but by releasing and *flowing towards* them. In this way the sensations you get from within your body can serve to guide you in labour.

PUPPET-STRINGS RELAXATION

Of course you do not always have someone to help you with relaxation. You can practise relaxation by yourself, using a method that I call the puppet-strings method.

Lie in whatever position you usually sleep. Make yourself really comfortable, well supported by pillows, and give a long, sighing breath out and relax. Imagine that strings are attached to all your joints. Think of one fixed to your elbow, being tightened gradually so that your elbow is pulled up with the string. Depending on the position in which you are lying, your elbow may be moved a lot or a little. Then let it go. Notice the different feelings. Now the angle of the string is different, so feel the pull in a different direction. It lifts your elbow higher and higher. Now the string is released. It may take a little practice, but try not to allow any parts other than those operated by the string to move. The hand hangs limp at the wrist. The shoulder is not lifted. Only the elbow is activated.

Now do the same thing with an imaginary string attached to the other elbow. Let it be pulled in various directions. Continue as if a string were fixed to one big toe, then the other one, the back of one ankle, then the other, the left knee, the right knee, the left wrist, the right wrist, the index finger, the middle joint of a finger, one shoulder, the other shoulder, your left hip, your right hip.

Then imagine two strings, attached to your right elbow and right wrist, for example, tightening one after the other till both are drawn taut; first the wrist string is released, then the elbow string. Experiment with the strings working in a different order. Keep your mind focused on the tightening string rather than on the muscle you are contracting. Only when the invisible string is taut should you turn your mind to analyzing which muscles are tightened.

Imagine one string fixed to the top of your head, another to the base of your skull. First one is pulled, then the other. One goes slack, then the other. You will find that you can make the strings pull in different directions and at varying angles. This saves it from being a repetitive exercise that you do from habit, not focusing on what your body is doing. It is important that any body movements you do bring awareness, an increased sense of working *with* your body. Mechanical exercises have no place in learning to relax.

STANISLAVSKY RELAXATION

There are acting techniques for increasing body awareness and learning which muscles contract and work together. The precise combination of muscles working together varies with each individual and the nature of the task, the angle at which you tackle it, the weight, dimensions and even the texture of the tools used. You will find that tasks you perform, even ordinary, everyday tasks, often cause you to change your breathing, and sometimes you hold your breath altogether. You may also discover that you tense up muscles that you do not need to use because you tackle a job in the wrong way or overwork at it, or because you are emotionally keyed up about what you are doing. All this is a valuable process of self-discovery as you can gradually learn more and more about yourself.

The method of relaxation that is based on Stanislavsky's acting techniques explores different sets of muscles in the body that naturally function together and the ways they work in response to different imagined activities and tasks and even thoughts and feelings. You think of certain situations – things you might be doing with your body – and mentally involve yourself in these situations as if you were actually performing them. Notice which muscles have become tense. Once the observation is made, switch off the picture in your mind and deliberately release those muscles. Start by sitting or lying against a firm support and let the pillows take the whole weight of your body. Listen to the sound of your own breathing. Breathe so that you can just hear yourself – in through your nose, and then out through your mouth. Allow the breathing to flow through your mouth, letting the breath out be long and slow. The sound is like a little sigh as you breathe out. You may notice that there is a slight pause after you breathe in as if you have reached the crest of a wave. Enjoy that slight pause. Then give a long breath out. And with each breath out, relax a little more.

SUGGESTED EXERCISES FOR STANISLAVSKY RELAXATION

The jaw Imagine that you have some very sticky toffee in your mouth, and chew it well. It is sticking to your teeth. Work this great hunk of toffee out of your teeth. Notice what is happening. Then rest and drop your jaw. Let it relax, quite soft and loose. Notice the different feeling of complete release of the jaw muscles.

The eyes We do not usually notice when our eye muscles become tense. Imagine that there is a fireman climbing a ladder to rescue a little dog stranded at the top of a house. Focus on the fireman as he climbs all the way up. Observe the feeling in the muscles behind and around your eyes. Follow him with your eyes – up and up – until he is at the top. He has the little dog under his arm and is bringing it down and down. Now he is at the bottom. Relax your eyes, and if you want to, let them close. Notice how different they feel.

The feet Imagine that you are at the seashore standing on a very pebbly beach with no shoes on. Making very slight movements, imagine that you are walking on the beach with the sharp pebbles underfoot, and really feel them under your bare feet. Pick your way carefully over them. Oh! That was a sharp one! Observe the tension in your feet. Now go on to the soft sand. Really feel the difference. Then imagine lying down and letting your feet relax completely.

The hands Can you recollect the feeling of making a snowball? Imagine that you are picking up snow and are patting the hard, cold mass into a firm snowball. You are hurrying so that you can throw it at someone. As you quickly make your snowball, notice the tension in your hands. Then drop them and let them relax beside your body on the bed or floor again and notice how warm, soft and loose they feel.

Taste Imagine that you are sipping some water. Place the glass to your lips. It is sharp, neat lemon juice! Really taste it. Notice what is happening in your mouth and the tension that is spontaneously produced. Now it is gone. Let the muscles of the mouth soften. Now you have a large, ripe peach. Take a good bite of it. It is very juicy and the juice is dribbling down. You need to suck it and draw in the juice. Smell it, too. Chew it, swallow it. Now it has gone. Notice the very different feeling in your mouth. Relax completely and think through what happened to the muscles inside your mouth and nose and to the other facial muscles as you imagined eating the peach.

Smell Muscles around the nostrils and in the cheeks and the mouth work together as we smell and taste things. Imagine that you have in your hand a bottle of liquid. Take out the stopper and take a good sniff – it is ammonia! Notice how you have become stiff down the back of your neck. Then deliberately relax. Breathe in fresh, pure, clean air. Let yourself breathe easily.

Here is another bottle. Do the same with this one. It is perfume this time: lily of the valley. You will find yourself drawing in the scent of lily of the valley in long, slow breaths, holding the fragrance as if it were suffused behind the surface of your face. Now the fragrance has gone and you are just breathing air. Relax.

Go on from this to recreate in your imagination actions that you usually perform without thinking, simple things like writing a shopping list, tying shoe laces or unlocking a door, and discover exactly how you use your body.

Visual imagery in childbirth

Preparation for birth is not merely learning techniques for "coping" with pain. It is much more positive than that, and at best enables a woman to draw on her own inner power. Ninety per cent of birth, like 90 per cent of sex, has to do with what is going on in her head. One woman experiences a long or physically difficult birth with elation. Another finds a straightforward birth distressing. It is in large part a result of the particular quality of the relationship between her and her caregivers. It is quite difficult to have a positive experience in an unsympathetic or hostile environment.

The mental images a woman has of labour and birth are vitally important, too: how she imagines all the intense physical sensations as they well up in her, and the meaning that these have as contractions sweep through her

"I enjoy windsurfing, so that's how I pictured myself while I was giving birth – an active image that fitted my strong, rapid labour exactly."

body and the baby's head descends. Pain may be seen as destructive and produce pictures of internal organs tearing and the baby being damaged. Or it may be seen as pain with a purpose, as the pain of strong muscles working and the body opening. It helps to focus on creative images, and to rehearse them ahead of time. It is good preparation to imagine being in labour, welcoming each contraction with relaxation, rhythmic breathing and a vivid mental picture that enables you to go *with* the work of your birthing body, instead of resisting it. It may be that these pictures inside your head are enough by themselves for you to get in tune with your labour. You may want an entirely internal focus and anything else may be distracting. But it often helps to have something that you can see and on which you can concentrate during contractions: a photograph, painting, the pattern on your partner's T-shirt or an object such as a beautiful piece of pottery, small sculpture or some intricate tiles – something that represents for you the energy and flow of birth. Sky and seascapes, a range of mountains capped with snow, a path through the forest, great trees with their branches spread wide, a waterfall cascading into a lake, a field of ripe wheat with the wind sweeping across it, a flower opening from bud to full bloom – perhaps a waterlily, rose or peony – are images that may be right for you. In some Mediterranean peasant cultures women have a flower beside them when they are in labour. It is the rose of Jericho, which looks dried up and lifeless but in the heat of the birth room opens up and spreads its petals wide. In southern Italy they call it "the hand of the Mother of God". It is both a symbol of the help that Mary gives them in childbirth and of the cervix that is opening wider and wider so that the baby can be born.

"A painting of Mary giving birth to her baby, his head crowning in a halo of light, was my visual focus."

In Mediterranean cultures, too, there is a tradition of ritual actions that provide a powerful sense for the woman in labour of everything being opened and released, so that she can feel her body opening in a similar way. In Greece grain or water may be poured, windows and doors flung wide and clothing unbuttoned. As labour progresses and contractions get stronger and longer, you may want very active images that express the extraordinary power that you feel unleashed in your body. It often helps to focus on imagined actions, and to feel that you are swimming over waves, windsurfing, climbing a hill and then skiing down a slope, swinging and flying or roller-coasting over contractions. You can use music in a similar way, selecting tapes that echo your images of birth and represent for you the elemental forces of earth, air, fire and water.

In many different cultures women are drawn to images of water. Contractions are like great waves bringing the baby to birth as if on the swell of the incoming tide. Women poets writing about birth use water imagery, too. For Kathleen Raine contractions are "waves that break on the shore of the world" and she calls to her baby, "Child in the little boat, come to the land". An ancient Armenian poem expresses the overwhelming feelings of giving birth: "The skies were in labour and the muscles of the earth and the ripe red seas were in labour".* For some women a poem, a chant, a prayer or a song can have special significance and help them keep on top of contractions.

If when you are in labour an image turns out to be unsuitable or irritating, simply discard it and choose others, or focus on your uterus squeezing in and hugging the baby, your cervix opening in increasingly wider circles, the tissues of your vagina fanning out, your baby pressing deeper and deeper to be born, and reaching down to lift your baby into your arms. The essential element in the use of images like these is to achieve focused concentration, rather than letting your thoughts be dispersed by pain, and interpreting physical sensations in a positive, creative way, instead of feeling under attack. A woman uses the power of her mind, in harmony with the power released by her uterus, to help her body work freely.

Breathing for labour

Relaxation and breathing are so closely associated that it is important to explore them as parts of a unity. You cannot breathe correctly for labour unless you are relaxed. As labour progresses you may spontaneously breathe more rapidly. If you breathe more

Having someone you love with you makes for the best atmosphere in which to relax.

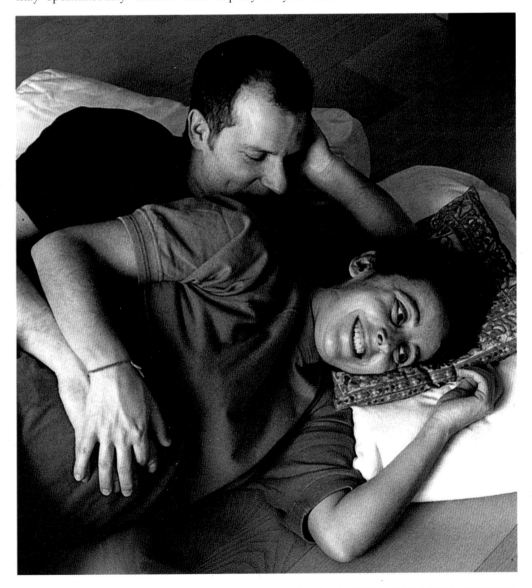

quickly and at the same time heavily, you will hyperventilate and flush carbon dioxide out of your bloodstream. This can make you feel uncomfortable and, if severe enough, you may even pass out. Ironically, when you hyperventilate, you feel that you cannot get enough air in, and you tend to gulp air which makes the hyperventilation worse. In fact, it is possible to correct the effects of hyperventilation by holding your breath for short periods, or by rebreathing carbon dioxide (by breathing in and out of a paper bag). This restores carbon dioxide levels and the symptoms disappear. The opposite – underbreathing or even not breathing at all – results in lack of oxygen and is more likely to happen if you have Pethidine to relieve pain. Although you can cope with this, your baby needs you to go on breathing. Overbreathing, "forgetting" to breathe, and holding your breath are all harmful to the baby during childbirth.

"As massive contractions swept over me I couldn't help holding my breath. My midwife said, 'Shout, moan, sing! That'll help!'"

In many cultures breathing in labour is deliberately regulated to help a woman work with the forces bringing her baby to birth. Among the Zulu, for example, breathing exercises are taught in pregnancy. A woman goes to the door of her hut each morning as the sun rises and takes careful, controlled, full breaths through each nostril alternately.* She uses the same breathing in labour. In other cultures breathing is regulated by background sounds, including prayers, music, the beating of hands, repeated phrases of encouragement or the swaying of attendants holding the mother.

BREATHING FOR RELAXATION
Smooth, easy breathing rhythms can also help release tension and create a state of pleasurable relaxation. In labour this is particularly important because, since contractions come like the waves of the sea, there is a strong natural rhythm built into the physiological activity. A woman can either resist this, trying to "switch off", escape from, or dominate it, or she can go with it and adjust her breathing to the compelling sweep of uterine power. She can only go with the rhythm if she can accept what is happening in her body and assent to it.

So the breathing I suggest for labour is not to do with "distraction techniques" and is no magic method of eradicating sensation or guaranteeing that you do not feel pain. It is simply another way of getting in tune with your body and especially with your uterus.

Rest your hands over the lower curve of your abdomen. In late pregnancy you have a lovely melon shape there. Breathe as slowly as you comfortably can. As the breath enters your nostrils, allow them to dilate, notice the slight pause between the breath in and the breath out, and then breathe out through a soft, relaxed mouth as if you had on a new, glossy and rather expensive lipstick. Enjoy that breath out. Notice what is happening to your abdomen. Feel it rising under your hands as you breathe in – a gentle swelling, like a wave building up. Then as you breathe out, the abdomen sinks back again and the wave recedes. Be aware of the slight pressure under your hands as you breathe in, and feel the pressure withdrawing as you breathe out and the abdomen goes back to its former position.

BREATHING DOWN YOUR BACK

You need someone to help you rehearse this. Try kneeling in front of a chair with your forearms and head resting on the seat and your knees well apart. Ask your helper to rest one hand firmly on each side of the base of your spine. Then breathe slowly right down your back, noticing the pressure against the hands as you inhale and how it gradually falls away as you exhale.

THE GREETING BREATH

When you are in labour, meet each contraction with your breathing, giving first of all a complete greeting breath. This is a deliberate, slow breath *out*. Imagine an early first-stage contraction lasting 45 to 60 seconds. Breathe slowly through the contraction, with the lower back spreading out and pressing slightly against the bed or floor as you breathe in, and the pressure being lifted as you breathe out.

THE RESTING BREATH

As a contraction fades away, you give a long, slow, complete breath out through your mouth – a resting breath. This is important partly because it offers you complete relaxation at the end of a contraction so that you can rest and get refreshed before the next one, and partly because it signals to everyone in the room that a contraction is over. If the midwife or obstetrician wants to talk to you, or ask you to turn over, now is the time, between contractions – never during them.

In strong labour you may want to give several of these complete resting breaths once a contraction finishes. Do whatever feels good. If you always respond to the end of a powerful contraction by one or more resting breaths you can be sure that, however difficult contractions are, you are giving your baby oxygen by breathing fully.

FULL CHEST BREATHING

You need a partner to help you practise this. Lie on your side with your back rounded, head and shoulders curved forwards, legs well apart and the upper leg drawn up and bent at the knee. Now lift your head as if stretching your spine all the way up the back so that you feel taller. Stretch your neck at the back, stretch all the way up your spine, and then simply let it drop back into place; let your head settle comfortably on your shoulders. See that there is a good space between your legs. Then give a long breath out and relax completely. Allow your eyes to close if they feel heavy.

Think of your back. Your spine is not stiff like a lamppost. It is constructed of small vertebrae in a curving shape like a string of sausages. We often act as if our spinal columns were very stiff. Yet think of the way a cat moves and how the movement ripples up and down the back. Now your partner rests one hand on each of your shoulders and massages with the flat of both hands from the top of your back right down to the bottom. The hands should be relaxed. Say if you would like the massage to be heavier or lighter, slower or quicker. Is it in the right place? It should feel good. Concentrate on relaxing towards the hands.

Then your partner rests the palms of both hands firmly above your waist on either side of the spine over the ribcage. They should be in a position that is comfortable for you and should not be pressing in on your waist (or where it once was!). Notice their warmth and strength. Breathe in through the nose and out through the mouth again so that the main level of breathing awareness is just where you feel the pressure and warmth of the hands, and listen to your breathing. Breathe right down to where you feel the hands, expanding your ribcage, so that it is swelling out under the hands as you breathe in, and then it falls away from the pressure of the hands as you breathe out. Listen to it for a moment. Can your partner feel the pressure, building up as you breathe in and falling away as you breathe out? This is full chest breathing. This kind of breathing can be very useful, once labour starts, to help you to cope effectively with the earliest contractions of the first stage of labour. You may be able to breathe like this all the way until you are about 5 cm dilated, concentrating on breathing into the area against which your partner is pressing the hands. When you are actually in labour you will not need the hands there because you will do it automatically and the contracting uterus itself will provide sufficient stimulus.

UPPER CHEST BREATHING

As contractions strengthen, you may want to lift your breathing above them, as if over the crest of a wave. Contractions come like waves and you may find that you can cope with them more easily if you breathe more lightly and more quickly. At this phase they may be coming every four or five minutes and lasting about a minute.

To practise breathing with these contractions, your partner rests the palms of both hands on your upper back just below your shoulder blades. You breathe so that your main level of breathing activity and awareness is where you feel the pressure of the hands. You may find that you want to breathe more rapidly, perhaps through parted lips. You should be able to hear a crisp little sigh or "huff" with each breath out. Now if you rest your hand over your upper chest you will feel it rising and falling at the same time, rather like a seagull floating on a wave. In labour the wave of a contraction will be underneath and you will be breathing over the top of it. Relax your shoulders; they are not doing any of the work. If you find that you can still breathe with your full chest, do so. Only "lift" your breathing if you really need to.

Practising for breathing

Prepare yourself to ride the waves of contractions during labour with the type of breathing that feels right for you. Breathe easily and without strain as contractions sweep through you. There are no rules about how you ought to breathe. When you are in labour your body will tell you what to do.

Full chest breathing is appropriate if you no longer find it easy to breathe all down your back. Your partner rests his or her hands at waist level and you concentrate on breathing down to where you feel the pressure.

Upper chest breathing is to lift you over the top of stronger contractions. Your partner rests his or her hands at the base of your shoulder blades and you focus on breathing where you feel the pressure.

Butterfly breathing can also be used to lift you over the top of stronger contractions. First rest your finger tips on your upper cheeks, feeling the space in your sinuses. Then practise breathing lightly and quickly in and out through your parted lips.

205

Practising for contractions

By simulating contractions you learn to respond to painful stimuli with the use of appropriate breathing techniques, so that you become able to work with your body in a positive way instead of fighting pain, which only increases tension and makes labour more difficult.

Simulating the action of the uterus

It is best to practise this technique with your partner, who acts as your "uterus" by pinching a little flesh on your inside thigh between his or her fingers. Be careful that this pinching is not over a varicose vein or so strong that it leaves you with a bruise. There is no need to press down on blood vessels. Simply lift a fingerful of flesh off the leg, gradually increase the pressure for 30 seconds or so, and then reduce it.

1 *If you need to, allow your breathing rhythm to get lighter and quicker as the pressure builds to the maximum. Then breathe slowly and fully as the contraction fades.*

2 *After a while it may be a good idea to change places with your partner. "Contractions" – like the real ones – can vary: some short, some long, some easy, some harder; some may even have double peaks. For your partner it may be the first real inkling of what labour can be like.*

BUTTERFLY BREATHING

This is a kind of breathing that you may never need to use, but which feels lifesaving in a speedy labour when contractions seem to hit you like huge waves in rapid succession.

When the going is hard, women tend to raise their chins in the air, tense the muscles of the neck and jaw, and start to gasp and overbreathe. Instead, let your head drop forwards on to your chest like a heavy flower on its stalk. Remembering to keep your shoulders loose, the back of your neck long, and your jaw released will help you to keep a steady rhythm and let your breathing "dance".

Butterfly breathing is the lightest, most rapid breathing you may want in labour. With most breathing techniques you are consciously using your diaphragm and lungs, but butterfly breathing is easier if you think of it as being centred in your mouth and behind your cheeks and not in the throat. If you centre your breathing in the throat, you will probably tense up your neck. Think of the space in your mouth, the space behind your warm, plumped-up cheeks. Either sit up in a chair or lie well propped up on the bed for this exercise. If you are lying flat, you can find yourself gasping and panting heavily when you are doing this breathing. So pile three or four pillows behind you, or try a squatting, kneeling, all-fours or standing position.

Resting the plump pads of the tips of your fingers against your cheeks will help you to concentrate on this area. Part your lips in a slight smile like the Mona Lisa. Relax your mouth and you will probably find that you are salivating a little. Breathe lightly in and out through your parted lips. Start gently, then allow your breathing to speed up till it is like little dancing waves.

Butterfly breathing may be quite difficult at first. You may feel that you are taking in or letting out too much air. Most people do to begin with, and find this the most contrived kind of breathing to learn. They think that they will never be able to manage it in labour, but then it comes quite naturally and they do not know how they could have coped without it. You may find that it helps to think in terms of a definite rhythm in which one beat is slightly accentuated: *one,* two, three, four; *one,* two, three, four; or *one,* two, three, four, five, six. If you do this, be careful not to expel a great deal of air on the accentuated breath or you will gasp in the following breath and start to hyperventilate. If you find it difficult to keep the rhythm, or find your throat getting tight, give a quick blow out through pursed lips and carry on with the light breathing immediately after.

After you have experimented with this breathing, try it once again, and this time notice especially if your shoulders or the back of your neck becomes tense. Drop your shoulders and relax. Under stress, it is tempting to breathe too heavily and sound as if you are a chugging piece of machinery. Try to keep your breathing as light as a whisper. When you rehearse, think of the sound of leaves in the forest floating to the ground, but bear in mind that in actual childbirth you will naturally make more noise than that. You will want to use this sort of breathing only when you are coping with the strongest contractions, at the end of the first stage. You may discover that full chest, upper chest or even breathing all down your back works well for you at this time. Do whatever feels right for you. When you reach this point, you may feel like a little ship in a storm at sea in the midst of huge waves and confusing cross currents. For most women this is the most difficult time of labour. Grantly Dick-Read used to call it "the pain period of labour". This does not mean that you may not feel pain at other times, but it is the time when you will need all your concentration and control.

SHEEP'S BREATHING

If we watch any mammal giving birth, a cat, for example, or a sheep, we notice that it does not take great breaths in and then "block" the birth canal by holding its breath. A sheep gives birth with rather light, quick breathing. Its breath is involuntarily held as it bears down and then it continues the light, accelerated breathing again.

During the second stage of labour, when the baby is travelling down the vagina or birth canal (see pages 252–253), most women feel the urge to push during contractions. As a contraction builds you move from full to lighter, quicker breathing, your cheeks plumped up. Then the surge of desire to bear down comes and you hold your breath. As soon as you can breathe again you do so, then feel you have to bear down again – and so on until the desire fades, your breathing slows down and then the contraction ends. Practise this with only a very slight push, with a hand resting over your perineum so that you can feel its gentle bulge forwards.

Different movements for labour

Once you are fairly confident about your ability to relax and breathe rhythmically, explore some different positions that you may want to use in labour. There is no reason why you should have to be tucked up in bed all the time. There are definite disadvantages to the supine position (lying flat on your back) for your baby, since the blood flow in the large veins in the lower part of your body may be obstructed by the heavy weight of your uterus and this can reduce the blood flow through the placenta to and from the baby.

Through the first stage of labour you will almost certainly feel happiest walking about or standing up. During contractions you will probably want to lean against a wall or your partner. If you have low backache, you can lean forwards on to a heavy piece of furniture. Once labour is advanced, it will be easier if you already know the positions in which you are likely to feel most comfortable. Avoid getting stuck in one position; the essence of labour is movement. Explore ways in which you can rock, circle and tilt your pelvis. You can try kneeling, leaning back over your heels or forwards on to a pillow placed on a chair or bed or over the top of the headboard;

a knee-chest position with knees placed either side of your body, rather like a frog; on all fours or squatting, with your back supported. Some of these positions are shown on pages 210–215.

Your aim is to give the baby as much room as possible in your pelvis by keeping your knees well apart and allowing the uterus to tilt forwards on to your abdominal wall and away from your spine. In this position the uterus assumes an egg shape, whereas when you are lying flat on your back it tends to be distorted from this natural shape. When you are upright you are also allowing gravity to help the baby down. In all these positions contract only those muscles you need to use to support yourself, and whenever possible use pillows, furniture or another person to help you.

You can relieve low backache in labour, especially common when the baby is in an occipito-posterior position (see page 263), by assuming a posture in which your abdomen can hang forwards, tilting the baby away from your sacrum, and by gently humping your lower back up and letting it drop down, or circling your pelvis – whichever feels right for you at the time. This position is also convenient for back massage and counterpressure, and because the longitudinal axis of the uterus is then in line with the birth canal it may help the baby

"It was agony to lie on my back during my labour, so although the midwife said it was interfering with the printout from the monitor, I knelt and held on to the bed. That way, I could cope much better."

to rotate into the correct anterior position. If the baby is lying in a posterior position, you will probably have bearing down sensations before you are fully dilated, and are more likely to be able to control the urge if you take some of the pressure off your rectum.

Pressure on the umbilical cord interrupts the baby's blood flow through it. Resulting decelerations of the fetal heart which last after the end of the contractions may be noted if you are having continuous electronic monitoring (see pages 330–334). Decelerations of the fetal heart will lead your doctor to consider undertaking a forceps delivery or Caesarean section for fetal distress. If you adopt a position in which your tummy is hanging forwards, however, such as on all fours, both the baby and its cord will be tipped away from your spine and the pressure on the cord may be relieved.

Incidentally, it is a good idea to adopt an all-fours position for delivery if the baby has large shoulders that might get stuck (shoulder dystocia). It gives the assistant more room to manoeuvre, as the baby's head can be extended and drawn out and up towards your anus. Thus the baby's shoulders are delivered nearer your front, and the rest will then follow easily.

Sometimes contractions are inefficient from the very start of labour and do not seem to pick up or, having been effective at first, become weak. In either case it is worth trying a position in which the uterus can most easily form a sphere. It may help to stand facing a wall, with your legs well apart, and leaning forwards with your hands resting against the wall.

Practising movements for labour

There is no reason to spend labour in bed. In fact, lying flat on your back diminishes the oxygen supply to your baby and prevents the uterus from contracting efficiently. While you are pregnant, try out different positions to find those that are most comfortable for you. Always keep your neck free and breathe with the movement, letting go of any tension.

Keep back flat

On all fours

To relieve low backache in labour, get down on all fours and place your hands flat on the floor, as wide apart as your shoulders. Remember not to arch your back.

Keep hands wide apart

Standing lunge

1 *Stand with your feet well grounded and wide apart. Place the flat of your hands against a solid surface, such as a wall. Try rocking and rolling your hips in this position.*

2 *You can step nearer the wall and lean your forearms against it. Rest your head on your forearms. Remember always to keep your shoulders and neck completely relaxed.*

Kneeling up

Kneel on the floor with your back straight, legs apart, ankles turned out and toes turned in towards each other. This position opens the pelvis and releases any tension in the back.

Kneeling forwards

In the same position as before, lean forwards with your forearms flat on the floor. This is a good position for opening the pelvis, too, taking the baby's weight off your back and relieving backache.

Hanging abdomen

Try kneeling on all fours, with your forearms on the floor, your knees spread wide and your abdomen hanging between them. In this position you may like to rock backwards and forwards. Keep your lower back flat.

Ankles turned out and toes turned in

Keep knees apart

Lying down

You can relax almost on all fours, but flopped forwards on to several pillows, a big floor cushion or bean bag to support the weight of your uterus.

Hold door handle

Squatting in labour

When you adopt the squatting position your pelvis is wide open and the baby's head pressed down. It is good to practise this position for labour on your own or with the help of your partner.

1 *You can use a door to practise lengthening up and letting go. Hold the knob with both hands, then lower yourself into a squatting position with your heels and legs wide apart.*

2 *Practise leaning forwards on to a chair or on to your partner, for support during labour. Place a rolled-up towel under your heels to help you tilt.*

3 *If a full squat is uncomfortable, you could practise a sitting squat. Place a soft towel or blanket on a bucket, low stool or pile of books and sit in a half squatting position with legs wide apart.*

Use a covered bucket

Supported squat

This type of squatting can be practised with your partner, who needs to support you as you adopt the squatting position.

Grasp forearms

1 *Stand facing your partner. Grasp each other's forearms. Then your partner bends her knees and leans just slightly backwards, with one foot placed in front of the other.*

Bend knees

2 *With your partner supporting and pulling against you, sink down, allowing your hips, knees and ankles to give thus transferring the weight into your lower back and seat bones.*

Release hips

3 *As your partner carries on supporting your weight, she enables you to lengthen up, lean forwards and sink your heels towards the floor, while releasing your hips.*

Practising movements for delivery

Try to explore different positions for delivery with your partner or the people who will be helping you at the birth, so that everyone has some idea of what to expect. Use a doll, a ball, even a grapefruit, as a substitute for the baby.

Supported kneeling

Kneeling opens up the pelvis fully and aids the baby's descent. You will feel most secure if you have the support of two helpers, one on each side of you.

Supported squatting

You may find it more comfortable to squat. Again, you will need two helpers, who can support your knees when you are bearing down.

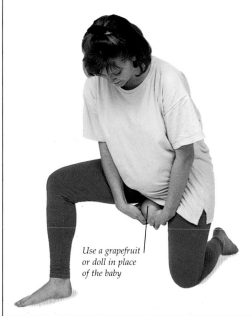

Use a grapefruit or doll in place of the baby

Half kneeling, half squatting

Kneel on one knee with the other leg bent, foot flat on the floor. This half kneeling, half squatting position is the easiest if you are planning to lift your baby out yourself. It should give you greater stability than kneeling or squatting and allows you to guide the baby out.

Kneeling upright

Kneeling with your body upright speeds up a very slow second stage. The midwife can deliver your baby from behind and pass her through your legs, or you may actually be able to lift her out yourself.

Knee-chest position

Kneeling on all fours, with your head down and bottom up, will slow down a second stage that is happening very fast. This position will help you to feel more in control, as well as allowing your vaginal tissues time to soften and stretch, so that they are less likely to tear as the baby is born. This can also be useful during the first stage to help turn a posterior baby, and during the transition stage to encourage dilatation of an anterior lip (by slowing down the urge to push).

Leaning forwards

This is especially good if the second stage of labour is fast, since it will slow you down a little. The midwife will guide your baby out, and then you can turn around and take the baby into your arms.

215

Practising for contractions and pushing

The experience of labour is difficult to imagine before you have had a baby. Will contractions be unbearably painful or hardly noticeable? Some women think of the contractions as bigger and bigger hills they have to climb, each hill having its own peak, until they reach the mountain range at the end of the first stage.

THE ACTION OF THE UTERUS
When the uterus contracts it is tightening up, just like any working muscle in the body. Make a very tight fist with one hand and raise your arm so that the big muscle on the inside of your upper arm, the biceps, tightens; then feel it with your other hand. You will notice that the biceps has become hard and is sticking out. If a man does the same thing, his biceps may stick out a good deal more than yours does, because his is probably a bigger muscle. The biceps gets hard as it contracts and it also protrudes. This is because the muscle fibres are shortened and thickened. The same thing happens, on a much larger scale, when the uterus contracts. Like your bulging biceps, the uterus bulges forwards in your abdomen when you have a really strong and effective contraction. The strong contractions are the best of all for helping the baby to be born.

Place your hand just above your pubic-hair line at the very bottom of the abdomen. The cervix lies under this area and it is here that you are likely to feel the strong, rhythmic pull as it opens, a pull that will feel tightest at the height of each contraction (see page 246).

You cannot do anything actively to help the baby down the birth canal until the cervix is wide open. A relaxed body, a mind at peace, and being able to move freely are the most important contributions you make to the birth process at this stage. Prepare yourself to respond with neuromuscular release whenever you want to. Your breathing techniques can help your relaxation and your relaxation can help to keep your breathing smooth and rhythmic.

SIMULATING CONTRACTIONS
Contractions are felt mainly as powerful pressure that comes whether or not you want it to, so when you are practising for them work with a partner and allow him or her to simulate the contractions, deciding when they start, how strong they become, and how long they last. Meet each contraction with a welcoming breath out and use the rhythmic breathing you have learned right through each one, with a long resting breath out at the end. Your partner sits beside you so that you have eye contact with each other. He or she pretends to be your uterus by taking hold of a piece of your flesh, the inner thigh, say, and squeezing it. He will find that grasping a small piece of flesh rather than a big area is the most

effective. He should be particularly careful if you have a varicose vein, lifting the flesh up off the leg instead of pressing down into the leg, and avoiding the area around the varicose vein. First he squeezes gently, and then tightens his grip to a strong pinch that lasts for about 15 seconds, after which he gradually releases his hold. The contraction should last about 45 seconds in all. This exercise will help him to be aware of what you are feeling and how you react to stress of this kind, so that he can give you emotional support and encouragement. If you do not want him to do this, because you cannot rely on him to be perceptive and sensitive, omit this method.

In between these mock contractions, you can discuss with him how each one felt, and perhaps how he can improve his performance and you can improve yours. In labour this rest space between contractions should be used to prepare you for the next one: do not waste time discussing the contraction that has just ended. It is a good idea to change places so that you become your partner's "uterus" and he can experience this firm gripping sensation and learn how to respond to it. This is important if he is going to be with you during labour and wants to be able to help you by breathing with you when and if contractions become difficult.

PRACTISING FOR STRONGER CONTRACTIONS

Switch roles again and imagine that labour is progressing, with longer and stronger contractions, each reaching its peak about halfway through. Always remember, however, that contractions vary and that it is no good wishing for a "textbook labour" if your own labour proves to be quite different. Some contractions have their peaks about a third of the way through; some may even have two peaks. The important thing is that if you go with your uterus, you tune in with it rather like an orchestra responding to a conductor. The conductor in this case is the uterus. You have

"My partner was very responsive. I never felt he was too tough on me. But it helped me prepare for strong contractions."

to be able to, as it were, "listen" to your uterus in order to react appropriately to it and be in complete harmony with it. For these stronger contractions your partner grips the flesh of your thigh for a minute or a even little longer.

When necessary during these longer contractions respond by lifting your breathing above the contraction – breathing more shallowly and more quickly (see page 204). Relax your shoulders and toes; then, as the contraction becomes slightly less intense, allow your breathing to become slower and fuller.

PUSHING

Bearing down or pushing is often described as an extraordinarily athletic activity, as if you could learn to do it the way you learn to do an aerobic exercise. It should not be like this. It is, rather, a spontaneous welling up of energy that culminates in a triumphant push and an opening of the vagina. A woman in the second stage of labour experiences mounting excitement. She feels that she is on the edge of a chasm with life at its most elemental surging up from the depths, until every nerve and every pore of her body tingles with urgent desire. She does not have to ask for any instructions. She does not have to ask doctors and midwives if she can "push now". The creative power in her body is intense and overwhelming.

However you are sitting now, rest your hands beneath the lower curve of your abdomen. Take a breath and hold it. Drop your chin forwards on your chest and at the same time allow the bulge underneath your hands to press downwards and forwards, so that from inside your abdomen you are pressing your hands out and moving them forward.

"It felt wonderful to swing into second-stage pushing. I know now what you mean by 'the birth passion'."

You probably feel your perineum moving forwards, too. Allow the movement to carry right down through you until you feel the tissues of the vagina spreading out, and then rest. Did you get that feeling of something moving forwards? When the baby is ready to be born, this movement helps its head to bulge further down the birth canal. Although it is useful to learn how to do this beforehand, especially if you practise it without straining and useless effort, most women who are free to do whatever they feel like doing have a spontaneous physical and emotional urge to do it anyway during the second stage of labour (see page 251).

Before going on to practise this pushing movement, make sure that your bladder is completely empty. You can adopt any of the positions suggested on pages 210–213.

One of the best ways of rehearsing pushing is on the lavatory since we also release pelvic floor muscles for defecation, so they are not put under unusual strain. If you happen to be constipated, as many women are in late pregnancy (see page 134), this movement will help to relieve the constipation and is an excellent way to encourage spontaneous, easy bowel movements.

Each time you practise you will feel more comfortable in an upright position. This will be an advantage during labour, too, as you are more in control of what is happening, can open up more easily for the baby to be born, and can see over the bulge to watch the birth if you want to. Gravity can help you in labour. If you are lying flat, or almost flat, you are pushing the baby uphill, because the uterus is almost at right angles to the vagina (see pages 244–245 and 252–253). In an almost upright position you can lean on your uterus and press the baby down.

After you have done this gentle pushing a few times, begin to work with your partner. To start, you might like to try sitting. Your partner sits near your head with a pillow over the forearm and supports your head and shoulders with it. This gives you a very wide base of support. With your partner's hands over your lower abdomen, you can both feel what is happening inside. Drop your head forwards on to your chest, so that you do not strain with your throat muscles and produce a grunting sound. Take a breath. Lean forwards and press from inside steadily out, slowly, gently; a little bit more; let it go; let the breath out and rest. While you are practising, your partner's hand pressed firmly against your lower abdomen gives you something to press against and guide you. It is easier to bear down when your baby is actually in the birth canal waiting to be born because you have something to press against. Allow your pelvic floor muscles to bulge forwards like a heavy sack of apples. When you have felt and noted the sensation this produces, lift your pelvic floor up again so that it is well toned and not sagging (see page 118). Think of it as smiling.

TRYING OTHER POSITIONS

When you are confident that you have the feeling of pushing with complete release of your pelvic floor muscles in this position, go on to explore other positions that may feel right when you are in labour. Experiment with every type of open position – on a mattress on the floor, on the bed, leaning over or against furniture, using cushions and other kinds of support, cradled by another human body – in which you can feel in touch with what is happening and free to let the energy of the uterus sweep through you to give birth. An almost impossible posture in which to do this is, as you can imagine, lying flat on your back with your legs in the air in the standard lithotomy position, or with your knees scrunched up to your chest while you try to roll yourself into a ball – both of which used to be standard positions for the second stage of labour and delivery in contemporary hospitals.

Since the eighties, however, there have been widespread changes in practice. Now, in many hospitals women are encouraged to find any position, and make any movement that is going to be comfortable for them during labour and, if they wish, to give birth on a sheet or mattress on the floor.

vagina instead of being placed on top of your abdomen. Most babies with severe chromosome abnormalities have extra fluid behind the neck, and this can be detected from a scan by an experienced radiologist at 12 weeks.

To assess maturity in late pregnancy In late pregnancy a scan is sometimes used to investigate whether or not a baby is ready to be born. The scan cannot show whether the baby's lungs have developed sufficiently and are mature enough for breathing after birth, but by accurately measuring the size of the baby's head the scan can establish the approximate age of the baby as well as its current stage of development.

To detect how the baby is lying If it is important to find out how your baby is lying in the uterus (for example, whether the baby is lying head down or is in the breech position), and the doctor cannot know this information for certain from carrying out a standard manual examination, ultrasound can tell this with accuracy. This knowledge may make all the difference to you if, for instance, you want to have your baby at home.

If the baby is shown to be lying in a good position, you can proceed with confidence in your plans for a home birth. However, if the baby is seen to be lying awkwardly, you will need to accept that it might be more sensible to go to hospital for the birth. Either way, you and your doctor can be guided by the information provided by the scan. The scan should not be a condition for you having a home birth. You are free to decline a scan if you wish.

To assess the condition and position of the placenta When there is bleeding in late pregnancy ultrasound can be used to locate the position of the placenta. The danger is that the placenta might be blocking the baby's way out of the uterus (this is a condition known as placenta praevia and it is described further on page 137). In fact, a scan done in the first few months of pregnancy often gives the impression that the placenta is lying low on the wall of the uterus, but as the pregnancy progresses and the uterus enlarges and stretches, the placenta usually proves to be in the right place after all. Sometimes a woman worries through the rest of her pregnancy because she is told that she has a low-lying placenta. Occasionally, bleeding in late pregnancy indicates that the roots of the placenta are becoming dislodged with pre-labour contractions, pointing to the fact that the baby's nourishment and oxygen supply would be cut if labour were allowed to proceed. A scan can show this clearly, and a Caesarean section can be performed to save the baby. Used in this way, or together with amniocentesis (see page 226), an ultrasound scan has undoubted advantages.

"I found the scans at sixteen weeks and thirty weeks really exciting because the images on the screen were so clearly explained to me that I could easily understand them."

HOW ULTRASOUND WORKS

You undress, put on a hospital gown, and lie on your back beside the scanner. Your abdomen is oiled and then a transducer is slowly passed over it in different directions. The transducer is a machine that picks up echoes from the different planes of your own organs and also the developing baby's tissues, and which then translates the information that it has picked up into the form of a map on a screen that looks like a television screen.

A scan done in the first few months of pregnancy gains in clarity if your bladder is full and therefore clearly visible, so you will probably be asked to drink a lot of water first and not urinate for an hour or so before the scan. Do not expect to see an immediately recognizable picture of your baby, even in late pregnancy; if a doctor is present, ask to have the picture interpreted, because it may look more like a map of the moon than a baby, and you may find it difficult to make out the different parts of the body.

Another technique involves the use of a specially designed intravaginal transducer which is sometimes used in very early pregnancy and also for other specific purposes.

IS ULTRASOUND SAFE?

As far as we know, ultrasound is safe, and is certainly much safer than X-rays (see page 110), which provided the only technological method of gaining information about the baby in the uterus before the scan was developed. On the other hand, it is known that high-frequency sound waves continued for a long time can cause damage to hearing in an adult. Questions have therefore been raised about the possible effects on the baby's hearing since, although the sound waves are bounced off the baby for only a short time, the baby may be vulnerable at certain stages of its development. Babies are not born deaf after having ultrasound, but no one yet knows if any of them will suffer delayed effects in later life.

Ultrasound does have other effects on the body that are not yet fully understood. It causes heat to be generated in body tissues, and tiny bubbles inside tissue may dance in reaction to the sound waves. This does not necessarily mean that diagnostic ultrasound at the level at which it is normally used in pregnancy is dangerous. But it does imply that we should be asking searching questions about possible long-term effects. It could be that ultrasound has some subtle harmful effects on especially vulnerable babies in the first 12 weeks of pregnancy, during the time that the major organs of the body are in the process of being formed.

Research on ultrasound carried out to date suggests that, in the words of the British Chief Medical Officer of Health, "All ultrasound exposure should be justified and limited to the minimum necessary for the diagnostic purpose. The greatest risk with ultrasound is from inaccurate interpretation of the image, rather than from any physical hazard of the ultrasonic field".*

225

SOME SAFETY MEASURES

It makes sense to expose pregnant women and the babies inside them to ultrasound only when a diagnosis is needed that cannot be made without ultrasound, and when that diagnosis would result in some change in the kind of care that is given. This rules out routine scanning at 16 weeks – now the accepted practice in many countries. It also rules out using ultrasound simply because parents would like to see a picture of the baby or to enable a woman or her partner to "bond" with the fetus. Many obstetricians are rather keen on this and believe that they can make a contribution towards ensuring that babies are well mothered by doing routine ultrasound scans. They do not realize that there are other – better and more intimate – ways of becoming aware of the baby (see page 237).

When ultrasound is used, the length of time you are exposed to it should be limited, and when you are discussing what you can see on the screen, ask for the image to be frozen. Understandably, a woman is fascinated by seeing her baby's movements on the screen; in Denmark the scanner is linked to a video camera so that the examination can be replayed later, the woman can see her baby moving, and there can be full discussion about it without exposing the baby unnecessarily to ultrasound.

Amniocentesis

Amniocentesis is a procedure that has been developed in order to detect any abnormalities of the baby's central nervous system (spina bifida and anencephaly) and some other genetic abnormalities such as Down's syndrome (mongolism). The sex of the baby can also be determined by this procedure, so you can discover if any sex-linked disorders might have been inherited.

HOW AMNIOCENTESIS WORKS

Under a local anaesthetic a hollow needle is inserted through your abdominal wall into the uterus, where about 14 g (half an ounce) of the water in which the fetus is lying is sucked out. This fluid has been swallowed by the fetus and passed out of its body through its mouth or bladder; it is full of cells from the skin and other organs which, when analyzed, can provide valuable clues to the baby's genetic makeup. The fluid is sent to a lab and spun in a centrifuge to separate the cells from the liquid. The cells are left to multiply and are then analyzed. Results are available in two to four weeks.

In the 1950s, when amniocentesis was first invented, mistakes were sometimes made and the needle penetrated placental tissues, causing miscarriage. But now ultrasound techniques are used to locate the placenta and the risks of damage to the placenta have been very much reduced. There still remains a 1 or 2 per cent chance, however, that amniocentesis may cause miscarriage. Because of this small but definite risk, there is no point in having amniocentesis unless there is a well-above-average chance of your baby being born abnormal. You will have thought carefully about the implications of discovering that something is wrong with your baby and have decided whether you would opt for termination. In some parts of the country, amniocentesis is offered to all women over 35, since the incidence of some disorders it is designed to detect rises sharply with age. You should be able to talk to a counsellor *before* an invasive diagnostic test to help you reach a decision. If an abnormality is revealed by the test, counselling should be immediately available to both parents.

There is a 1 to 2 per cent risk of miscarriage when amniocentesis is performed after 16 weeks. Experiments have been done with amniocentesis as early as nine weeks, but the miscarriage rate then is between 3 per cent and 7 per cent, depending on the skill of the operator. Since less fluid is available at that stage of pregnancy, the laboratory is unable to grow a cell culture in up to 21 per cent of cases, so the amniocentesis has to be done again.*

When amniocentesis is done between the 14th and 16th weeks of pregnancy, when many women have felt the first fetal movement, the decision to terminate a pregnancy is a distressing one to make and the termination is riskier than one that is performed earlier in

Ultrasound transducer

Placenta

Amniotic fluid

Hollow needle

Uterus

Amniocentesis
This can be performed under ultrasound. When amniocentesis is done under guided ultrasound there is a much reduced chance of the needle touching or harming the baby in any way.

pregnancy. The woman who is going through this experience needs generous emotional support from her partner and family. Amniocentesis is sometimes performed late in pregnancy if it looks as if the baby may possibly be born pre-term or if there is a complication such as placenta previa (see page 137) It this case the risks of continuing the pregnancy must be weighed carefully against the risks of delivering a child with immature lungs. The amniotic fluid can reveal vital information as to whether the fetal lungs are mature, that is, whether they are now strong enough to allow the baby to breathe normally after birth. If the lungs are discovered to be still immature, then labour will not be induced, nor will the pregnancy be terminated via Caesarean. Instead, appropriate drugs (corticosteriods) and some more time will be allowed. Results of amniocentesis for lung maturity are available immediately.

Chorionic villus sampling

Chorionic villus sampling (CVS) entails taking a sample of tissue from the part of the outer membrane around the embryo that will later become the placenta. This is in order to diagnose whether or not a fetus will have a genetic handicap. One of the handicaps this process of testing cannot detect, however, is spina bifida. CVS can be carried out before 12 weeks – even as early as 10 weeks – so that an abnormal fetus can be terminated much earlier in pregnancy.

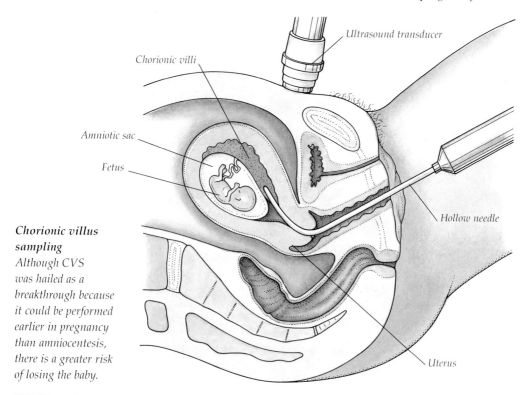

Ultrasound transducer

Chorionic villi

Amniotic sac

Fetus

Hollow needle

Uterus

Chorionic villus sampling
Although CVS was hailed as a breakthrough because it could be performed earlier in pregnancy than amniocentesis, there is a greater risk of losing the baby.

The risks of CVS, however, outweigh any of the benefits. There is a high incidence of infection, bleeding and miscarriage following CVS. It has also been linked to limb defects. This was not discovered by a medical researcher, but by a woman who had CVS and gave birth to a child with deformed limbs. After meeting another woman whose baby had been diagnosed with similar abnormalities after she had CVS at the same hospital, she reported it to a genetic counsellor. She was told by doctors that there was no connection. But she continued to ask questions. A study was then conducted, which suggested that there was an association. The earlier the CVS the more likely a limb deformity will occur, probably as a result of interfering with the blood supply to the limb.* Amniocentesis in the second trimester of pregnancy is safer than CVS.

Umbilical vein sampling

At the end of the Seventies, fetoscopy – photographing the baby with a telescope introduced into the uterus – was the latest technique for finding out exactly what was happening to babies known to be at risk. Unfortunately, the risk of miscarriage after the procedure proved to be as high as 5 to 10 per cent. Fetoscopy has now been superseded by umbilical vein sampling (cordocentesis), hailed by Dr Stuart Weiner of the University of Pennsylvania as opening up "a whole new area of fetal medicine".*

In umbilical vein sampling, a very fine needle is passed through the mother's abdomen and uterus into the fetal vein in the umbilical cord and blood is withdrawn so that it can be tested. Intrauterine blood transfusions can also be given in this way, and drugs can be injected directly into the baby. Because the fetal vein is frail in early pregnancy, the technique cannot be performed until after 18 weeks.

Umbilical vein sampling is now being used in some clinics in addition to amniocentesis and ultrasound; it is also used when there is Rhesus disease (see page 113), in order to diagnose haemophilia in a baby, and to check for metabolic disorders as well as any infections such as toxoplasmosis and rubella.

Dr Kypros Nicolaides, of King's College Hospital, London, estimates that when the method is used by experienced doctors, the risk of losing a baby is only 1 to 2 per cent – the same as that for amniocentesis and chorionic villus sampling in that hospital. He emphasized to me that "the greatest risk of any operative technique in pregnancy is always the skill and experience of the operator".

ETHICAL DILEMMAS

The developing science of antenatal diagnosis presents ethical dilemmas. In many countries it is unregulated. In some countries no counselling is offered. In others, telephone counselling is available. Some firms offer do-it-yourself tests for conditions such as cystic fibrosis – a disorder of the lungs and digestive system. Making decisions about whether or not to have screening, and if so, exactly what to screen for, is becoming increasingly complex. Would you want to know if a child you were bearing, or yourself, or other members of your family, run an increased risk of having heart trouble in middle age, developing breast cancer at some stage or Alzheimer's in old age? If you did, how great would the risk have to be for you to go through genetic tests? And how great the risk for you to decide on termination of a pregnancy? How accurate would tests have to be? Suppose there was nothing you could do to prevent an illness from developing or to treat it effectively if you or your child did get it; would you still want to know? Would you want to have this knowledge if future employment prospects and insurance depended on test results indicating that there was no additional risk?

"I didn't want these tests, but I knew that everyone would blame me if I had an imperfect baby that I could have aborted."

The decision to terminate pregnancy is implicit in screening procedures that are now readily available, such as those for Down's syndrome and neural tube defects. You may feel absolutely sure about what you would want if it turned out that there was a high probability of the baby being handicapped. But now screening is becoming available for conditions that do not produce serious handicap, which are not life threatening, and which may develop only in adolescence or later. How can you weigh up the pros and cons of such tests? You may want to discuss these issues with your partner, a close friend or your doctor or midwife, who can put you in touch with a genetic counsellor.

The genetic counsellor may be of real assistance in helping you establish your priorities. She will give you the facts that are known and discuss your options. She will not advocate termination, although she will support you if that is what you want. She will not persuade you to go on with a pregnancy, but will support you if that is your choice. It is up to you. You cannot predict your reactions to a positive test result. Even if you are certain that you would not terminate a pregnancy, you may wish to know beforehand that a baby is not going to be perfect, so that you can plan ahead, or you may prefer not to have screening, and to wait and see.

The last few weeks

Your baby is almost ready to be born. The firm body is nestled in the cup of your pelvis, and the little arms and legs are plumper as the last layers of fat form to help the baby's temperature-control system function efficiently after birth. Sometimes the baby gains as much as 226 g (8 oz) in a week at this stage of pregnancy.

PHYSICAL SENSATIONS

You may feel fewer big body movements but an insistent kicking underneath your ribs on one side or the other. If your abdominal wall is thin you may even be able to hold your baby's foot. There may be other strange movements, perhaps a sudden urgent knocking which continues intermittently for half an hour or more. This can be so pronounced that you may worry in case your baby is having something like an epileptic seizure. But it is definitely not that. The baby may have hiccups, perhaps because he was gulping amniotic fluid; or he may have lost his thumb which he was contentedly sucking, and is "rooting" to find it again, with quick, darting movements of the head from side to side, just as after birth he will search for the nipple. The baby's head feels like a melon or coconut pressing through your bulging perineal tissues.

There may also be odd sensations in your vagina. Sometimes there is a sharp buzz like a mild electric shock or a tickle. The baby may be lifting and lowering his head against your pelvic floor muscles which is another movement that he will do naturally after birth too, when put down on his front in an alert state. There are times when your baby is sleeping or drowsy, and other times active – often in the evenings.

MIXED EMOTIONS

Conflicting emotions are characteristic of these last weeks. You may be tired of being pregnant, but on the other hand the state you are in now is a condition you know and understand, whereas in front of you there is an unknown challenge. So sometimes you want the baby out and long to get on with the labour. But at other times you feel safer as you are, and anxious about the future. Some women say that as the birthday draws nearer they feel irritated with the pregnancy. This produces an emotional state that makes them welcome the start of labour. Other women relish these last weeks.

ANTENATAL DEPRESSION

It is common to feel low some time in the last six weeks of pregnancy. If you have been practising and preparing for a natural birth you may experience a kind of stage fright and be convinced that you are going to forget everything when you are actually in labour. You may also be feeling physically tired and heavy with the weight of your burden.

Antenatal depression, though usually shortlived and spasmodic, is a fact of life for some women. It may suggest a need for more rest. You may feel very different if you lie down to rest in a darkened room in the middle of the day, have some early nights and adjust your activity to slower, gentler rhythms if possible.

If you find yourself becoming depressed at this stage of pregnancy, have a talk with your childbirth educator who, probably a mother herself, will understand what you are feeling.

Thinking ahead to labour

You will probably be thinking a great deal about labour in the last few weeks, wondering what it will be like. One of the things you can find out is the position your baby is in; remember to ask when you are being examined by the doctor or midwife. The ideal position for a straightforward labour (and by far the most common) is head down and anterior. Some babies present in different positions, as posterior or breech, for example. Delivery may not be quite so straightforward with the baby in these positions (see pages 262–276).

THE BABY WHO IS PRESENTING AS A POSTERIOR

If your baby is lying head down with its back against your spine, limbs towards your front, it may either be because it is still rather small or you have such a roomy pelvis that it can still move freely. Women who think they are due but who really have another two weeks or so to go before delivery can have a baby who is still moving like this – sometimes posterior, sometimes anterior. Pre-labour and early-labour contractions usually work to turn the baby into an anterior position in a matter of hours.

If your baby seems to have settled in a posterior position, you may find that you can coax it to change during one of its waking periods by very firm hand pressure. The posterior baby is usually lying with the ball of the head on your right side. You want to shift the baby's body around and over towards the left. Treat the baby as if it were a sleeping kitten that you are trying to scoop off the middle of a sofa and move over to the left side. Curve the side of your hand around the most solid section of its bulk and firmly, little by little, edge it over. Keep the fingers of your other hand over your navel. If you are successful the saucer-shaped dip there (the space between the arms and legs of a posterior baby) will become – at least temporarily – a hard, convex curve (the back of a baby in an anterior position). You will be able to detect the change as your navel will probably stick out. Talk to your baby as you move it. This is not simply a clinical exercise, but a bit of maternal persuasion.

Once the baby is stretching the uterus to its utmost it is a tight fit and you will probably not be able to move it. Wait and see whether the first-stage contractions will do it for you, and explore the positions and movements that aid rotation while you are in labour.

Towards the end of pregnancy, especially with the first baby, it is natural to feel a kind of stage fright as the great day approaches (opposite).

Helping a breech to turn You can try to tip the baby up out of your pelvis yourself by adopting a position with head down and bottom in the air for 15 minutes three times a day (before meals). Some babies turn a somersault once clear of the pelvis – even after 37 weeks.* A knee-chest position, leaning over a firm bean bag on your front with your head on the floor and your hips as high as possible, or lying in this position on a steeply sloping, cushion-padded ironing board propped between the bed and the wall or a solid piece of furniture, offers a range of options – none of them, it must be admitted, very comfortable in late pregnancy! But if you are able to turn the baby, it may make the difference between a vaginal and a Caesarean birth.

THE BABY WHO IS PRESENTING AS A BREECH
Most babies tip head down – in the vertex or cephalic position – between the seventh and the eighth month. If your baby is still presenting buttocks first (breech) after 36 weeks, the doctor may try to turn the baby – a procedure known as external version. There is little point in doing it earlier, as the baby often turns back again.*

How external version is done You empty your bladder and then lie down on your back with your knees drawn up. The doctor will probably do an ultrasound scan to find out exactly how the baby is lying and will listen to the baby's heartbeats before and after turning the baby. You may be asked to lie on a sloping examining table with your legs up and head down for about a quarter of an hour before the manoeuvre, so that the baby is encouraged to move clear of the pelvis. Spend this time relaxing as deeply as you can; use abdominal massage to help you release your tummy muscles and use your breathing to help you as well. The uterus often contracts when the doctor's hands are pressing on it, and this makes it more difficult to turn the baby.

When you feel the doctor's hands on your tummy, release and flow towards the touch. Give a long, slow breath out and let your lower tummy bulge out in a great wave as you do so. If the version is successful and the baby turns, walk around for an hour or two so that there is the best chance of fixing the baby head down. Some babies turn back into the breech position. Seven times out of ten, external version at 37 to 39 weeks is successful.* But if the baby tips back again you will have to accept that it prefers this position; discuss with your doctor the sort of delivery you will have (see page 267).

Being "overdue"

Concern about the best things to eat, the position of the baby and whether labour will be straightforward can be preoccupying in the last few weeks. If you actually go *past* the estimated date of delivery you may really begin to worry; you are now consigned to the category of the woman who is "overdue".

THE ESTIMATED DELIVERY DATE

The date that you are given at the beginning of pregnancy for your baby's birth (EDD or EDC) is only a statistical mean. Studies show that only 5 per cent of babies arrive on that day. If you look at the 95 babies out of 100 who do not put in an appearance on the "correct" date you find that three out of ten babies come before the EDD and seven out of ten come *after* it. This is partly because women's menstrual cycles are of different lengths, and ovulation – and hence conception – may occur at different times within it. But by the time you reach the end of your pregnancy you may not be able to prevent yourself from fixing on the expected delivery date as your goal. If it comes and goes and nothing happens, you may become very depressed. Each day that passes seems like a week, and each week

---

CHOOSING WHAT TO PACK

Now is the time to think about the comfort things you want available during and after birth. Select a small number of items that you think will be most useful, and gather them together in a lightweight, easily carried case. Choose from the following:

Comfort aids for birth
- Cotton pyjama top, short nightdress or baggy T-shirt.
- Face cloth.
- Two small sponges to be dipped in ice water and used for sponging your face, wetting your lips and sucking between contractions.
- Lip salve or vaseline for dry lips.
- Lavender and other essential oils.
- Talc or massage oil to avoid skin friction when massaged.
- Cassettes and cassette player.
- Candles, matches.
- Swimwear so that your birth partner can come with you under the shower if you wish.
- Camera and plenty of film, including fast film for night-time if you do not want to use a flash / video camera.
- Small spray bottle for moistening your face with cold water.
- Baby's hot-water bottle or a picnic thermal pack to be heated up in water for use as a hot compress in the small of your back, for example, or between your legs.
- Rolling pin with cloth tied over it to iron away backache.
- Honey to keep your strength up in early labour.
- Paper bag to breathe into in case you hyperventilate.
- Beautiful object to use as a visual focus if you wish: a painting, photographs or sculpture.
- Nourishing snacks for your birth partner.
- Notebook to serve as logbook.
- Hairbrush and ribbons or bands if your hair is long; comb.
- Books, magazines, playing cards, chess, scrabble, crosswords.
- Herb teas or glucose drinks.
- Bendy straws.

Comfort aids for after the birth
- Calendula and hypericum cream from a homeopathic pharmacy, for a sore perineum.
- Bottle of witch hazel lotion with which you can soak the sanitary pad next to stitches.
- Sanitary pads, largest size and belt.
- Soft toilet paper.
- Cotton nightgowns and robe.
- Nursing bras.
- Toiletry bag, and makeup if you wish.
- Earplugs.
- Writing paper and envelopes.
- List of telephone numbers.
- Coins for the telephone / cellular telephone.
- Deodorant (you will perspire heavily in the first few days after birth).
- Baby clothes.
- Clothes to wear going home.
- Baby seat for car.

more like a month. Unless you plan for activity and recreation during this time, your morale will drop to rock bottom. If you find that you are getting despondent, remind yourself that, although very few babies are born on the day predicted for their birth, nine out of ten do put in an appearance within ten days of the expected date. There is nothing abnormal about a baby who is nine days "late". Many women, however, are made to feel "under sentence of induction" if they go as little as a week past their expected date. Some obstetricians induce labour when the woman goes even a few days beyond the estimated date, and this is done without further investigation. If your pregnancy is normal and you are in good health, being ten days "late" is a very poor reason for induction.

Whether induction (see pages 324–328) is really necessary or not depends entirely on your baby's wellbeing towards the end of your pregnancy. Your baby's wellbeing, in turn, depends on the condition of the placenta.

THE AGEING PLACENTA

At the end of pregnancy the placenta looks like a piece of raw liver about the size of a dinner plate and the thickness of your little finger. Like every other human organ, it has a youth and an old age. An elderly placenta works less well. If labour does not start at the right time (which may be anywhere between two weeks before and two weeks after the estimated date of delivery – and very occasionally later still) the placenta may fail to support the baby in the uterus. The baby is then deprived of nourishment.

This is why obstetricians become concerned if a pregnancy is prolonged much past the date worked out for the birth. Even so, a baby who is thought to be overdue may prove at birth not to be postmature at all. There are various ways in which the baby's condition can be assessed. Some are tests which doctors do to you; however, probably the most reliable method is one that you can do for yourself (see page 237).

URINARY OESTRIOL TESTS

Some doctors still try to test whether the placenta is functioning well enough by measuring the output of oestriol in your urine or blood. (Oestriol is a form of the hormone oestrogen that is very important for the baby's growth.) The level of oestriol produced by the placenta rises during the course of your pregnancy. But just before labour starts, the level of oestriol drops.

The proportion of oestriol in your urine varies by as much as 30 per cent with different readings, however, and there are day-to-day variations even when everything is normal. When levels of oestriol output are compared with the information provided by an ultrasound scan to assess the baby's growth, there is often a discrepancy. Recent research has shown that the measurement of placental proteins and hormones is unlikely to be beneficial.*

ELECTRONIC FETAL MONITORING AND ULTRASOUND

Ultrasound may be used to check both the flow of blood through the umbilical blood vessels (Doppler flow studies) and the volume of amniotic fluid. Electronic fetal monitoring (called a non-stress test) can reveal whether the baby's heartbeat shows the usual variations when the baby is active and at rest. If the baby's heartbeat is normal, induction of labour has no advantage, and may be harmful.

FETAL MOVEMENT RECORDING

One of the most accurate ways of knowing if a baby is doing well while still inside the uterus in late pregnancy is something you can do for yourself. This is to note the baby's movements. In the last weeks of pregnancy, until it engages, the baby usually wriggles, dips and turns, bangs and kicks, and moves like a porpoise from side to side in great sweeps of activity that you can actually see through your clothing. Once it has engaged it often moves less because it is a rather tight fit. Even so, a vigorous baby moves even after it has gone down into the pelvis, although the movements then tend to be just the knocks from knees and feet. You feel as if you have a rolling coconut in your groin or just behind your pubis (the head turning), and later the strange buzzing sensation of the engaged head bouncing against the pelvic floor muscles (see page 231).

You may not normally be aware of most of these movements while you are busy but as soon as you sit down to rest, or lie down hoping to sleep, you cannot help noticing them. They are a good sign that your baby is healthy. Studies of fetal activity show that every baby has its own individual pattern of waking and sleeping inside the uterus, and by late pregnancy you will have probably noticed what your baby's pattern is. Sometimes you may be wide awake and expect to feel a kick; and if nothing happens it can be disconcerting. In fact, the baby is most probably fast asleep; if you have had an alcoholic drink or taken sleeping pills, your baby will probably be affected by them too.

Mothers do vary in the extent that they observe fetal movements. Sometimes this awareness is related to the amount of amniotic fluid, since the fluid cushions movements. If you are preoccupied and concentrating hard on something you may also be less aware of fetal activity. If you are still working outside the home, or busy inside it, there may be too much going on for you to notice any fetal movements. Each woman's experience of the movements is fairly consistent if her baby is thriving in the uterus, bearing in mind that the nature of movements changes after the baby has engaged, as described above. If for any reason it is thought by your doctor or midwife that your baby may be "at risk" (usually because you have not put on weight for two or more weeks, your tummy has not got bigger during this time or because you are "overdue"), you can use your own sensitive awareness about your baby's movements to keep a check on its wellbeing inside you.

The experience
of birth

What happens in labour **240**

Different kinds of labour **262**

Giving support in labour **277**

Dealing with pain **295**

Toward the medical control of birth **314**

Gentle birth **343**

What happens in labour

Language shapes the way we think. It is never neutral. The language used by men about women's bodies – especially their genitals – is often degrading. In some languages the only words available for parts of women's bodies express disgust. In Swedish, German and Dutch, for example, a nipple is a "breast wart". In Polish and Swedish the vaginal labia are called the "shame lips" and the pubic symphysis is the "shame bone". In Japanese pubic hair is the "shame hair". Terminology like this must make it difficult for women to feel positive about their bodies, in particular the organs involved in childbirth, which are associated with a sense of shame and pollution.

Today the language that is used about childbirth is medicalized and imposes a medical view of birth. This does not mean that you should not understand medical terminology about your body and the process of labour. But it does mean that it is important to find words for your own personal experience of pregnancy and birth too, both negative and positive aspects of it.

Women in the childbirth movement have been working to create a language of birth that is not medically dominated. They have invented or adapted words like "rushes" for uterine contractions and "visualization" for the mental pictures that help a woman to adjust to the different sensations of birth. Some have analyzed the inappropriate and often sterile or destructive language that is employed by obstetricians, and sometimes nurses and midwives, too, to describe the stages of the birth process.

The medical model for childbirth incorporates an image of the pregnant woman as an ambulant pelvis, and for a woman having her first baby this pelvis is "untried". During labour she becomes a contracting uterus, and the birth process is an equation between the "powers", the "pelvis" and the "passenger", for the baby is seen as an inert passenger through the skeletal structure. Metaphors of war and conflict are often employed: obstetricians talk about "the aggressive management of ruptured membranes", "the oxytocin challenge test", "a trial of labour" and "the trigger factor for labour", and as the baby is about to be born its head "hits the pelvic floor". Midwives sometimes urge a woman to push in the second stage by telling her to "get angry with her body" or even to be "angry with the baby". A woman may be made to feel that she is being blamed for failing to function effectively: she is in "false labour". Her cervix is "incompetent", "sloppy" or "rigid". There is "failure to progress" because her uterus is "lazy" or the fundus is "boggy". Some terms, such as "elderly primigravada" and the term "abortion" when it is used to mean miscarriage, have all but disappeared from medical vocabulary because they were so obviously offensive. But there are plenty still around.

In this chapter, as we explore the feelings of birth and the ways in which you can adapt to your physical sensations, I shall try to use not only medical words but also those that convey sensory meaning and that express the personal experience of birth.

The stages of labour

There are three stages of labour. During the first stage the cervix is being drawn up into the main body of the uterus and dilating (opening). In the second the baby is pressed down through the birth canal; this stage culminates in the birth. During the third the placenta and membranes are sloughed off the lining of the uterus and expelled.

Having said this, it is important to add that for many women labour is an overwhelming and dramatic experience, and you are certainly not sitting around thinking in terms of neat stages. There is no fanfare of trumpets to tell you when the first stage is really under way or when the second stage has started. Some women have a clear physiological message, such as the breaking of the waters and sudden strong, regular contractions, leaving them in no doubt that labour has begun and that this is unmistakably it, and when they reach the end of the first stage they know with equal certainty that they are now in the second stage and have to push. For a great many women, however, the different stages of labour shade over into each other. The experience is rarely as tidy and compartmentalized as birth books seem to suggest, and the third stage may even pass completely unnoticed as you hold your newborn baby in your arms and marvel at him or her.

THE BABY SIGNALS THAT IT IS READY TO BE BORN

The *baby* initiates labour by sending endocrine signals to the placenta to produce enzymes that stimulate production of oestrogen. These signals consist of catecholamines (see page 346). Simultaneously, the same hormonal signals help the baby's vital organs to mature. If labour is induced artificially, the timing may not be right either for the uterus to work most effectively or for the baby to be ready for life.

THE BUILD-UP TO LABOUR

Labour starts with the gradual softening and ripening of the cervix at the base of the uterus. This can take days and days or can happen overnight, especially if you have had a baby before. Once the cervix is soft and stretchy the uterine contractions – which are occurring anyway in late pregnancy – tend to draw it up bit by bit, so that it gradually changes from being a long canal hanging down in your vagina to being a dip in the bottom of the uterus, the tissues having been pulled up into the lower segment of the uterus.

You are not considered to be in labour while all this is happening. Your labour has not started in medical terms until you are having regular contractions that are effectively dilating the cervix; it is

Muscle bundles
The uterus is composed of spiral muscle bundles which in early pregnancy start to unfold into an open-latticework formation at the top of the uterus. If you think of the uterus as a clock, the muscle bundles are spaced out most between 9 and 3 – that is, over the fundus of the uterus. By the end of the pregnancy these bundles of muscle have unfolded much more and are stretched lengthways.

Early pregnancy

Late pregnancy

work that has to be done before it is possible for the cervix to open wide. Usually this means you are at least 3 cm dilated (see page 251) before you are considered to be in labour. In fact many women already have a partially dilated cervix by the time they begin to realize that they are having contractions.

It is obviously more pleasant for you if your body is working for you while you are carrying on with your work, shopping, eating, sleeping and seeing your friends. You cannot possibly be tensing up and fighting your body when you are busy doing all these things and leaving your uterus to work undisturbed and unremarked on. So carry on normal living for as long as is comfortable.

THE FIRST SIGNS OF LABOUR
Three things can indicate that labour has started or is about to start: you see a show, the waters break or contractions begin.

A show This is the bloodstained mucous discharge that appears when the cervix is beginning to stretch. Until the start of labour this mucus has acted as a gelatinous plug in the cervix, sealing off the uterus. Its appearance is a good sign that there is some definite activity around the cervix. But it can come out two or three weeks before you actually go into labour and contractions are established, or it may appear when your labour is so far advanced that you may not notice it. So, although you can take it as an encouraging sign, do not rush off to hospital. Go on with your everyday activities or, if it is night, have a hot milk drink and go back to sleep.

The bag of waters breaks When the membranes surrounding the baby have been pressed down like a wedge in front of its presenting part (usually the head) and pressure has built up, the bag pops. It may do this quite suddenly with a rush of water or, and this is more likely, with a slow trickle of water. In fact, you may not be quite sure whether the bag of waters has burst or you are wetting your pants.

If you are not sure, forget it (if you can) and carry on as usual, unless you are still several weeks away from your EDD, in which case you should ring the doctor or midwife. If it is more than three weeks before your baby is due it may actually be best for you to be in a place where special care is ready for the baby at delivery.

You will probably have been told to ring the hospital or your doctor or midwife if the waters break and you lose a lot of water at once. This is because, if labour is slow, taking 24 hours or more from the rupture of the membranes, there is a chance of infection. If labour starts within 24 hours, however, there is no increase in infection.*

The other concern is that if the baby's head does not fit neatly into the cervix the waters might sweep the cord down through the cervix (prolapsed cord), which in turn results in blockage of the oxygen supply to the baby. If, therefore, you know that your baby is breech before you go into labour, or that the head is still high, you should be prepared to go to hospital if the waters break. Although a prolapsed cord is rare, prompt arrival at hospital and quick action, which could include a Caesarean, may save the baby's life.

Obstetricians may wish to stimulate the uterus once the membranes have ruptured. If your baby's head is well down, it is a good idea to give nature a chance. There is an 85 per cent chance that contractions will start naturally within 24 hours. Many obstetricians will allow more than 24 hours if all is well with the baby and you let them know that you really wish to start labour naturally if possible. Involve yourself in some gentle activity or get a good night's sleep. Say "no thank you" to vaginal examinations. They increase the risk of infection. Say "no thank you" to any offer of induction before at least 24 hours have passed. Research shows that induction leads to longer labours, greater need for painkilling drugs, more operative vaginal deliveries and more Caesarean sections.*

You do not have to worry about having a "dry" labour, with the baby travelling down an unlubricated birth canal, as there is no such thing. Your amniotic fluid is completely re-formed every three hours. Actually, a "wet" labour is more likely and can be uncomfortable, since a continual leaking throughout labour is cold and unpleasant. If you are leaking, wear a sanitary pad and change it frequently. If you are in a bath or birth pool you will not notice any leaking, so you will be much more comfortable.

The contractions start Contractions usually feel like a tight elastic belt slung under your bump and around into the small of your back, being drawn tighter, gripping for 15 to 20 seconds, and then being released. This sensation occurs again after ten minutes or even sooner. They might be the Braxton Hicks "rehearsal" contractions, which some women experience in the last three weeks or so of pregnancy. These tend to be called "false" labour. All this means is that you thought you were in labour, with good reason, but were not. These contractions are probably softening your cervix so that it can open.

Using gravity to help your labour

*If you stay more or less upright in early labour, and continue to move
around, the downwards force of gravity will help to push the baby out.
Your contractions will be more effective, too, and should
prove less painful than if you were lying down.
These exercises will help you do this effectively.*

Squatting

*If you find squatting comfortable,
crouch down between your partner's
legs and lean back against him,
using his knees for support. Then
you can rock or rotate your pelvis.*

Supported lunge

*With firm support from
your partner, and one foot
raised on a chair, stool or
low table, you can move
into a supported lunge.*

Bending forwards

*You can lean over a bed or
windowsill and rock your
pelvis while your partner
applies counterpressure to
the small of your back.*

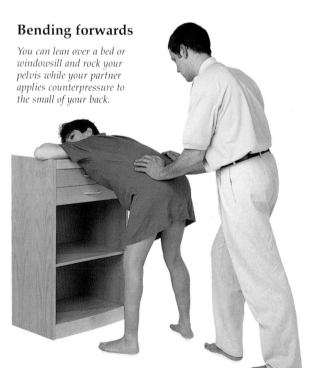

Supported dance

*In a standing position,
supported by your
partner, you can both
move together in a
slow dance.*

Supported kneeling

You may find that you are more comfortable when in a kneeling position, rather than a standing one, with an arm supported by a bed, chair or pile of firm cushions.

Kneeling over

You can also kneel in front of your partner, leaning forwards over his knees while he applies gentle pressure to the base of your spine.

Sitting down

You can sit on a chair leaning forwards slightly over its back, with your partner behind you giving firm counterpressure.

Pelvic rocking

Try rocking your pelvis backwards and forwards or making slow, circling movements as if you were belly dancing.

245

If you want to be fairly sure about being in labour, time your contractions over a period of 30 minutes or an hour; make a note of the interval between the start of one and the start of the next, and also note down the length of each contraction. The contractions need to come closer and closer together and to last longer (40 seconds or more) before you can be confident that labour is being established.

During contractions the muscle fibres at the top of the uterus tighten, pressing in and down on the centre, and producing an upwards pull on the cervix. When the baby's head is pressed down by a contraction, the muscles and fibrous tissues of the cervix are drawn apart. In a straightforward labour most of the physical sensations caused by contractions come from this area in and around the cervix, apart from a hardening and swelling felt at the top of the uterus.

Once contractions are going well, they have a regular rhythm, a wavelike shape and last longer and longer, while the interval between them is reduced. You may feel your contractions as firm squeezes that make you want to gasp when at their tightest, like hot sunlight pouring through your pelvis or like rushing ocean waves.

THE FIRST STAGE OF LABOUR

The hormonal changes that the baby has started now stimulate the beginning of a quite remarkable process. The uterus produces prostaglandins and as a result contractions like those that you have been having in late pregnancy get bigger and also come closer together. So the contractions of early labour may feel like Braxton Hicks contractions, but heftier and also more regular.

These more efficient contractions press the baby's presenting part down to the base of the lower segment of the uterus and against the cervix. This then becomes progressively more stretched and thinned out as the muscle fibres are pulled up into the upper segment. The effacement and stretching of the cervix trigger the production of oxytocin from the posterior pituitary gland, and this stimulates the uterus into a steady rhythm of contractions. Labour is under way!

MOVING AROUND IN LABOUR

Going to bed in the first stage of labour and becoming more or less immobile can slow down labour or interfere with it starting effectively because the presenting part may not be pressed down against your cervix. When you are upright and moving around, you have gravity to help you: everything is being pressed down.

It was not until the end of the 18th century in Europe that women began to lie down in order to give birth. Before that time they had walked around during much of labour, used birth stools to sit on or sat up in bed or on a chair. Birth stools were designed like horseshoes with the open part at the front, were low on the ground so that the woman squatted and sometimes provided support for her lower back as well as handgrips. As a result, the woman was in a physiologically excellent position for childbirth.

Mauriceau, then the obstetrician to the French court, introduced the lying down position, and it soon caught on because people sought to imitate the manners of the court. When forceps were first introduced, obstetricians found that they were easier to use on a woman who was lying flat. Still later, the lithotomy position, in which the patient lies on her back with her legs fixed to raised stirrups, and which was first devised for surgery on gall stones, was introduced. This highly artificial posture is often very uncomfortable for the woman, pressing her uterus against the big blood vessels in the lower part of the body. This interferes with her circulation, causing hypotension (low blood pressure), and also with the production of urine; it can also sometimes cause distress to the fetus.

Research on the effect of different positions in the first stage of labour* has shown that most women prefer to be up and about, not lying in bed, and that contractions are stronger and labour shorter with the woman in an upright position. The uterus is working nearly twice as efficiently to dilate the cervix.

Keep walking around between contractions. Try pelvic rocking and circling as if you were belly dancing – through contractions, too, if it feels good. If dilatation is taking a long time, soak in a warm bath or squat on a low stool under the shower.

WHEN TO GO TO HOSPITAL

Unless you feel strongly that you need to be in hospital during this time, or your doctor or midwife has advised that there is a special reason why you should come in as soon as there are any signs of labour starting, it is best to stay at home and carry on as usual. This is partly because of the psychological effect of going to hospital, being admitted and prepared and getting into bed. If you have only just begun labour, all this can stop it entirely. There are many women who have rushed to hospital with regular contractions that are still more than five minutes apart, and who have then gone out of labour and have either had to wait around with their morale dropping steadily or have had an intravenous oxytocin drip inserted in an arm vein to stimulate the uterus into action.

Remember to continue to eat and drink. Labour may last a long time, and both you and whoever is going to be your companion in labour are going to need your strength.

Knowing that your contractions will be coming one every two minutes and will last about one minute or longer just before the baby is born may give you some perspective on your labour when it is just starting. Having contractions every five minutes can be tiring, and some women experience this for 12 hours or more, usually when the baby is in a slightly awkward position, facing the mother's front instead of her back (see page 262); but the baby cannot possibly be born when contractions are coming this far apart, so if you are happier at home, stay there. Keep a careful record of what is happening, time the contractions now and again, and be ready to go to hospital as soon as the membranes rupture or contractions come more often than every five minutes. Of course you must bear in mind the distance from your home to hospital and the difficulty of getting there. If you are going in your own car, it is as well to have done a trial run beforehand at the rush hour to see how long it can take and to be sure that you know the way, even in deep snow, hail or fog, and also any short cuts that may be convenient. Your partner should drive steadily, but not fast, and should certainly not brake suddenly at corners or at lights. Decide early what you will need to make the journey comfortable and whether you would prefer to be in the front or back seat of the car. If you are calling an ambulance, find out well in advance how to do this and if you are relying on getting to hospital by cab have a list of numbers pinned up by the telephone in case one is not immediately available.

ADMISSION PROCEDURES

When you arrive at the hospital, a midwife will take you to a little room where you will be "prepped" (prepared) for labour. She will ask you questions about how labour started, if the waters have broken and if so when, how often contractions are coming, and so on. She will do some of the things you are already familiar with, such as requesting a urine sample, checking your blood pressure, feeling the position of the baby through your abdominal wall and listening to the fetal heart. She or a doctor will feel through your vagina and into your cervix, to tell if you have started dilating. If you are already partially dilated, he or she may break the waters (see page 317). This is done routinely in many hospitals at 3–4 cm dilatation, and sometimes before this phase has been reached. If you want your membranes to remain intact until they rupture spontaneously, say so before your internal examination.

It used to be hospital practice to shave a woman's perineum, and in some hospitals every perineum was required to be as bald as a hard-boiled egg. Still today some attendants like the hair surrounding the vagina to be clipped short. Women have spoken out strongly against the unnecessary, uncomfortable and degrading practice of perineal shaving; research has also shown that it is entirely useless in avoiding infection and, however carefully done, always results in some injury to the skin.

Some midwives still give an enema to empty the lower bowel, but there is no point in doing this unless a woman is very constipated. In the hours before labour starts, most women have loose motions. In this way the lower bowel is cleared naturally.

After you have been examined you will be asked to don a hospital gown; it is usually done up at the back, but if you hope to have your baby at the breast immediately following delivery you will find it easier to wear the gown with the opening at the front. Many women prefer their own clothes. Select something made of cotton rather than a synthetic fabric, since hospitals are often overheated.

Whatever you wear should be short and loose, so that you can move about freely. An external or internal fetal monitor may be attached to assess your baby's heart rate and response to contractions, as well as the strength of the uterine contractions. It is routine practice in many hospitals to do an "admission trace" of the fetal heart sounds for 20 or 30 minutes. There has been no research into the value of this, so it should be your choice whether or not you have it.

In some hospitals your partner may be asked to wait outside while you are prepared, but most take it for granted that a couple will want to stay together. It can seem a very long time to be separated, and if your partner has been helping you cope with contractions up till now, it is good to go on having the same kind of support. It also gives the midwife a chance to talk with the partner, which means that she is meeting you not as an isolated patient but in your relationship with someone who is important in your life. If you have chosen to have other people there too (a doula, friend or relative), they should also be able to stay. Labour is not a good time in which to have people coming and going. You will be able to relax knowing that you are with someone who understands you and is giving continuous emotional support.

A doctor may come into the room at intervals to assess progress or to discuss your case. If you have any questions, take this opportunity to ask them. If you are planning a natural birth, want to walk around in labour or have any other particular wishes, remind the doctor or midwife of these and ask if they have been or can be noted on your chart.

COUNTDOWN FOR BIRTH AT HOME

If you are having your baby at home, plan ahead and make sure that any major chores do not pile up. When you think you are in labour, start to prepare for the birth. Put a plastic sheet (a shower curtain also works well) on the bed and if the bed is not already at right angles to the wall move it to this position. Put out the things that the midwife has asked you to have ready on a small table or, better still, a trolley, arranged on a freshly washed towel or pillowcase, and cover them with another piece of cloth. Arrange the lighting so that the midwife can direct some light on to your perineum for delivery and so that the other lights can be dimmed or turned out when required. Put the baby's clothes out and a change of clothes for yourself. Boiling water will be used mostly for tea, but is also useful for washing your perineum after delivery.

Turn your mind to what you are going to eat and drink for the next three days and also what you may want to offer visitors. You will have been wise to have stocked up your food cupboard and freezer well in advance. If you put anything in the oven at this stage, take a timer with you when you go to the bedroom and pin a reminder in a prominent place, or your labour may well be accompanied by the smell of burning food.

Call the midwife to let her know that you may be needing her later, and pin all important telephone numbers within easy reach by the telephone. The midwife will probably ring to check how you are doing and encourage you to contact her whenever you wish.

TRANSITION

Towards the end of the first stage of labour, when you are between 8 and 10 cm dilated, you are in transition. For most women the very end of the first stage is stormy and challenging. Contractions follow each other relentlessly, with hardly a pause between, and they tend to become arrhythmic, with sharp peaks and sometimes with more than one peak to each contraction. The buildup of energy with each may be so sudden and tumultuous that there is no time for slow breathing. You must adapt straight away and may need to breathe much more lightly and quickly if you are to soar over the top of the peaks with your breathing. The very length of the contractions may demand every bit of concentration and determination that you are able to summon, and you will need strong emotional support and unfailing encouragement.

At the same time other physiological signs may occur that can be quite unsettling, until you remember that they are indications of progress, and that if you are aware of three or more of them, then you are likely to be 8 cm dilated and hence in transition. Feeling hot then cold, then hot again, your cheeks flushed and your eyes shining bright, suggests that you are in transition. So does a fit of hiccups or belching, or you may even feel nauseous and actually vomit. Perhaps your legs feel icy cold and begin to shake uncontrollably. One of the surest signs is feeling that you have a large grapefruit pressing against your anus or that you want to empty your bowels. You might have a catch in your throat that stops your easy, rhythmic breathing, or you involuntarily hold your breath or start to grunt. You may suddenly feel that it is all too much hard work, and that you really cannot go on and would like to go home and forget all about having a baby. Or you may become irritable with everyone and hypercritical of the help your partner is giving.

Not all women experience these signs, but a sufficient proportion do to make it a good idea for your partner to memorize them, so that at the right moment he or she can say: "I think you are in transition". You may have forgotten that you are having a baby by this time and are simply concentrating on the work of handling each contraction. You are also likely to feel that you are not making any progress at all and have lost all sense of time. Since in transition you may get an urge to push before you are fully dilated, you may be told to continue breathing and not to hold your breath until you absolutely must.

Pushing powerfully and for a long time against an incompletely dilated cervix can make it puffy and swollen, so that the opening actually closes rather than opens wider. This is why you may be asked not to push until you cannot avoid pushing. This is wise advice, because then you can be quite certain that your body is really ready to push, and you will also enjoy the surrender to the great sweeps of energy that come with the contractions in a way you cannot if you are just pushing because someone has told you to do so.

Transition may be very brief – just a few contractions – or it may last an hour or more. It is likely to last longer if the baby is in an occipito-posterior position (see page 262). The cervix has to dilate to 10 cm before the baby can be pressed down through the opening. At full dilatation (10 cm or the width of the palm of a large man's hand including the thumb joint) the cervix is open enough for the baby's head, its largest part, to ease through. There are spaces between the baby's skullbones, the fontanelles, which can close up as the baby slides down the birth canal, so shaping its head to make the journey much less arduous, even for a 4 kg (9 lb) baby. This is why, especially in first labours, the baby's head is moulded, sometimes into a rather peculiar shape; this gradually disappears in the first week or so after the birth (see page 362).

THE SECOND STAGE OF LABOUR

This is the most exciting stage of labour. During the first stage of labour the cervix has thinned out and opened. At the end of the first stage it is open to 10 cm, making the uterus and vagina one birth canal. Contractions ease the baby's head down further and there is often a lull during this phase.

Pushing Women are often told to start pushing as soon as the cervix is fully dilated. This does not shorten the second stage of labour. In fact, if a woman does not have an overwhelming urge to push it may be because the baby's head has not yet fully rotated into the best position for birth. If she starts doing deliberate breathing exercises and straining to push the baby out, or is told that she ought to push, it may not be what her uterus wants to do. Forceful bearing down can push the head down too soon and result in deep transverse

Dilatation of the cervix
The cervix has to be 10 cm dilated (widened) before the uterus can press the baby out. The time taken to reach full dilatation varies enormously: some women are 3 cm dilated before they realize they are in labour, some take many hours to reach 5 cm.

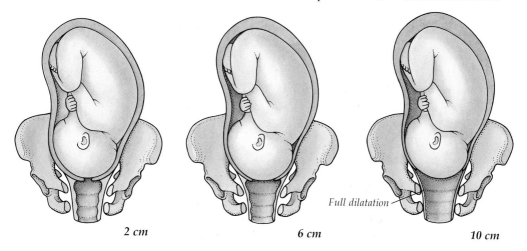

2 cm *6 cm* Full dilatation *10 cm*

arrest. That is, the baby actually gets stuck.* The woman has wasted all her energy in this harmful activity and may not be able to push energetically when it is the right time for her to do so. Sometimes she has lost the synchronization between her uterus and her actions and then never gets the desire to start pushing again. Many of the forceps deliveries and vacuum extractions that occur are performed for this reason.

Focus on the idea of *opening up* for the baby to come out. Wait to push until you feel that you cannot avoid doing so, or until the baby's head can be seen on your perineum. If you experience a pause at the onset of the second stage of labour, trust your body and enjoy this "rest and be thankful" phase.

Then follows a wonderful time when you can begin to push. The second stage of labour is often described as if it were sheer, grinding, hard work, but you will want to do it. You will probably have an overpowering urge to bear down and press the baby through the birth canal. This is passionate, intense, thrilling and often completely irresistible, and for some women it is the nearest thing to overwhelming sexual excitement. Pushing is not something you decide to do with a rational part of your mind, but a force that sweeps through your body and culminates in the delivery of your baby. Let your body take over at this stage.

The journey through the pelvis

About 80 per cent of women have good, well-rounded pelvises for childbirth. Problems may be encountered if your pelvis is narrow: an android pelvis, for instance, is shaped like a triangle at the brim, which is hard for the baby to negotiate. Even when the pelvic shape is not ideal, the uterus works to press the baby into a neat package that, given time, can often make the journey easily.

Basically, the baby consists of two balls that move against each other. The ball with the largest diameter is the baby's head. The other ball is the baby's trunk with the limbs well tucked in. The action of a uterus that is contracting well results in the baby being moulded into the right shape for the journey down the birth canal.

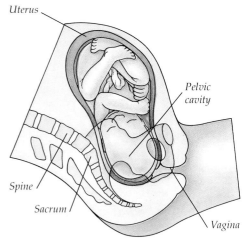

1 The vagina is almost at right angles to the uterus. The baby has to negotiate an angle similar to a foot putting on a Wellington boot. There are several bones that may hold up the baby's progress. The sacrum is the big bone at the base of the spine that forms part of the pelvic brim. Once the baby's head has travelled below the pelvic brim, it is in the pelvic cavity.

Normal female pelvis

Android pelvis

There are a few women who do not feel much of an urge to bear down during the second stage of labour. Sometimes women who have had other babies do not experience any strong pushing urge. The whole process of labour may be much gentler; the mother seems not to need to do that much bearing down because the baby is going to be born very easily anyway.

There are three to five urges to bear down with each second-stage contraction, although sometimes we talk about these contractions as if they were all push. Frantic pushing results in your becoming desperate, straining to press the baby just that little bit further. This is not necessary, because surges of desire to bear down come with each contraction, and it is important to go naturally with each as it comes; allow yourself to hold your breath, bear down and open up with the surge, which usually lasts five or six seconds, no longer. Only you can know when these surges are there. Some people think it is a good idea for a woman to hold her breath for as long as she possibly can in the second stage and only then is she really working hard. However, research suggests that directed pushing, prolonged breath-holding and sustained bearing down is not only exhausting for the mother, but can also be dangerous for the baby because it reduces the oxygen content of the blood.* So trust your spontaneous feelings and do what comes naturally.

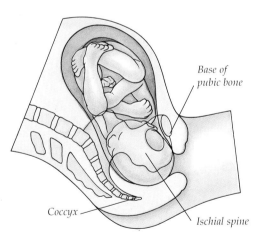

Base of pubic bone

Coccyx

Ischial spine

2 *Once the baby has negotiated the pelvic brim, it moves on to the pelvic outlet. This is bordered by the coccyx (the tiny bone at the base of the spine) at the back, the bottom of the pubic bone at the front, and the ischial spines, which are the two projecting crests on the side walls of the pelvis. The coccyx slips out of the way as the baby's head comes through the pelvic outlet.*

3 *It is usually the downwards pressure from above provided by good and powerful contractions that will ease the baby's head down, so that as it comes through the steepest curve at the beginning of the vagina the muscles at the back of the baby's neck extend. This means that the baby is usually facing downwards just before birth and as it is born.*

YOUR BABY'S HEAD APPEARS

When the top of your baby's head can be seen for the first time, it looks like a wrinkled walnut in the vagina, not like a baby at all. Your partner will probably see this before you can, and will be able to tell you the colour of the baby's hair. With the first baby the second stage make take one or two hours. With the second or subsequent baby it may take only ten minutes.

Then there comes a time when the widest part of the baby's head is at the birth opening and does not go back in between contractions. You feel stretched to your utmost. At this moment of "crowning" it is important not to go on pushing, even though you feel very much like it. Otherwise you might tear the perineal tissue. The doctor or midwife may perform an episiotomy if they think you might tear (see page 320). If you want to avoid having one, say so, and before the head crowns start to breathe the baby out instead of pushing it out (see page 208), and in this way it may slip forwards. The midwife or obstetrician will check to see that the cord is free of the neck and may insert a mucus catheter in the baby's mouth and suck any mucus out.

The baby's head slips under your pubic bone and extends, the chin being automatically lifted off its chest. As the head emerges, damp and sticky with mucus, it is often a violet or purple colour. This is nothing to worry about: the child has not yet taken that first great gasp of air that will oxygenate its blood.

The baby may be covered in vernix, a cold-cream-like substance that coats the baby's skin in the uterus and makes it look as if it has been spread with cottage cheese. The head has been moulded by the journey down the birth canal, so it may be an odd, pointed or bumpy asymmetrical shape, and the forehead may recede and the baby be almost chinless. The nose is often flattened like a prize-fighter's and there are little red marks between the eyes and on the eyelids.

At delivery, the baby's head is facing downwards but the shoulders are still turned sideways inside you. Once the head is free, it turns to come in line with the shoulders. You may need another push for the shoulders. The doctor or midwife may press the baby's head down so that the shoulder nearer your front slides out first. Tell them if you would prefer them not to touch. A shoulder slides out next. At last the whole body slithers out and your baby is born!

There is often a great gush of water, and the baby may be already breathing and crying, limbs lashing, and face puckered up with what looks like rage. The lower end of the body seems very small in comparison with the head end, apart from the genitals, which often look extraordinarily large. All this is normal. If the baby is not yet breathing, attendants suck out the respiratory tract, hold the child's head downwards, and may give oxygen. If you are propped or upright, you can reach your baby, provided he or she is lying over your thigh, between your legs, or on your tummy, and you may want to reach down and take your baby in your arms.

THE THIRD STAGE OF LABOUR

Although you may not feel the contractions, your uterus continues to contract after the birth of the baby. This makes the placenta separate from its lining, since the placenta cannot contract. As the uterus squeezes down into a firm, hard ball the placental mass is then automatically peeled off. This process has been compared to stretching a piece of rubber on which a postage stamp has been stuck; when the rubber moves, the stamp becomes detached. The sinuses in which the placental blood vessels were rooted are closed by the tight squeezing of the uterus, and these contractions also prevent excessive bleeding from the uterine wall.

When the placenta has detached itself, the midwife or doctor may pull on the cord (see page 322). Take a breath, hold it and bear down at the same time to help this process. You can ask that instead of having cord traction, you can push and do it by yourself.

There is a squelchy, slippery feeling as the placenta slides out. It is then carefully examined by the person who delivered the baby to see that every part is there. Pieces of placenta left inside the uterus could cause unnecessary bleeding, pain and infection in the postpartum period. Although the placenta looks like a large piece of raw liver, it was the tree of life for your baby. You may be interested to examine it and see the difference between the rough side, which was against the wall of the uterus, and the smooth side, which lay towards the baby like a soft, velvety cushion, and to note the network of blood vessels that provided your baby with its life-support system.

If you need stitching, it is usually possible to have the baby with you throughout this procedure. Suturing (the technical term for stitching) is done under local anaesthetic and may take a long time, sometimes as long as an hour, since careful embroidery has to be done and the underlying layers of muscle must be correctly aligned. So keep your baby in your arms or near enough to touch.

The midwife will help you to put on an ice pack to reduce swelling and a sanitary pad, since there will be some bleeding now and for several days, resembling the height of a heavy period. The length of time during which there is a bloodstained vaginal discharge (lochia) varies greatly among women. Some new mothers bleed for just a few days after the birth, others for as long as five or six weeks.

BEING TOGETHER

In many hospitals the staff tidy up at this point. They wipe and weigh the baby, examine you to see if you need stitches, give you a wash, change your gown, shorten the baby's cord and reclamp it. But practice is changing fast and many hospital staff now give the parents the opportunity for a quiet time with their baby in the period immediately following the birth, only doing the basic essentials and leaving the couple alone for an hour or so to start to get to know their baby. Being together should always come first. Tidying up can be done later. It is far less important.

A home birth

Pauline chose a home birth because friends who had recently become fathers and had hospital births, didn't feel totally included, and she believed a home birth would entail much less stress for the baby.

She is 7 cm dilated by the time she needs to call her midwife, Nicky. Her husband, Clifton, lies beside her on the bed giving her loving support.

Then she kneels by the bed with a heating pad on her lower back. Nicky tells her, "Make as much sound as you want but keep the tones low". Pauline says this really helped. "I felt in control all the time. I felt safe, and I had my own space".

The baby is born still inside the bag of waters. Nicky says, "Pauline was brilliant! Completely focused on the task at hand". She tells her, "It's coming now. It's lovely – well done!" and then she prepares her for not pushing with the next contraction to enable the baby to be born gently.

Then in the space of one contraction, the baby's head advances, inside the membranes; the head slides out facing the mother's back and rotates to align with the shoulders, which are still inside. Next a shoulder and arm slip out, and are followed by the other shoulder; then finally the whole body emerges.

A glistening, transparent veil of membrane envelops the baby. Supporting the baby's back, the midwife takes the membrane off the baby's head so that she can take her first breath. Nicky rests the baby between Pauline's legs and Pauline exclaims, "Oh, it's a girl!"

The baby cries and is a perfect colour. Pauline picks up her daughter and cradles her in her arms, cord still uncut. After all her striving to bring this child to birth she is radiant.

Everyone is laughing and admiring this beautiful baby. Pauline is still bleeding quite heavily, so Nicky gives her a quick injection of syntocinon in order to stimulate the uterus to contract. Then she clamps and severs the cord.

When the baby's searching mouth indicates that she is ready to suck, her mother offers her the breast, and after nuzzling and licking as she explores this new sensation, she latches on. The parents share together the miracle of birth in an atmosphere of timelessness and peace. These are moments that they will never forget.

Different kinds of labour

However much other people may advise you not to have any preconceptions about your labour, just to be ready for whatever comes, it is difficult not to have some, because it is almost impossible to prepare yourself to cope with a situation that you have not imagined in advance. So it is useful to think ahead to the major variations on the theme of childbirth that you might confront. However, it is still vital to keep in the forefront of your mind the normal, rhythmic and harmonious pattern of a straightforward labour. Otherwise all the medical technicalities may seem quite bewildering, and you may interpret each uncomfortable physical sign as an indication that something has gone wrong. This chapter looks at some different types of labour, all of which can throw you unless you understand what is happening.

LABOUR WITH A POSTERIOR BABY

When the back of the baby's head presses against your sacrum, the baby is said to be in an occipito-posterior position. Most women have some backache in labour, but women with posterior babies may have it all the time, so that the labour can be described as a "back labour". Few women with posterior babies do not have backache, which can be the most tiring and stressful thing about a labour – especially if, as is often the case when the baby is posterior, it continues *between* contractions as well as during them.

Another characteristic of labour with a posterior baby is that it starts very slowly, often over a period of several days, and contractions are usually felt as one big one followed by a feeble one. Plan for morale-boosting activity during a long first stage. Do not go into hospital too soon. A walk in the park or the country is probably better. Eat and keep up your strength in early labour and have plenty of fluids, remembering to empty your bladder regularly. Your partner also needs stamina in a back labour, to keep you going by giving you total attention during difficult contractions.

If the baby is in a posterior position the membranes should not be ruptured artificially. It is much easier for the baby to rotate if it is still floating free. When the membranes are ruptured the baby often drops down into the pelvis in a posterior position and is fixed rather like a cork stuck in a bottle.

The baby will probably rotate at the very end of the first stage or at the onset of the second and things will be plain sailing from then on. About 5 per cent of posteriors do not rotate and then the hard work has to be continued in the second stage and you may need obstetric help (see pages 334–340) to deliver the baby. But chances are that the baby will swivel around by itself and then be able to complete the journey down your birth canal with ease.

Presentations for birth

When the baby is lying head down and curled into a neat ball (occipito anterior), the uterus can usually work well to open the cervix and press the baby down into the birth canal to be born. There are other positions that the baby may adopt and these can sometimes lead to problems during labour and giving birth.

Right occipito anterior
This position is a common presentation for labour.

Left occipito anterior
The most usual presentation is with the baby facing to the left.

Full breech presentation
With this position the baby is able to flex during labour.

Frank breech presentation
This type of presentation makes flexion difficult.

Footling breech
In this type of presentation the baby's foot is born in advance of the rest of the body.

Left occipito posterior
This position can cause backache in labour.

Right occipito posterior
More common than LOP, this also causes backache in labour.

Common abbreviations
Left occipito anterior = LOA
Left occipito posterior = LOP
Right occipito anterior = ROA
Right occipito posterior = ROP

WAYS OF DEALING WITH A BACK LABOUR

You may find that some of the things described on the following pages are helpful in the first stage of a back labour.

Heat A hot-water bottle wrapped in a towel, or a hot compress (in the form of a facecloth or small towel wrung out in really hot water) applied to where you feel most pain may bring relief. A hot shower with the water pulsing on your back also helps.

Cold Use a packet of frozen peas or sweetcorn from the freezer wrapped in a cloth, or crushed ice knotted into a polythene bag to numb pain and relieve muscle spasm.

Changes of position Keep upright and moving around for as long as possible. In this way you tip the baby down to press through the pelvis and birth canal instead of right into the small of your back. Crouching, leaning forwards, leaning forwards with one foot placed on a chair beside you, kneeling, squatting, getting on to all fours with your lower back arched and lying on your side with your back well rounded, your head and shoulders curved forwards and a pillow between your legs, may all be positions in which pain is eased. They may also encourage the rotation of the baby's head. Research has shown that an all-fours position helps babies to rotate from posterior to anterior. It can be combined with pelvic rocking. Seventy-five per cent of babies turn when women with posterior babies adopt a hands-and-knees position. But babies do not turn when women sit upright.*

Movement If you want to get a tight ring off your finger you do not just pull it. You wiggle it. In much the same way, you may be able to help your baby's head rotate by rocking your pelvis forwards and backwards, from side to side, by circling it, doing these movements with one foot up on a stool or chair, going up and down stairs, rocking from foot to foot, walking slowly with big strides and exploring all the movements that form the intricate steps of a birth dance. Spontaneous movements that are comforting and that feel right not only relieve pain but can also help the baby's head rotate.

Pressure Ask your partner to provide firm pressure, either right over the place where your pelvis joins your spine or to the left or right of this if pain is more to the side. He or she should use the heel of one hand, with the other resting over it, and press his body weight down through his arm. Or you may prefer the feel of knuckles.

Stimulus on pressure points may help you handle the pain more effectively. One place where deep pressure of a thumb or finger may feel good is on your bottom, level with the top of the slit between your buttocks and a little more than the width of your palm out towards the leg on each side. Experiment to find the spot: it feels

Relieving your back labour

*One of the greatest threats to a woman's morale in childbirth
is having constant backache. With the help of your partner you
can practise the techniques below. They will help you to take
the edge off pain in labour and find the energy to cope with it.*

*Press gently on
either side of the
buttocks*

Firm pressure
Pressure above and to either
side of your buttocks can
greatly relieve a tender and
aching back. Make sure
your partner presses evenly.

Pelvic pressure
By pressing his pelvis
against your lower
back, your partner
can make you more
comfortable while
having a rest
himself.

*Use your full
weight to
press down*

*Move the rolling
pin slowly and
evenly*

Pressing the sacrum
Your partner can apply firm
pressure to your sacrum by
leaning over and allowing
his full weight to pass
down through his arms.

Using a rolling pin
Your partner can also roll
a rolling pin wrapped in a
warm towel slowly and
evenly over your lower back.

tender, but pressure on it is satisfying. If you are in a position in which you are tilted forwards, your partner can apply pressure to the spot on both of your buttocks at once.

If you are on your side your partner will be able to reach only one, but even this may help. These areas are called "pain prevention points" in one system of psychoprophylaxis.

Pressure points Your partner can exert pressure on parts of the body far away from where you are feeling pain, but where a really strong stimulus can offer almost miraculous relief. Known as *shiatsu* or acupressure, this can be particularly effective in childbirth when used on the feet. One pressure point is just below the centre of the ball of the foot. Another point is between the fleshy pads under the big toe and next toe. Your partner holds one foot firmly, exerting very strong pressure with a finger or thumb on the chosen spot, and providing light counterpressure with the rest of the hand over the top of the foot.

"It was extraordinary how pressure on the balls of my feet relieved the pain during the labour. I wouldn't have believed it possible, but it really did. The pain receded into the distance and instead I felt exhilarated and in an odd way could enjoy the contraction."

There are many acupressure points on the buttocks, too. Kneel forwards over the seat of a chair or lie three-quarters over on your side so that your partner can "map" the places on your buttocks where it feels good to have strong, steady pressure. Try, for example, pressing just under the curve of the buttocks, and beneath the bony pelvis at either side of the buttocks. Another place where pressure can be very effective is on the inside wrist, between the tendons. Care should be taken to press only with the fleshy pad of a finger or thumb – but not with the nails. It is surprising how strong the pressure from finger and thumb can be on the right spot, and in all these places continuous pressure will produce a tingling, buzzing sensation. Acupressure for up to 10 seconds at a time followed by a pause, and then repeated, in a steady rhythm, can provide effective pain relief during powerful contractions, whether they are felt in your front or back, and wherever the pain is centred.

Massage Massage may feel better than pressure, or can feel good alternated with pressure. The massage that suits most women best is firm, slow and steady, moving the flesh and muscle on the bone. You can use powder, cornflour or massage oil to avoid skin irritation, and your partner should have some cream to rub into his or her hands if the massage is to be applied for a long time.

Another effective way of giving massage is to use a rolling pin. Knot a face towel or hot compress around it to get more grip. Your partner can sit on the bed with his pelvis against your lower spine and lean back against you, too. This provides welcome rest for someone who after several hours of working to relieve backache may develop back pain himself!

Immersion in water A birth pool or deep bath is enormously helpful in backache labour and may take away pain entirely. Do not lie back in the water. Try a hands-and-knees or floating squat position instead. Not only is warm water comforting and relaxing, but it also enables you to move smoothly and easily. If you leave your head loose, you can change position frequently without any strain, one movement flowing into another as if in a slow, luxurious water dance.

Labour with a breech baby

This type of labour sometimes starts with the waters leaking. This is because the baby's bottom does not fit the opening cervix as well as the oval of the crown of the head, so part of the bag of waters becomes wedged between the baby's bottom and your cervix. Ring the doctor if this happens to you and the baby is not yet engaged. The risk is that the cord might slide down and be caught between the baby and the cervix, so that the oxygen supply to the baby is cut off.

If the waters do not break, keep walking around through the first stage, until they break spontaneously. If a breech baby is left in its bag of waters there is less chance of pressure on the cord.

After the waters have gone, the best positions are on all fours or on your side. You may have backache and if so your partner could exert pressure with the knuckles over the small of your back.

Foot work
Applying pressure to certain parts of the feet can relieve pain from contractions. One spot is just below the centre of the ball of the foot; another is between the fleshy pads under the big toe and the next one.

The second stage of a breech labour

You may be moved to the operating theatre before the second stage starts, in case you should need an emergency Caesarean section. Sometimes your partner is shown to the waiting room at this time. If you want to stay together make this clear.

Many doctors prefer to deliver breech babies with the woman in the lithotomy position (see page 247), since they feel that they have most control over the birth this way. But you will probably be more comfortable squatting, on all fours, dangling, standing or standing and bending your knees during contractions.

It is usually best to let the second stage proceed with no voluntary exertion on your part until the body is born and the head is about to slip out, so that the baby's body is born on contraction waves only. (It may be easiest to do this if you are on all fours.) Concentrate on total release: breathe, rather than push, the baby out. If the baby has both feet up by its head the doctor or midwife may slip a gloved hand in to draw down a leg and turn the baby into a "footling" (see page 263). Relax and breathe as this is done. Once a foot is down the baby can then take the curve of the birth canal more smoothly, as its legs are no longer splinting its spine.

If you are not having an epidural (see page 309), an injection of local anaesthetic is given in your perineum if an episiotomy is to be done (see pages 320–322), before the baby's head is delivered. It takes one or two minutes to be effective. Most obstetricians do a large episiotomy with a breech so that the head can be delivered

Exploring birth movements in water

It is easy to move in water and you will probably do so quite spontaneously. But it helps to explore in advance different positions for birth, such as squatting and kneeling, with the people who will be helping you at the birth.

Kneeling slide

1 *Kneel forwards, grasping the rim of the pool with your arms extended. Slide forwards and backwards, lifting your head and bending your arms as you pull forwards and extending your arms as you slide backwards.*

2 *At the height of a contraction it may feel good to drop your head down in the water and blow out.*

3 *Then lift your head as you pull forwards and slide back with your arms extended.*

Squatting and forwards slide

1 *Squat in the water with your arms and shoulders supported by the rim of the pool, feet well apart so that your pelvis is at its widest.*

2 *Slide down in the water with your legs extended, and back up to a squatting position again.*

Squatting and backwards slide

1 *Squat in the centre of the pool, knees wide apart, arms extended and holding the rim of the pool.*

2 *Drop your body forwards, legs extended behind you, and grasp your partner at waist level, while he supports your upper arms.*

269

Forwards and backwards slide on front

1 *Kneel in the water with your arms supported by the rim of the pool. Keep your knees well apart so that your pelvis is at its widest.*

2 *Slide down in the water with your legs extended, and back up to a kneeling position again.*

Forwards and backwards slide on back

1 *With arms spread wide and supported by the pool rim, sit with your legs across the width of the pool so that your feet are resting on the opposite side. Extra padding behind your head and neck makes this more comfortable.*

2 *Slide forwards and backwards, using your feet against the side of the pool to propel you.*

Supported kneel

1 *Kneel leaning forwards, knees wide apart, with the rim of the pool under your upper arms. In this position the cervix is tilted forwards, which is helpful during the second stage of labour.*

2 *Swing back to an upright kneeling position with your legs wide apart.*

Rim support

Lie on your side, with your head and arms resting on the rim of the pool.

Head cradling

Lie back in the water with your head cradled in your partner's hands. He should use a light touch, so that you can still move your head quite freely as and when you wish.

unimpeded. But if you give birth with breathing instead of pushing, your tissues may fan out well and an episiotomy may not be necessary. Since there is unlikely to be an opportunity for discussion at the time, when things will be happening fast, talk about this earlier on in your labour (between contractions). Otherwise the doctor will probably do an episiotomy.

Once the episiotomy is done, the doctor delivers the head using hands or forceps to cradle it. You will be asked to push for the head and will probably need to bear down only once.

Sometimes women help to deliver their breech babies by leaning forwards and lifting the baby's legs up, while the doctor or midwife controls the delivery of the head and supports a shoulder. I first saw this done by mistake when a helpful midwife told a first-time mother to put her hands down and touch her baby while its head was still inside her. The mother was so excited that she held the baby's legs, lifted them, and as she did so the head slipped out without an episiotomy.

Epidural anaesthesia (see page 309) is often used for breech deliveries and has largely replaced general anaesthesia. It means that you only feel a pulling sensation, are awake and aware and can hold your baby as soon as it is breathing well. An increased number of obstetricians routinely do Caesarean sections (see page 336) for all first-baby breeches. Discuss this with your obstetrician.

Doctors who prefer to do routine Caesarean sections for all breech babies explain their practice by saying that vaginal delivery lowers a baby's IQ. In fact, it is doubtful whether there are any long-term benefits for the baby of Caesarean section over vaginal birth. Carefully controlled follow-up studies of the health and behaviour of 2- and 8-year-olds who were born bottom-first have revealed that the mode of delivery makes no difference at all.* When thinking ahead to the kind of birth you will have for your breech baby, it is important to remember that the pelvis is not a rigid, confined space.

Standard breech birth
Breech babies can be born vaginally as long as the pelvic outlet is wide enough for the head to pass through it.

First of all
The buttocks are usually delivered first, and are followed by the baby's legs.

Turning the baby
The baby turns so that the shoulders can emerge as easily as possible.

Drawing the head down
The baby's own weight draws the head down and its legs are then lifted to deliver the head.

Breech birth in the squatting position

If you stay more or less upright in early labour, and continue to move around, the downwards force of gravity will help to push the baby out. Your contractions will be more effective, too, and should prove less painful than if you were lying down.

Massage
Pressure applied above and to either side of your buttocks can greatly relieve the pain of a tender and aching back.

1 *The mother is supported by her helper standing behind her. The baby's buttocks emerge first.*

2 *After the baby's buttocks, the body and legs are born and are caught gently by the midwife.*

3 *The baby simply uncurls and drops into the midwife's hands. The baby's body is supported as the head is born.*

4 *The mother can then sit back and take her baby into her arms the moment after birth.*

During pregnancy the joints relax, bones move more freely on each other and the pelvis actually expands to make more room for the baby. Moreover, both the width and the size of the opening from front to back are increased in 28 per cent of women when they switch from lying down to a squatting position.*

In Dr Michel Odent's practice most women with breech babies have vaginal births. He likes the woman to be upright: "Our only intervention will be to insist on the supported squatting position for delivery, since it is the most mechanically efficient. It . . . is the best way to minimize the delay between the delivery of the baby's umbilicus and the baby's head . . . We would never risk a breech delivery with the mother in a dorsal or semi-seated position".* If the first stage of labour goes well without any intervention, a woman has every chance of a vaginal birth. But if first stage contractions are inefficient yet painful, and dilatation does not progress, a Caesarean section is decided on.

SHORT, SHARP LABOUR

It is wrong to assume, as do some textbooks, that a short labour is bad for the baby. In many apparently short labours the cervix is dilating gently (see page 241) over a period of days before the woman realizes she is in labour. Some short labours can be delightful. But however easy it might be physically, a violent precipitate labour is emotionally demanding and may leave you feeling drained and shocked.

If, from start to finish, your labour lasts less than an hour or two, you may need a great deal of active help from your partner, as well as his or her emotional support: in effect it is like starting straight in at the very end of the first stage. Your partner needs to concentrate with you and it may help to maintain eye contact and breathe with you. A partner who becomes anxious or excited may hyperventilate if everything is happening quickly. So remind each other to keep the breathing butterfly-light over contraction peaks.

When you feel the baby pressing like a grapefruit against your anus it may be easiest to avoid pushing if you turn on your side with your knees drawn up, or onto all fours. Whatever position you choose, push only when you have to and for as short a time as you can. Open your mouth, drop your jaw and relax your lips. Continue breathing in and out through a relaxed mouth and concentrate on releasing all the tissues around your vagina as they fan out and open wide.

If the baby is coming very fast in the second stage you will probably need to blow as well as breathe quickly to stop yourself from pushing. If you feel as if you really must push, blow as if you were extinguishing a candle flame to reduce the intensity of the push (see page 208). You will not stop the push altogether, because the expulsive power of the uterus is there whatever you do, but you can limit it to a certain extent. Some women feel after a labour of this kind that they want the baby inside them again; they wish that they could go back to the beginning, because everything happened so fast that they cannot make sense of it. Some even feel "cheated". If this is so with you, talk through each event of labour with your partner after the birth, fitting the pieces together, and reliving the birth in your thoughts until you can see its shape.

LONG-DRAWN-OUT LABOUR

A lengthy labour can be psychologically taxing as well as physically exhausting. You need constant confident emotional support from someone who loves or knows you well and does not leave you. Yet unfortunately a prolonged labour tends to make a male partner anxious about what is happening, unsure of his role and often feeling that he ought to leave it all to the professionals.

A long-drawn-out labour can seem prolonged for two reasons: firstly, you may be unable to differentiate clearly between the lead-in to labour proper – sometimes called the "latent" phase – and active labour. Secondly, active labour in turn may then be prolonged because contractions are faint and infrequent, or because the contractions are not achieving dilatation of the cervix as they should.

In these cases, psychological support from your partner and midwife, accurate information and a chance to rest are vitally important. Even if the contractions seem to be ineffective and dilatation is slow until you reach 4 cm, everything may seem to co-ordinate suddenly so that from then on labour goes like a bomb. Over 90 per cent of women having a lengthy latent phase go on

"Throughout the entire labour I was conscious that I could only go with the contractions. I felt it was like running in a marathon."

to have a normal labour and delivery if given the chance.* So do not immediately assume that if labour takes several days to start it is going to be like that right through. Have relaxing hot baths, sleep or rest in different beds if possible, so that you have a change of scene, and automatically take up different positions. There may be a couch, an easy chair or even a rug to lie on as a change from your usual bed. Do not to go into hospital until you think you would feel happier there. Even if you have a long first stage, the second stage may be completely normal.

The progress of your labour is assessed in terms of the rate of dilatation of the cervix (see pages 241–242). Provided that the baby is all right and its heart tones are regular, *slow dilatation at the onset of labour does not harm the baby*, however tiring you are finding it. Slow dilatation in the early phase is not the same as complete lack of progress over several hours once active labour has started (that is, after the cervix has dilated about 3 cm); then the baby may be exposed to special risk and the heart rate may slow down.

Do remember that it is difficult for people to be accurate about dilatation: you may be examined by someone who says you are 5 cm dilated, but an hour later someone else says you are only 4 cm or perhaps 5 cm dilated, when by then the first person examining you would have reckoned you to be 6 cm dilated.

WAYS OF DEALING WITH A LONG LABOUR

In hospital it is often difficult to walk about and alternate periods of rest with sessions of activity. But if you can do this, it is the best natural way of helping a uterus that is contracting ineffectually to start working far more efficiently.

Be sure that you are taking enough fluids, since you can forget to drink and become dehydrated. You may be given an intravenous "cocktail" of dextrose solution to keep up your strength and ensure that you do not become dried out. If this is the case, get into an upright position beforehand so that you are not then stuck lying down with an intravenous drip in your arm. If you have to stay in bed, take up positions in which the long axis of the uterus is in line with the birth canal. You can do this by kneeling or squatting, and it is one of the most effective non-invasive actions you can take. You can do this *before* taking drugs for pain relief (see page 306–313), having an epidural (see page 309) or accepting hormone acceleration of labour (see page 328).

Sometimes fear or anxiety seems to prevent a uterus from functioning well. If physical difficulties have been ruled out, work together with your partner on facing up to any worries that may be on your mind. Both of you together can create a psychologically positive atmosphere by concentrating on the reality of the baby who is coming to birth and on the visual image of the cervix opening up. In parts of New Guinea, when labour is long drawn out the woman is urged to confess any hidden anger she may feel because it is thought that labour will proceed smoothly and easily once she has got rid of negative feelings she is bottling up.

The general obstetric term for a long-drawn-out labour is "failure to progress". It is one of the main reasons why Caesarean sections are done. In the words of two obstetricians, "In many cases failure to progress is really failure to wait".* However hard the uterus is working it cannot push the baby out unless your cervix is soft and opening up, and in most long-drawn-out labours the cervix simply needs time to soften and open up.

DYSFUNCTIONAL LABOUR

One thing that may hold up labour is inco-ordinate uterine action. Unfortunately it is possible to have massive contractions and yet for the upper segment of the uterus not to be able to draw up and pull open the lower section. It is as if one part of the uterus is working against another part. The result is dysfunctional labour and failure to progress. With this kind of labour, floating or crouching in a birth pool or in a deep bath, with lights dimmed, might help. If there is still no progress, an epidural and augmentation of labour with an oxytocin intravenous drip set up may be the answer. The obstetrician usually decides on augmentation because an epidural itself has the effect of prolonging labour. If you choose an epidural, you will have time for a rest and then, if you wish, the anaesthetic can be allowed to wear off a little so that you can push the baby out yourself.

Giving support in labour

It is now accepted that there is a place for fathers in the birth room and that couples often want to be together. There is still some way to go before many hospitals are as welcoming to several companions, or to a woman partner, as they are to the baby's father. They may allow only one person with the woman. Any woman should be able to choose exactly whom she wants with her for this important experience in her life. If the baby's father cannot be with his partner, or if she feels he is not the right person to help her, she may want another person, such as a doula – a woman who is experienced in giving one-to-one support in childbirth – or a woman friend or relation, instead of, or along with, the father. In many cultures it is not acceptable for the husband to be present. In others, women appreciate having their partners there simply to know that they can rely on them and that they are loved, and gain strength from this. In the past, women in childbirth have always been supported by other women. A woman should not be deprived of companionship because her male partner cannot offer the support she needs, or she does not want him with her, or because religious or cultural tradition prohibits it. Although this section is addressed mainly to fathers, it is also meant to give guidance to anyone helping at the birth.

Research has shown that the presence of an experienced doula or other woman reduces the need for pain-relieving drugs, shortens labour, makes the birth an easier and happier experience, and results in fewer babies needing intensive care.*

Whoever is going to support a woman in childbirth, it is important to learn in advance exactly how to help most effectively. Childbirth education classes can be useful in teaching how to give emotional and physical support, in exploring emotional aspects of birth, and in understanding the stresses felt by a birth partner. Massage, help with breathing, all the techniques learned in antenatal classes for couples, can be really useful. Or they may not. You may not want your partner to do anything but give quiet encouragement. Although you may want to be held, you may not want to be touched. Some fathers, especially anxious ones, get too busy and do not realize that a woman may need her own space. This becomes intrusive and can have a negative effect on the progress of labour.

THE FATHER AT THE BIRTH

The man who knows what he can do to help is in a much better position than the one who is merely invited into the birth room but has no idea of what is going on. He has every opportunity to be an informed and knowledgeable participant. It is not just a question of holding his partner's hand, although this can be a way of giving emotional support, but also of being able to judge where and when she needs guidance and encouragement with relaxation. He has also learned how to breathe "over" the contractions so that he can breathe with his partner at times when she needs extra support. He knows how to rub her back and do gentle, light massage over her lower abdomen when the uterus is opening up, and how to apply firm pressure to her shoulders, arms and legs.

It can, however, be one thing to learn how to give support in the friendly atmosphere of a small childbirth class, where couples are working together, with much discussion interspersed with laughter, and quite another to put that learning to use in a large, impersonal hospital. Confronted in labour with masked figures in white or green whom he has never met before, whose names he does not know, in a strange, clinical environment, the father can feel out of place, in spite of consent by the hospital to his presence at the birth.

This is why it is a good idea for him, as well as for his partner, to have toured the hospital and especially the birth room beforehand. Women sometimes say that it was when they were approached with some unfamiliar piece of equipment in birth that they began to tense up, and that if they had known what it looked like and how it worked they would have found it much easier to remain relaxed. Also, men who have been giving good support to their partners before an apparatus of this kind is used sometimes give up, since they feel that the machinery is controlling the labour.

This is understandable, because when an intravenous drip stand or monitoring equipment is brought to the bed it is difficult for the man to get close to his partner, and because a monitoring belt that fits around her abdomen may make it impossible for him to massage that area. In most hospitals, too, once the labour is monitored and speeded up, a nurse will stay with the patient all the time, so the intimacy that the couple had in earlier labour is lost. This can lead to them feeling that experts and machinery have taken over.

The kind of support you can give

The most important thing for a companion helping a woman during the long first stage of labour is to be relaxed. This is difficult in an exciting situation, but any anxiety is immediately communicated to the woman in labour. If labour is different from what you expected, that can worry you more than it does the woman, who is enveloped in the force sweeping through her and who may shut out irrelevant stimuli. You, however, may be made anxious by the doctor's tone of voice, the midwife's remark to a colleague, or by the (quite normal) appearance of blood-stained mucus during a contraction. Ask for information, because if you are in doubt about anything, it is better to find out early rather than late. Speak slowly and quietly. Move slowly and deliberately. Touch your partner without haste, resting a relaxed hand on her body and, when you lift your hand away, do so slowly. If you are massaging her, stroke very slowly.

The late first stage, *with contractions* *coming every two* *minutes, may feel like* *a whirlwind (opposite).*

DISTRACTIONS IN THE BIRTH ROOM

When helping your partner to achieve focused concentration on what is happening in her body during contractions, never break that concentration by chatting to anyone else, watching a machine or allowing yourself to be distracted by what is going on around you. As well as causing the woman in labour to become anxious and tense up, modern equipment can often be so fascinating that you may become so involved with watching a monitor, for example, that the woman takes second place and feels that emotional support has been withdrawn. You should not allow yourself to forget that, however sophisticated the machinery, it is the woman who is actually having the baby. Once labour is well under way, your attention should be focused entirely on her, and encouragement by word, touch or look should be given with every single contraction.

On the hospital's side, too, an induced or speeded-up and monitored labour becomes an interesting clinical exercise. Midwives, doctors and students may come in to watch. Teaching may go on at the bedside. Discussions about the equipment sometimes take place while the woman is busy with a contraction and would appreciate silence so that she can concentrate better. Although you cannot insist that everyone be quiet during contractions, you can indicate politely by your own silence and attention to her that you are not available for conversation, and encourage her to enter a "circle of solitude" with you and the baby coming to birth.

Occasionally machines break down and engineers arrive. This can be very distracting for the woman in labour. Fortunately she is not dependent on the monitor or other pieces of equipment to have her baby. Give her your full and undivided attention during the labour. Be on the same level, not towering over her. Use eye contact to give her emotional support. If she is coping well, she may like to close her eyes and handle contractions without looking at anybody, but if the going gets hard, suggest that she open her eyes and that you go through it together. This is likely to be of special help at the end of the first stage of labour, after her cervix is 6 cm dilated.

POSITIVE SUPPORT DURING CONTRACTIONS

Everything you say should be positive. Avoid saying "You're not relaxed here" or "Your shoulders are tightening". Say "Your feet are beautifully relaxed. Do the same with your hands" or give her positive suggestions such as "Pull your shoulders down and now let them go". When she is doing well, tell her so. This helps most as contractions reach their peak. It can be useful to hold her shoulder firmly during big contractions and if she has practised relaxation techniques that help her flow out towards your touch (see pages 186–194), these will keep her shoulders loose and so prevent her from hyperventilating. Between contractions talk to her about where she likes to be held. She may find it helps her to work with her contraction if you describe to her what is happening as the uterus goes into action: "You are opening up wider and wider. Your cervix is being pulled up and open, and the baby's head is pressing right down". Ruth Wilf, an experienced American midwife, suggests that if the woman seems out of touch with her body the support person should quietly discuss with her, between contractions, any negative thoughts she may be having. This gives you something to work on during the next contraction. Create an image for the next one – the baby pressing down, the cervix opening up – and use your hands to suggest gradual opening. After the next contraction ask, "How was that compared to the last one?" The woman may be able to suggest other things you can do to help her focus her concentration.

UNDERSTANDING LABOUR'S PROGRESS
The woman also needs information on what is about to be done by her birth attendants. Being in labour can be disorienting. Fear of the unknown is the main reason why women panic, and a request for pain-relieving drugs is usually one for reassurance. A woman may be distressed because she does not realize the progress she is making. She loses all sense of time and each contraction is so enveloping that she cannot see the pattern of her labour. So be clear about the progress of labour and prepare her for what is about to happen. For instance, if the waters have not broken by the time contractions are coming every two minutes, you can be fairly sure that they will break

"I couldn't have done without my partner. I really needed his strength, especially as it took me a long time to push the baby out."

soon. If she does not want to have an amniotomy (see page 317), make this clear to the doctor. If she has one, prepare her for the renewed strength of contractions after it and discuss with her how she might change her breathing to cope with them. In the second stage remind her that the hot, throbbing, tingling feeling is a sign that the baby is about to be born and will soon be in her arms.

Know when to be quiet. This depends very much on the empathy between you. Talk when it helps, but keep quiet when you can give other forms of emotional and physical support. Facial expression, gesture, touch and massage are all very important. One of the best ways of helping is to rest a hand on her shoulder with the other hand at her wrist as she goes through the contraction. If she has backache, she will welcome firm pressure or massage over the sacrum, or slightly to one side of it (see page 192).

HOW TO HELP WITH BREATHING
Breathe with your partner through difficult contractions. Do not wait until she is tense to start the breathing. Begin with a relaxed breath out together. Keep closely in rhythm with her own breathing at the beginning of the contraction so that there is a partnership. Do not impose a radically different level or rate of breathing on her, or it will become a fight between her breathing and yours. If she starts to drag through the contraction with heavy, gasping breaths, this is

the time to try to differentiate your breathing from hers. When you think that it is appropriate, try moving your hand in a light, butterfly-wing movement in order to stress the lightness of breathing that is necessary when the uterus is at its tightest.

Help her enjoy complete relaxation between contractions. This is especially important in stressful labours, as otherwise the woman carries her tension from one contraction to the next and the effect is cumulative. When she is relaxed, you can talk together about how to meet the next contraction. Avoid complicated anatomical and physiological terms. When you speak about the uterus or cervix, remember it is "your" uterus and "your" cervix, just as it is also "your" or "our" baby. Any words used during contractions should be simple, rhythmic and repetitive.

COPING WITH PAIN

Labour companions are often unsure whether or not they should mention the word "pain". For some it is taboo. It is imperative to acknowledge pain when it exists and not to pretend that it is not there. To do so is to deny a woman the validity of her own experience and to say in effect: "You aren't feeling what you think you are feeling, and if you are, there must be something wrong with you or with your labour". If she tells you it hurts, agree and say, "I understand" or "Yes, I realize that". It might be the moment to add, "Your uterus is working very hard" or "The baby is pressing right down" and also to help her see the pattern of her labour. If she is more than 6 or 7 cm dilated she is now at the most difficult part of labour. Show her with your hand how far she is dilated. Help her to change position, freshen her up with a face wash, brush her hair and use massage to help her. Give her your total, undivided attention. Emotional support of this kind can often take the place of drugs for pain relief.

"We didn't plan on my husband being there for the birth. But the doctor took it for granted he would come into the room. He was pleased as Punch and afterwards couldn't stop talking about it!"

The most undermining thing that you can possibly do to a woman in labour is to encourage her to start feeling sorry for herself. The woman who is told by her helper, "I can't bear to see you in such pain", or words to that effect, is actually being deprived of emotional support. Even the expression on a helper's face can give that message, sometimes even more clearly than words could do. We would not think much of someone who leaned over the side of an ocean liner and called to the person in the water, "It looks terrible down there. The waves are so huge and, poor thing, you look as if you are drowning. Do you want an injection?" Yet this is the equivalent of the sympathy and the offer of "something to take away the pain" that some attendants offer to a woman in labour. The woman who has prepared herself for labour often wants help to enable her to cope with the mountainous waves rather than the offer of a drunken stupor or sensation-free childbirth. If she wants drugs for pain relief, this should always be entirely her own decision. If she does ask for narcotics or an epidural, she should do so freely, certainly not because she has been persuaded or coerced.

STAYING TOGETHER

If you feel queasy or that you must have a break, tell your partner you will be back in a moment and stroll out. Women especially need support when they are being examined, when drugs for pain relief are offered or when there is any intervention, and for you to go out then is the worst time. This is one point in labour when the woman can herself speak up and state her preferences. She could say, "I'd very much like my husband to stay, please. Don't send him away. I really need him" or "I don't think I'll be relaxed if he goes out". She could add, "He's learned about what happens and understands it pretty well. He's being a wonderful support!"

START – STOP LABOUR

Some labours seem to come to a full stop for a time and a woman may be stuck at 4 cm dilatation or more for several hours. This is a sign for a change of activity and a change of scene. Lying flat on one's back is not a good position for labour, from either the woman's or the baby's point of view. Make sure that she does not slip down in the bed. When she is lying on her left side or is upright the blood flows freely to the placenta, allowing more oxygen and nutrients to get through to the baby than when she is lying flat on her back, and it is also easier to cope with backache.

It is not a good idea to lie still for long periods, so suggest that she may like to roll over on to the other side occasionally or to sit well up. If she is sitting, supported by four or five pillows, there is not the same problem of decreased blood flow to the placenta. It is also fine if she wants to squat, kneel, stand or adopt any of the many positions which women spontaneously choose in labour (see pages 210–215). But the variety of possible positions is very much limited if intravenous drips and machinery are in use.

If labour comes to a stop, encourage her to get up and move around. If she is already walking around, suggest a bath or a shower, perhaps a back massage, and then rest in bed with hot-water bottles placed around the areas where she aches. Jamaican folk midwives give the woman a sponge-down and then wrap her in hot towels and offer a drink of hot thyme or mixed-spice tea when labour fails to progress. Perhaps we could learn something from this.

A full bladder can cause unnecessary pain. It used to be thought that it could also hold up labour, but there is no evidence to support this. For her own comfort, remind the woman to empty her bladder every hour and a half, or more frequently if she feels she needs to do so. If progress is slow, help her to feel that her natural pace is the right pace. Each labour is different and having a baby is not a competition to see who can do it fastest or conform to a norm. Especially when

A water birth

Jane's third baby was born under water. She decided to give birth at home with a midwife who was experienced with water birth, and to rent a birth pool. When she sank into the water she experienced instant pain relief.

The birth went smoothly and she breathed the baby's head out by herself while the midwife watched and waited. The cord was loosely around the baby's neck, and her midwife unwound it under water and lifted the baby to the surface. They waited for the cord to stop pulsating and then Stewart cut it.

She squatted and pushed out the placenta while still in the pool. Her midwife said, "It was such magic, being there!"

285

When a woman labours in a birth pool in a calm and peaceful atmosphere, other family members are quite naturally included. Children can do things to help: pressing a damp facecloth against the woman's brow, stroking her shoulders – or just giving her a cuddle.

For everyone the presence of children contributes to the normality of the birth experience. Children who share in the experience of birth in a loving environment where there is no fear learn that birth is an important transition in the life of the family, witness the power of a woman's body in the act of creation, and celebrate the birth of a new brother or sister.

*It is easy to move in water and
a woman often switches between
forward leaning and other
upright positions without even
thinking about it, because it
feels right at the time. This
movement helps the rotation
and descent of the baby's head.*

*One position a woman may
like to adopt as she pushes the
baby down is a supported squat,
her upper back against the side
of the pool and her partner's
arms under her shoulders. It is
important that he does not press
on nerves under her arms and
that he holds her securely without
gripping her. Her knees are
spread wide so that her pelvis is
open. She feels her pelvic floor
muscles and the tissues of her
perineum fanning out as the
baby presses through, until at
last the top of the head can be
seen glistening in her vagina.*

*Then she has another
passionate urge to push and the
head begins to slide forwards.
The midwife watches, leaving
the baby to uncurl naturally, her
hands poised to support the body
as it emerges. Gently, carefully,
intermittently pushing and
breathing, the mother eases the
head out. Only one more push,
the shoulders are free, and the
whole body slides out.*

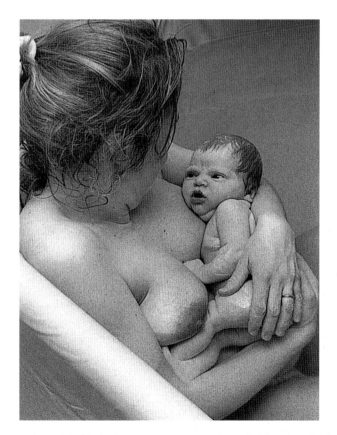

The baby is lifted gently from the water immediately into the mother's arms, either by the midwife or by the mother herself. The cord is not clamped and cut until it has ceased to pulsate, thus enabling the baby to receive the blood that rightfully belongs to her.

With eyes wide open, in the quiet, alert state that often follows birth, this baby gazes at her two brothers who welcome her with delight. As her mother cradles her in her arms they start the first of many "conversations" together and join in the dance of interaction which is the basis of all later socialization.

labour is long, affirm your confidence in her own body rhythms. Between 8 and 10 cm dilatation the woman may feel lost and tossed in the sweep and turmoil of contractions following on from each other almost without a break. Keep eye contact and breathe with her through each contraction. Letting her know that you trust her own natural rhythms is nowhere more important than at this point, when many women are made to feel that it is a race to the finishing line. Your partner's legs may feel very cold and begin to shake, and you can help her by firmly massaging the inside of her thighs.

THE LULL

There is often an apparent pause in labour for 20 minutes or more when the woman's cervix is just about fully dilated. She may have no urge to push, and may feel no contractions, yet her attendants are alert for the start of the second stage. They expect action but nothing seems to be happening. They may worry that the uterus is not going to do its job of pushing the baby out, and some try to get the woman to push even though she does not feel like it, so that she gets exhausted. They may also call for oxytocin to stimulate contractions.

If the woman feels rushed and that there are anxious eyes upon her, she becomes tense and anxious herself. Reassure her that there is all the time in the world. This is a normal part of the unfolding birth process – the "rest and be thankful" phase when the baby's head is still not deep in the pelvis. The head usually drops lower naturally if the woman is able to rest and refresh herself.

So help her stand up, and perhaps take a shower, offer her a sponge bath, and put some music on the tape recorder. She may want to walk around, gently rocking and circling her pelvis, perhaps enjoying slow belly dancing movements. You can stand cradling her body against yours as she does so, holding her shoulders, elbows or wrists, and move with her. After half an hour or so – occasionally an hour or more – contractions pick up, and with renewed energy and excitement she enters the expulsive stage. She has had a refreshing interval before the drama of the second stage.

"It is not a question of just being there for her sake, but for your own. You don't know what you're missing if you are not at the birth."

SUPPORT IN THE SECOND STAGE

When the woman begins to push the baby out, she can be in any position that feels comfortable to her: held firmly in your arms or cradled by your body, or with something solid to grasp or over which she can lean. She needs to be free to round her back, roll her shoulders forwards and rest her chin on her chest during contractions. You can help by providing physical support if she wants it and, perhaps, by reminding her to keep her head forwards at the height of each pushing urge (without making any attempt to force it forwards). From time to time give her a sip of water or juice through a bendy straw, or ice cubes to suck.

Do not say "push". Say "open up" instead. Straining wastes valuable energy and results in unco-ordinated expulsive efforts. If you suggest she does not push at all unless she feels she has to, she will push in the right way at the right time.

Avoid clock-watching. It can be as disastrous to have one eye on the clock as it would be if you were watching the clock while trying to make love. A birthing woman needs to feel secure in a world without time or standards of performance, simply able to be herself and experience the intensity of what her body is telling her to do. If the pushing urge is strong and difficult to control, and it looks as if everything is happening too fast, help her to lie on her side or get down on all fours, as this may reduce the impulse. Encourage her to put her hands down and feel even before any part of the baby's head is oozing through the vagina, then use a mirror for her to see the top of the head as it crowns. If you see that the crown is moving forwards, but she is still holding her breath, say quietly, "Breathe". She should breathe out and go on breathing in and out with a dropped jaw.

SHARING IN THE BIRTH

Many women are anxious that they might be too small. Reassure your partner that there is room, and her feelings of openness and flexibility will help to make room. The power of suggestion is so great that each word and phrase used can affect her ability to work with her body.

When you are with a woman in childbirth, you share with her a journey into the unknown. The helper is like the lookout on a yacht sailing at night, watching for the coastline and helping to steer her through. She needs your constant presence – to be left alone is the most frightening thing of all. Giving support in labour needs vigilance, skill, patience, an understanding of a woman's rhythms, her responses to stress, an awareness of what she is thinking and how she is feeling at each moment and your complete commitment to this task. Sometimes it demands endurance and courage. It can be hard, exhausting work. But yours, too, is the excitement, the deep satisfaction and the joy when a child is born.

Surprise delivery

If you are alone with a woman who is giving birth the most important thing is to stay calm yourself and give her quiet and confident support. Drop your shoulders and relax! Tell her she is doing well. Hold her in your arms and help her to feel secure.

MAKING THE WOMAN COMFORTABLE

If the room is cold, heat it. The baby will need a warm environment after birth. If you can, place a pile of newspapers or a plastic sheet or tablecloth under the mother. She may like to sit or kneel on a firm cushion or bean bag. Cover whatever she is on with a sheet if there is one available. Find some big towels, a blanket or something else warm to wrap the baby in. Offer the woman sips of water if her mouth is dry. Put pillows or some firm support behind her back, shoulders and head to allow her to sit up, kneel or squat comfortably or for her to lean over unless she prefers some other position. Her own feelings about this are likely to be right. If traces of faeces appear at her anus, wipe with cotton or toilet paper down and away from the vagina. Wash your hands and scrub your nails thoroughly.

If she is pushing, gently remind her to "open up" and not to hold her breath or push unless she feels she needs to. Just before the head crowns, suggest that she pant, so that from then on she *breathes* the baby out instead of pushing it out. She can then push gently *between* the contractions if the birth is slow.

If a loop of cord is around the baby's neck as its head slides out, hook a finger around it and lift it carefully over the head. Take care not to pull the baby or the cord, since this may detach the placenta from the wall of the uterus. If a membrane is over the baby's face, lift it off. Either you or she can then catch the baby. Lift the baby up on to the mother's upper thigh or tummy, with the head slightly down so that any mucus can drain away safely.

AFTER THE BIRTH

Cover the mother and baby with a coat or blanket, or better still a duvet, which is both light and warm. Then put a bowl between the mother's legs to receive the placenta as soon as she feels more contractions. There is no need to cut the cord. Enjoy the peace as you admire the baby together and wait for the placenta. Make the woman comfortable. She may be shivery and appreciate a hot-water bottle and a cup of tea. When the baby is ready to suck, lift it to the breast so that the nipple is well back in the mouth.

If you are in a car, away from any help or home comforts, there is no need to do anything about the placenta or cord. However, if you have a plastic bag or some newspaper, you can wrap the placenta in it and keep it at the same level as the baby.

If you are at home, boil shoelaces or soft string for tying the cord, and scissors for cutting it. If the placenta does not come after about 20 minutes, ask the mother to kneel and give long, slow blows out. It may slip out then. Never pull on the cord. Put a bowl under her buttocks and pour warm water between her legs. She can keep her uterus contracting and reduce bleeding from the placental site by massaging it firmly and putting the baby to the breast.

Tie the cord about 10 cm (4 in) and again about 15 cm (6 in) from the baby, and cut with a pair of sterilized scissors or a new razor blade between the ties. Check that there is no bleeding from the cord stump. If there is, make another tie nearer the baby.

The greatest heat loss from a newborn baby is from its head, so cover the head. Keep mother and baby cuddled together and cover both of them. When birth comes by surprise it is unlikely that anything will go wrong. This is nature at its most efficient.

Dealing with pain

"I've got a very low pain threshold. I can't stand going to the dentist, so I can't think what labour is going to be like!"

"The idea of the pain really worries me. I've never really experienced severe pain, and I can't imagine what it's like to be in pain for hours and hours and hours."

"What is labour pain like? I mean, is it like breaking your arm or a bad headache or period pains or indigestion – or what? If I knew what it was going to be like I could face it better."

These three statements express what many women who are pregnant for the first time feel, but perhaps do not acknowledge or put into words: fear that pain is going to be overpowering, a sense that they have never experienced pain that tested their inner resources, and ignorance of the kind of pain that is likely to be felt.

PUTTING PAIN IN ITS CONTEXT

People often think that pain is just a matter of a "high" or "low" pain threshold. There are very few women who think that they have a high threshold and can bear pain as well as other women. In fact, the idea of a pain threshold being like a wall, with some of us possessing high walls and others low ones, is a myth.

It is now known that the pain sensation threshold is exactly the same in all human beings.* In one study in the United States, members of Italian, Jewish, Irish and other ethnic groups were all given electric shocks ranging from mild to fairly strong, and every single person said pain occurred at exactly the same point. Yet obviously people do not *react* to pain in the same way and there are times when a pain, which you once bore easily, becomes too much to take and you cannot stand it any more. Toothache that you can cope with without difficulty when you are busy and preoccupied can be absolutely shattering when you go to bed, lie down and try to go to sleep. So you cannot judge the degree of pain by seeing how an individual reacts in a laboratory situation.

People may see a pain-producing stimulus as a test of their power to *endure* pain, and may not always be ready to admit to being hurt. In the Sudan, for instance, a young man who cannot bear pain loses social esteem and is unlikely to find a girl to marry him. As in many cultures, the ability to bear pain stoically is part of a code of values.

In every society there are cultural stress points, situations that are seen as threatening and thus predispose people to feel pain. When we know what makes people anxious, we can begin to understand these stress points. In many societies some painful stimuli may be linked with pleasure. Take lovemaking, for example: slightly painful stimulation may be sought because it is sexually exciting. The borderline between pleasure and pain can be indistinct.

The context within which pain occurs is important. As an experiment,* electric shocks were given to test people first when they were feeling relaxed and cheerful, and then when they had been made to feel anxious. The electric shocks were felt as much less painful when the subjects were feeling cheerful. In another study,* as many as 35 per cent of a doctor's patients experienced marked pain relief when given a placebo, an inactive substance that they believed was a painkiller. It has also been found that the degree of pain tolerated bears a direct relation to the rate of increase in pain, rather than to the level of pain reached.* A person experiencing a pain stimulus that gets worse rapidly feels it more than someone experiencing just as strong a stimulus that takes longer to reach the same point. It may help to have time to *adapt* to pain.

This may have particular relevance to very rapid labour, especially an induced labour (see page 324), when the pace is more than a woman can cope with. We sometimes talk about labour as if a long labour were difficult and a short one easy. But speed alone can give no indication at all of how a woman experiences her labour.

Pain perception involves not only a recording of the stimulus by the brain, but also a judgment as to its significance, and its place in the scheme of things – the meaning of the total situation in which the stimulus occurs. The experience of pain in labour is profoundly influenced by the values of the society in which the woman grew up and everything that she learned about birth when she was a child.

So labour pain is partly a product of personal and social values about the meaning of childbirth. The way we eat, sleep, empty our bowels, make love, have babies and die makes these experiences more than simple biological acts. They all express ideas, for the most part shared, about good and evil, beauty and ugliness, the pure and the polluting, what is considered to be healthy and what diseased and what is normal and what abnormal.

SOME PHYSICAL CAUSES OF BIRTH PAIN

As the first stage of labour progresses, nerve fibres that record pain are stimulated because the muscles of the uterus are squeezed tightly. A similar thing happens if you contract a muscle in your leg or arm very tightly and hold it taut for a minute or so. When you consider that the uterus is the largest muscle in your body, it is not surprising that this squeezing hurts. Pain of this kind is a sign that a woman is having good, strong contractions.

When the uterus contracts firmly the flow of oxygenated blood into the muscle and of deoxygenated blood out of the muscle is slowed down until the contraction is over. For this reason, there is a temporary build-up of waste products, which are released again in the interval between the contractions. Relaxing and taking slow, complete breaths as soon as each contraction is over enables you to provide the necessary fresh oxygen for this hard-working muscle so that it is able to continue to function effectively.

As the cervix is stretched to make space for the baby to pass through, localized pain is felt at the place where the cervix is dilating. This pain, at the very bottom of your abdomen, is common in straightforward labours and a good sign that your cervix is opening.

When pelvic ligaments and joints are stretched as the bony pelvis spreads wide and the baby descends, nerve fibres that run through them are stimulated, resulting in pain as your body opens up. This kind of pain from stretched ligaments, although difficult to handle, is a sign that your body is working well.

A baby who is not curled up, head down, in a neat ball with its chin tucked into its chest, may take longer to pass through the cervix and down the birth canal, and the pressure produced by the back of its head sticking into the small of the mother's back, or the unflexed head pushing down through soft tissues, can cause pain. This also happens sometimes if the baby is very big.

As contractions become stronger and more frequent they usually have the effect of rolling the baby round and down into a better position. So this kind of pain may disappear entirely once the way is clear and you can push. You can help your baby to rotate into the best position by being upright or on all fours. Upright positions such as standing, kneeling or squatting enable you to use gravity to your advantage. An all-fours position lets the baby drop away from your spine so that it can turn more easily against your springy abdominal wall.

"The backache was bad, but I kept thinking of what you said, 'The baby is opening the gate', and suddenly her head turned and from then on it was easy."

PAIN RELIEF IN OTHER CULTURES

There are two myths about the ways in which women in the Third World give birth. One is that labour is always horrific and dangerous, but that women do not cry out because of strong taboos against showing that they are in pain. The other is that the women all have completely painless births, and just squat down in the fields and have their babies before getting back to work again. The truth is probably somewhere in between the two extremes. In many Third World countries healthy women have straightforward labours while other, malnourished women suffer a great deal.

Most cultures have methods of relieving pain in childbirth, so there is obvious recognition that it exists. But the ways in which pain is relieved and labour made more comfortable are radically different in the technological Western countries. We can give complete relief from pain and remove all sensation from the waist down with regional anaesthesia. This is what an epidural does (see page 309). We have other forms of pain relief that partially remove pain or that eradicate the memory of it. We rely on pharmacological substances to do this for us. Herbal medicines are used in the Third World and some of them have narcotic or mood-altering properties, just like modern drugs, although it is much more difficult to prepare the right dose when you are using plants. There are also other kinds of help that are much favoured in these countries and that used to be employed in the West but tend to be ignored in hospitals today. They include religious and magic rites, counterstimulation, massage, hot and cold compresses, changes in position and emotional support from others sharing the experience with the woman in labour. These supporters hold her, stroke her, rock her back and forth and live through the birth *with* her rather than do things *to* her as a patient.

Much of what is done by birth attendants in other cultures provides simple, practical help based on the handed-down experiences of generations of women. It is also intended to have a psychosomatic effect, helping the baby to be born by positively influencing the mind of the woman in labour. This kind of practical help in labour may be forgotten or misunderstood in our modern hospitals. Yet there are advantages in being able to cope without drugs if possible, because all powerful drugs have side effects and they all go through the mother's bloodstream to her baby.

IMAGINING YOUR LABOUR IN ADVANCE

In preparing for birth it is a good idea to work out how you might like to be helped in order to be more comfortable, and also how you can use your mind to help your body through relaxation, focused concentration and ideas and mental images that produce a harmonious pattern between what is going on inside your uterus and the way you think about it. You may find that all this is difficult to conceptualize before you have your first baby.

Trying to master your body or running away from the sensations you are experiencing can actually produce pain, because you are bound to become tense and then chemical messages are sent instantaneously into your bloodstream which affect your whole metabolism. This causes changes in skin, blood pressure and heart rate, breathing, digestion, and defecation, as well as changes in muscle tone. Psychosomatic factors can even change the action of the uterus itself in ways we do not yet fully understand. A woman who is very anxious may have a long labour because her uterus does not work efficiently or stops contracting altogether.

"My mind was full of sea images. It was as if I was an island with waves rushing and swirling and opening my body in readiness for birth."

WHAT LABOUR FEELS LIKE

In a normal labour any pain experienced is quite different from the pain of breaking a leg, for example, or being injured. The physical feelings produced by a strongly contracting uterus are powerful and challenging. They are likely to involve a combination of sensations – a very tight squeeze, a pulling open of tissues, and the firm, downwards pressure of the solid ball of the baby's head through a passage that is being slowly stretched wide. In films you sometimes see a pregnant woman suddenly double up, her hands clasped over the top of her abdomen. The director is telling viewers that labour has started. But it never happens like this in reality. Instead there is a sensation of being gripped by tightening muscles low down in your abdomen or in the small of your back. All the sensations are at hip level. Nor is the feeling a sudden one. A contraction has a wavelike shape, building up to a crest and then subsiding and disappearing until the next contraction. There is always a rest period between them, often lasting a minute or more, even in the stormy late first stage. As contractions get stronger, longer and closer together the tightening may extend right around your body, so that it feels more like a circle of thick, wide elastic across your pelvis which is being steadily drawn in, held firm and then slowly released again. Or you may be conscious of expansion during contractions and aware of the top of the uterus spreading and rising, tilting forwards in your abdomen, while the great muscle squeezes its lower part open and thereby presses the baby down.

PAIN WITH A PURPOSE

Feelings that you experience during labour may be painful, but it is pain with a purpose and thus different from the pain of injury. Contractions are not painful in themselves, and in fact the uterus contracts strongly and rhythmically at intervals in the second half of pregnancy, usually without causing any pain. It is the peak of the contraction, when the muscle is working hardest and is making most progress, that is most likely to be perceived as painful, and this may last as long as 30 seconds or as little as 15 seconds.

The idea of a pain that is *qualitatively* different from other kinds of pain is difficult to accept for anyone who has not experienced it. Yet sheer physical effort, like that involved in running a race or climbing a mountain, produces just that kind of "functional" pain, the ache of muscles that are working very hard. If the athlete thought only of pain instead of about winning the race, she would give up. If the mountaineer thought that her aching muscles were the sign of some dreadful physical injury instead of the natural result of working them so hard, she would forget all about her goal and lose the feeling of triumph when she reaches the summit.

Pain in labour is the by-product of the body's creative activity. Contractions are *not* pains. They are tightenings that may be painful, especially when they are being most effective. There is an art in approaching each new contraction, in thinking "Splendid! Here's another one!" and later, as you approach the end of the first stage, when they are at their strongest, "Oh, this is a really good one!"

When you are in the thick of labour, your whole self is involved. It is almost impossible to think about other things or to hold a part of yourself back in any way. The intensity of labour can be frightening, especially for the unprepared woman who does not know what to expect, or for one who wants to keep it all at the level of a learned skill, doing her exercises in much the same way as she might carry out a three-point turn in a driving test. This is why preparation merely for handling contractions is never enough. You also need to prepare yourself mentally and emotionally for the overwhelming nature of the sensations and feelings of labour.

HYPNOSIS

Some women find that hypnosis is an effective method of relieving pain in labour, and it has the great advantage over chemical anaesthetics of not reducing the baby's oxygen intake. In fact, about a quarter of women who have had hypnosis in childbirth say that they experienced no pain, but results do vary and most women who have hypnosis need chemical pain relief as well.

The common belief that hypnosis involves some kind of magic trickery and that you can be made to do anything the hypnotist wishes is actually very wide of the mark. Hypnosis is a state of increased suggestibility that is induced by deep relaxation and concentration, and you can prepare yourself with a good practitioner so that you can, if you wish, use *auto*-hypnosis.

With hypnosis, some women become immune to pain and may have a forceps delivery or be stitched up after an episiotomy without a local anaesthetic. It has been calculated that two out of every hundred women can be so deeply hypnotized that they could even have a Caesarean section without feeling any pain.*

If you agree to have hypnosis in childbirth you are usually trained in progressive relaxation to remove anxiety and taught to think positively about childbirth. If you want to try auto-hypnosis, the hypnotist will suggest that you put yourself to sleep and wake up when you wish. After the birth the doctor may suggest that in the future you only be hypnotized by someone for a therapeutic purpose, so that you need not be afraid of being put into a trance by anyone using hypnosis for their own purposes or for fun.

It could be claimed that all good childbirth classes teach an element of auto-hypnosis. Childbirth educators do not usually like to admit this. Yet in many ways thinking ahead to labour constructively when one is deeply relaxed is equivalent to using the power of suggestion. Whether or not you decide to try hypnosis, you can use auto-suggestion and positive fantasies about labour and your beautiful baby in a creative way to prepare yourself for childbirth, in the knowledge that this is completely safe.

ACUPUNCTURE

Another way of reducing pain in childbirth is by acupuncture. It derives from a completely different system of beliefs about the human body from that of Western medicine. Hair-fine needles are used to stimulate 12 lines of energy called "channels" flowing beneath the skin. This energy keeps the blood circulating, warms the body and combats illness. Acupuncture is used antenatally, for example, to relieve nausea and vomiting, cure constipation, encourage a breech baby to turn, and start off labour. Acupuncturists also sometimes use moxibustion, the burning of a small pellet of mugwort at certain parts of the body, to turn the baby. In labour, electroacupuncture may be used at points in the ear for analgesia, and with this technique the woman herself can control the degree of stimulation.*

In Beijing nowadays acupuncture is performed in preference to epidural anaesthesia for 98 per cent of Caesarean sections.* It is also sometimes combined with small quantities of drugs.

The advantages of acupuncture are that it is non-invasive, easily administered by someone trained in the method and instantly reversible, and babies are in better condition at birth than after pethidine has been given. Some studies show that acupuncture shortens the first stage of labour for women having their first baby. Women say that they feel more in control of labour and delivery than when they have taken drugs for pain relief.*

TRANSCUTANEOUS ELECTRONIC NERVE STIMULATION
With TENS, a pulsed wave of variable intensity is passed through electrodes attached to the skin surface. This seems to stimulate the production of natural pain-relieving substances in the body (endorphins and enkephalins). The electrodes are attached in the first stage and the woman operates a switch like a push-top pen or two dials as she feels a contraction build up. She feels a tingling sensation when it is switched on. The electrode pads are

"One advantage of the TENS machine was that it gave me something active to do, and that helped me get through a long, tiring, first stage."

usually stuck on her back, but can also be used on the abdomen or in the groin. The disadvantage of TENS is that it cannot be used in water. It is being offered in increasing numbers of hospitals.

REFLEXOLOGY
Similar to shiatsu, reflexology is a form of acupressure. It consists of manual pressure on reflex points in the feet, hands and face to stimulate subcutaneous nerve endings. The idea behind it is that it causes the brain to release natural endorphins and other chemicals that help to reduce pain. In childbirth, reflexology involves massage and gentle pressure on the feet.

AROMATHERAPY
At its simplest level aromatherapy is a matter of breathing in pleasant smells that help you feel good about yourself. It can provide you with a positive sensory environment for birth. This is useful if you are having your baby in hospital, where it can erase any off-putting hospital smells and where doctors and midwives can relax and enjoy it, too. There has not been much research into the benefits and risks of aromatherapy in pregnancy and birth. The essences used are highly concentrated and molecules that can cross into the bloodstream may reach the baby. If we demand rigorous trials of drugs, most of which are derived from plants anyway, we

should also be insisting on research into the effects of aromatherapy. Plant essences stimulate sensory cells in the nose, which send chemical messages to the limbic area of the brain, which cause neurochemicals to be released into the bloodstream. These essences are energizing – imagine smelling an orange, a lemon, eucalyptus or a sprig of rosemary – or relaxing – imagine breathing in lavender, sweet geranium or the scent of an old-fashioned rose. Essential oils also stimulate the production of endorphins, the body's natural analgesics, which are similar to morphine, so that you are less likely to need medication for pain relief.

Essential oils can be used in different ways. You can put a few drops on a pillow, handkerchief or hot, damp flannel. They can be mixed with a vegetable or nut oil (soya, jojoba, apricot kernel, wheat germ, sunflower, almond, and avocado are all good) and massaged into the skin. They can be added in concentrated form, or mixed with a dispersal oil, to the water of a bath or birth pool. You can use them in a warm foot bath. Or they can be burned in a porcelain vaporizer over a candle or in an electric vaporizer.

As you inhale essential oils notice how your face becomes softer and your breathing slower and fuller. The breathing of fear, anxiety or panic is rapid and jerky. When you are relaxed and confident, breathing is rhythmic, and each breath is complete, with a slight pause between the breath in and the breath out, and another between the breath out and the breath in. During pregnancy you can experiment with different essential oils to discover which ones work best for you and enable you to breathe easily, and which refresh and reinvigorate you and help any tensions flow out of your body.

Lavender can be put directly on the skin. It can be mixed with one or two other essences, such as chamomile, sweet geranium, cedarwood, frankincense, myrrh, jasmine, neroli, rosewood, rosemary, peppermint (but do not use peppermint if you are also taking homoeopathic medication), melissa or mandarin. Some of the essential oils are overpowering if you use more than one or two drops, so sniff the bottles first before you concoct your recipe to make sure that it is well balanced. Some good combinations – all relaxing – are lavender and orange, lemon grass and orange, geranium and orange, ylang ylang, sandalwood and jasmine. Rose, neroli (very expensive) and sandalwood in jojoba oil can be massaged into your forehead, face and neck.

"The obstetrician came into the room and asked, 'What's the wonderful smell? Oh, I like that!' The aromatherapy made a relaxing atmosphere that we all enjoyed."

Clary sage should not be used in pregnancy, since it can stimulate uterine contractions. This is why it may be helpful if the cervix is dilating very slowly in labour, if the introductory phases of labour are lasting a long time, or if you are two weeks or more past your due date and want to give some gentle encouragement to your uterus to start contracting. Some books about aromatherapy and reliable sources of oils and advice are listed at the end of this book (see pages 412–414).

HOMOEOPATHY

Unlike conventional medical treatments, homoeopathy aims to treat the whole person, including the mental and emotional states that have an adverse effect on physical wellbeing. There are 2,500 homoeopathic remedies, many of them derived from plants, but others from metal (gold, silver), animal products (cow's milk, snake venom), allergens (pollen, house dust) and drug extracts (aspirin). The principle behind the remedies is that like is treated with like, but in minute quantities. The more diluted a remedy, the more effective it is.

A homoeopathic labour pack might consist of 7-gram (¼ oz) bottles of the following remedies:
• Arnica leopard's bane at 30c. It helps reduce bleeding and bruising.
• Hypericum St John's wort. This promotes healing of skin.

These two can be taken together, starting when labour begins and continuing for at least five days.
• Staphisagria stavesacre at 10 ml (2 tsp). This is said to be a remedy for trauma to the urethra, and also a treatment for postnatal "blues."
• Hypericum and calendula pot marigold can be combined in a 10-ml (2-tsp) tincture, which helps to soothe and heal skin that has been bruised or grazed. Mix ten drops with 20 ml (1½ tbsp) of sterile, cooled water and just stroke it in wherever you feel sore.*

When you go to a homoeopathic practitioner, the case history will take about an hour, and this readiness to listen may be one element in the success of homoeopathy. On the other hand, there are homoeopathic veterinarians, so results cannot all be chalked up to the placebo effect. Some homoeopaths are medically qualified. Others work closely with GPs, and all will refer to them when necessary. Homoeopathy is available on the NHS and you can ask to be referred to a homoeopath through your GP.

BACH FLOWER REMEDIES

These remedies, which are another form of homoeopathy, are designed to treat emotional states, not physical conditions. They can be used in pregnancy and during labour as antidotes to stress, fear and lack of confidence. Tinctures are available in homoeopathic dilutions and the plant essences are preserved in brandy. There are 38 remedies for different emotional states, such as depression, shock, apprehension and irritability, and because our emotions are often complicated they are often used in combination. The general "rescue remedy" is recommended for those "distressed by startling experiences". You can get further information from the address on page 413.

USING WATER

You probably already know how soaking in a warm bath can relieve pain, whether you have experienced backache, aching muscles from strenuous exercise or a state of physical tension, or menstrual pain. Many women have discovered that being immersed in water can be comforting in labour. Lying in warm water increases venous pressure so that veins can return blood to the heart more efficiently. It also enhances cardiac action and slows the pulse rate. Total relaxation in the warmth and comfort of a bath may help the uterus to contract more effectively. But it does more than this. Water both counteracts the force of gravity and any pressure a woman may feel against her back and buttocks, and also reduces pressure felt from inside the body, so there is a further pain-relieving effect.*

Sometimes pain is so much reduced and dilatation proceeds so fast as a woman surrenders herself to the water that the baby slips out while she is still enjoying the bath. This is quite safe, since the baby only takes a breath when lifted clear of the water, and for a few minutes after delivery blood is still pulsating through the cord, thus providing the baby with oxygen. After the baby has left your body, the midwife will rest a finger on the cord so that she can feel the blood pulsating through it. You may like to do this too.

WATER BIRTH

The waves of huge contractions are easier to ride if you are immersed in water.

If you would like to use water in labour and birth discuss it with your midwife or doctor. Some hospitals are not happy about births taking place under water, but encourage it for labour. Some obstetricians have expressed concern about cross-infection, particularly with HIV, from using birth pools. There is no reason

Paracervical block is a series of injections of local anaesthetic around the cervix. It affects the baby immediately, and in three out of ten babies the heartbeat becomes slower (a condition known as bradycardia).* Some babies have died as a result. Paracervical block is rarely used in Britain for this reason.

Spinal anaesthesia is given by injection into the cerebrospinal fluid in the lower spine. The effect is to numb the woman from waist to knees. It takes about five minutes to work. If you have a spinal you may have to lie flat for around eight hours after delivery to avoid a post-spinal headache and should be careful not to lift your head quickly. Spinals are considered potentially dangerous because blood pressure drops so that the oxygen supply to the baby is reduced. Labour may slow down, and a forceps delivery is usually necessary. However, they give effective pain relief.

Pudendal block is an injection numbing the nerves in the perineum given at any time after full dilatation, and is often used before an episiotomy or a forceps or vacuum extraction.

Epidural anaesthesia is injected into the space just outside the dura, the outer membrane around the spinal cord. Top-up injections or a continuous drip of anaesthetic are given through a fine, plastic tube, which is left in place. The continuous drip allows the anaesthetist to use a lower concentration of the drug, which reduces undesirable side effects. An epidural may be given with you sitting up and curled forwards or lying on your left side curled up into a ball – a difficult position when you are in strong labour. An epidural takes about half an hour to set up.

"I had to look at the machine to see when I was having a contraction . . . I did want to feel him slide out, and not feeling that was terribly disappointing."

An epidural can provide complete pain relief and can even be used as an anaesthetic for Caesarean section. It removes sensation from the waist or sometimes from your navel down, either completely or partially, while allowing you to stay conscious. For a painful, prolonged labour it seems the perfect answer. Many women say how marvellous the epidural was, but it should be your own choice – no one should be put under pressure to have one. Some hospitals give epidurals to all first-time mothers, unless there is no time for it.

An epidural should not be given if there has been bleeding from the placenta, if you have low blood pressure, if you are taking anticoagulants such as Warfarin to avoid blood clots or if you have a skin infection where the needle is to be introduced. An epidural tends to prolong labour, so stimulation of the uterus with an oxytocin intravenous drip is often necessary. It is also important to remember that epidurals do not always work. It may be difficult to inject into the right place, or the anaesthetic may take on one side only, so that you get the odd feeling of contractions occurring in only half your body, which can be disconcerting. The usual practice is for the anaesthetist to try to adjust the placement of the epidural so that finally you can get good pain relief.

The anaesthetic is similar to that used by dentists, and you feel it like liquid ice numbing your tummy, bottom and legs. Even though it anaesthetizes only part of you, it must be given by a skilled anaesthetist and under sterile conditions. If by mistake the needle punctures the dura, you end up getting a complete spinal: you are more heavily anaesthetized and may have a bad headache that can last a week or more after the birth.

An epidural lowers blood pressure, sometimes drastically, so that other drugs may have to be given to raise your blood pressure again. Because of this, an epidural is sometimes offered to a woman whose blood pressure is already high, even though she may not be having a painful labour. In one study 39 per cent of women having epidurals experienced low blood pressure (hypotension), although it did not last longer than one hour. The proportion went up to 47 per cent when women were also receiving an oxytocin intravenous drip (see page 325).* When your blood pressure suddenly drops, you feel sick and faint and may vomit. This sudden lowering of blood pressure affects the baby too, since the oxygen-bearing blood supply is pumping more weakly and slowly through the placenta. If your blood pressure drops and causes fetal distress, you will wear an oxygen mask to get more oxygen to the baby. Epidural techniques and drug dosages vary in different countries. In the United States, a continuous infusion pump is almost always used and bupivacaine is usually kept low with the aim of reducing side effects. But because drug cocktails are often given, there are new side effects from these other drugs. To reduce the risk of a sudden drop in blood pressure, intravenous fluids are given very fast before the epidural. This increases the woman's blood volume. In Great Britain if blood pressure drops significantly another drug is given to raise the blood pressure. Excessive intravenous fluids cause water intoxication. This means that the body becomes overloaded with fluids. One result is that women often have swollen legs and feet for some days after an epidural.

Having an epidural may start a whole train of other procedures which you did not bargain for. You may receive oxytocin to augment labour and have continuous fetal monitoring. There is also an increased risk of finishing up with a Caesarean section.* This appears to be greatest if a woman is given the epidural before she has reached 5 cm dilatation. Because you have no feeling in your

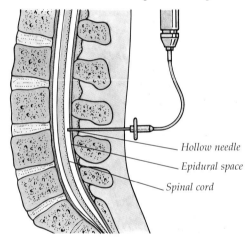

Hollow needle

Epidural space

Spinal cord

Epidural
An epidural is the most effective pharmacological pain relief. The needle does not enter the spinal cord. It stays short of it in the epidural space.

bladder, it will need to be emptied by catheter. And because you may not feel any urge to push, the obstetrician may rotate the fetal head with forceps or manually.*

Since there is an increased chance of a forceps delivery once an epidural has been given, you may want to refuse a top-up and let the anaesthetic wear off as you reach the very end of the first stage of labour . If you have not felt the first-stage contractions at all and then suddenly have to cope with the long, hefty ones as you approach full dilatation, the experience can be overpowering.

Do not push just because you are fully dilated. Always breathe your way through contractions, which you can feel as waves of pressure, until the baby's head is well down on your perineum. If you push because you think that you *ought* to be pushing, you are more likely to have deep transverse arrest of the baby's head, because with an epidural the natural tone of the pelvic floor muscles is lost, and it is these muscles that help the baby's head to rotate as it descends against them. If you have deep transverse arrest you will inevitably need a forceps or vacuum extractor delivery. An epidural multiplies the chance that your baby will get stuck in an occipito-posterior (see page 263) or transverse position.* Obstetricians often tackle this problem by setting up an oxytocin intravenous drip in order to make the uterus work harder, with a view to avoiding the need for an assisted delivery later on. You can however, do something yourself about this, and will reduce the risk of deep transverse arrest by more than half if you wait until the baby's head can be seen before starting to push. It may take two hours or longer from when you are fully dilated for this to happen.*

One side effect of having an epidural is that your temperature rises which can make you feel very uncomfortable. Being over-heated can in turn have an adverse effect on the baby during labour. Moreover, when a woman has a fever in labour, investigations are made to find out if she and the newborn baby are suffering from an infection, and the baby may be treated for infection "just in case". This may entail observation in the special care nursery, and the baby may even be given intravenous antibiotics.

Epidurals may have long-term side effects for you, too. A small proportion of women have problems with backache, migraine, neckache or numb areas of skin after an epidural.*

An epidural anaesthetic passes into the baby within ten minutes, and studies are still being carried out on the possible effects of an epidural on the newborn.* Some studies suggest that the baby becomes nervous and jittery while others show that the baby is very drowsy after delivery,* but this may vary according to what drug and dosage are used, how long the epidural is in place and the condition of the fetus before the epidural is given. If you decide to have an epidural, bear in mind that some of the difficulty you might have in coping with the baby in the week or so after the birth may be connected with the effect of the anaesthetic on the baby, and does not mean that you are an incompetent mother. You will soon be over this difficult period and the interaction between you and the baby will rapidly become much easier.

Mobile or "walking" epidurals To achieve an epidural so that the woman retains some feeling in her legs and can move a little, the drug bupivacaine is given in smaller doses than when full anaesthesia is required. There are three ways of doing this.

1. The first dose of anaesthetic – half as much as usual – is injected into the subarachnoid space where cerebrospinal fluid circulates. A very fine spinal needle is used. This reduces the risk of the mother suffering a post-dural puncture headache but the problem is that this space is more difficult to find than the epidural space, and if mistakes are made there is a risk of meningitis.

2. Opioids and local anaesthetics are injected into both the subarachnoid and epidural spaces. Again, when a drug cocktail that includes opioids is given the bupivacaine can be cut by almost half.

3. Epidural top-ups are injected when needed, or the drug is given by continuous infusion pump. Having top-ups reduces the drug dose by 35 per cent compared with an epidural infusion.

Advantages of lower drug doses are that a woman can move around in bed, and possibly walk. But spinal opiates can make her feel dizzy, her legs may feel rubbery and she is unable to walk about. She should therefore have someone with her all the time and should not leave the labour room. There is less need to catheterize her bladder, and a mobile epidural may reduce the risks of long-term backache and the need for assisted delivery.*

WHAT WOMEN THINK ABOUT EPIDURALS

My own research into epidurals reveals that women are sharply divided in their opinions about them. In my study of women's experiences many were very happy with their epidurals and said things like "It was a miracle!" and "It was pure magic". However, 18 per cent of women very much regretted having had the epidural and said, in effect, "Never again!"* *Women praise epidurals when:* it was their own decision, and theirs alone, to have one; they felt that they were among friends; the epidural provided effective pain relief; there was minimal other intervention; and the mother managed to push the baby out herself. *Women are highly critical of epidurals when:* they felt that they were not able to make a free choice about having one; they did not feel that they were in an emotionally supportive environment; the epidural was not effective; delivery was

"If I had known what I do now about epidurals I wouldn't have agreed to it, but it was presented as entirely risk-free and without side effects."

by forceps; and there were side effects – they felt sick and giddy, suffered headaches or had long-term problems, such as pain or numbness, which they attributed to the epidural.

Caudal A caudal is like an epidural, except that it is injected into the epidural space around the sacrum and blocks only that particular area, rather than the larger area blocked by an epidural. A greater dose of anaesthetic is necessary for a caudal than with an epidural, and a caudal is not of much use in the first stage of labour. It is usually given for short-term pain relief to a woman having a very difficult second stage of labour.

THE FUTURE OF DRUGS IN CHILDBIRTH

Hospitals should provide an environment and the kind of personal care in which each woman is free to accept or reject pain-relieving drugs as and when she wishes to do so. Whatever drugs are given to you in labour, their effects and possible side effects on you and the baby should certainly be fully explained and your consent should always be obtained beforehand.

Unfortunately, drugs are often used in place of loving emotional support and encouragement and one-to-one care. Fear, anxiety, loneliness and the feeling that you are part of a factory for producing babies all increase the experience of pain. Understanding what is happening inside you and what is being done to help you and your baby, being able to move freely, having non-pharmacological ways of handling pain, knowing what you can do to help yourself, feeling you are among friends and having someone you love with you all make pain much more easy to bear.

Pain-relieving drugs almost invariably have an effect on the progress of labour, and often prolong it or make an operative delivery more likely. This may be a price worth paying. It is up to you to decide. Nobody else should make the decision for you. Modern obstetric anaesthesia, used only when necessary, is fairly safe for the baby, but little is really known about the subtle effects, short- and long-term, on the child. One consultant anaesthetist warns that "numerous questions about the effects of drugs given to the mother on mother–baby interaction and future child development require an answer",* and stresses that long-term studies should be carried out to assess exactly what risks are being taken. For the present this remains a largely unexplored field of research.

Towards the medical control of birth

You have the right to decide what happens to your body before, during and after childbirth. You are not bound, either in law or out of politeness, to agree to procedures and investigations to which you object. If things are done without your consent, it is a form of assault on your body. But your consent is implied when you are forewarned about an obstetric intervention and concur by remaining silent.

You are also entitled to full information about anything that is being done to you and your baby, and can reasonably expect to be able to ask questions about it and to be given straightforward and honest answers. You may also want time to think through any of the alternatives that are available to you, and should not be rushed into agreeing to any treatment that is proposed. If you do not ask questions, then the professionals may well take it for granted that you do not want to know any more, and even that to offer further information might make you uncomfortable.

If birth is to be a fulfilling and satisfying experience the important thing is to feel in control of what happens to you and your baby before, during and after the birth. Once you are secure in that knowledge you can "let go" and allow your body to work freely. You are not fighting it or trying to rein in the power that is released from your uterus. Women are sometimes blamed for approaching birth with expectations that are "too high". But research into psychological outcomes of birth reveals that feeling cheated or let down has nothing to do with having had rosy expectations of birth that are destroyed by the grim reality of labour. In fact, women are more likely to be disappointed in their birth experiences when they did not expect much anyway. How you feel about the birth afterwards has to do with human relationships. You are much more likely to have a positive birth experience if you are able to get the information you want, discuss everything fully and share in all the decisions that are made.*

"I was made to lie flat on my back for hours. I felt like a lump of meat, being poked and prodded as if my body didn't belong to me."

YOUR RIGHT TO CHOOSE

In all medical procedures it is a question of carefully balancing the relative risks of a policy of intervention on the one hand and one of "wait and see" on the other. To be able to make an informed choice you may value the counsel of skilled professionals, but ultimately you make the decision. This applies to both *where* and *how* you have your baby. If you want natural childbirth, go all out to get it. Plan for it, prepare yourself for it and do everything you can to create the right setting for it to take place. But also be flexible, so that if something in your physical condition, or that of your baby, indicates that modern technology can be used with advantage, you will not miss out on its undoubted benefits, even if this means that the birth of your baby is less "natural".

A woman having a baby has responsibilities as well as rights. One of the most important of these is the responsibility to give the baby the best possible start in life. Some obstetricians believe that whenever a machine or a procedure is available which permits greater medical control of childbirth, it ought to be used. An equally valid view is that one should be selective in the use of technology, employing it where necessary, but bearing in mind that birth is also a psychological experience that affects the relationship between mother, father and baby – perhaps for a long time after.

THE BEST ENVIRONMENT FOR BIRTH

The highest-quality childbirth and the best welcome for the baby must include emotional as well as medical aspects of birth. If you accept medical help, it does not automatically follow that you relinquish concern about the psychological dimensions of the experience. Technology need not, and should not be permitted to, ruin a woman's personal experience of childbirth. When machines are used in place of warm and friendly human relations they seem to take over. But when they take second place to emotional support and encouragement, and you feel free to reach your own decisions about how much aid to accept, they can be a useful adjunct to good care, especially when the risk to a baby is considered to be higher than usual.

Many couples can bear witness to ways in which sophisticated modern apparatus made them feel more secure in childbirth and helped rather than hindered. But for this to happen the environment provided for birth has to be a very special one, and all those coming into contact with the expectant parents need to be able to give of themselves, not only lending their technical skills. For it is only in such a setting that there can be trust, honesty and self-confidence.

THE GROWING USE OF TECHNOLOGY

Obstetricians are discovering new ways of controlling a process that in the past was left to nature. Many now say, "Why stand by watching and intervene only when something goes wrong?" and believe that, instead, labour should be regulated from start to finish. To do this effectively they need to be able to monitor exactly what is happening in the uterus and to the fetus at every second, and to intervene at any point to ensure that cervical dilatation, the strength of contractions and the biochemical state of mother and fetus conform to a predetermined norm. This is called *active management of labour.**

Many inventions are appearing on the market that obstetricians, eager to reduce the perinatal mortality rate, want to buy for their units. Some women hate this intrusion of machinery into what they feel should be a natural process, and question its benefits for labour and for the baby. Others find security in knowing that labour is controlled by the obstetrician with all his machinery; they like knowing exactly when the birthday will be, and are relieved to know that the labour will not last longer than 12 hours at the most. In some hospitals the love affair with technology is gradually giving way to a new concern about the quality of human relations. But there is no standard recipe that will suit all women. The vital element is *personal* care.

Common procedures in labour

The usual way to assess the progress of labour is by vaginal examination. Dilatation of the cervix is estimated by inserting two gloved fingers through the vagina into the os, the mouth of the cervix. The examining fingers can also detect how soft the tissues of the cervix are, whether the baby is head down, how far the head has descended and which part of the head is presenting.

The drawbacks to vaginal examinations are that they disturb the labouring woman's concentration, may be painful, can feel threatening and also introduce the risk of infection. However, some women like to be told that the cervix is dilating well and ask for an examination. Especially when a woman is in an undrugged state, an experienced midwife who has remained with her should be able to assess the progress of labour by observing the whole woman – her facial expression, her movements, her breathing and any other sounds she is making, rather than relying on frequent vaginal examinations.*

When you arrive at the hospital, you may be given an amniotomy, linked to a fetal monitor, and hooked up to an intravenous drip. During the second stage an episiotomy may be performed to hasten delivery. Some women experience many kinds of intervention

Rupture of the membranes

When membranes are intact they act as a cushion in front of the baby's head. When these membranes have ruptured, the baby's head is pressed against the cervix.

Intact membrane

Before

Ruptured membrane

After

during the course of their labour, and unless you specifically tell the obstetrician or midwife that you do not want your labour controlled in this way, there is a chance that you will have at least one of them.

ARTIFICIAL RUPTURE OF THE MEMBRANES
Artificial rupture of the membranes (ARM for short), or amniotomy, has come to be accepted as a normal routine in most hospitals and is frequently performed as part of the "prepping" done after you are admitted. It should not be done until you are in active labour (more than 4 cm dilated). The membranes surrounding the fetus are punctured with a small tool rather like a crochet hook, which is introduced through the open cervix. Routine amniotomy is now open to question, however (see below).

When the membranes are allowed to rupture spontaneously they tend to do so towards the end of the first stage of labour.* In 12 per cent of women the membranes remain intact right through to delivery. Some membranes rupture spontaneously when the midwife or doctor touches them during a vaginal examination. Since there are no nerve endings in the membranes, their rupture is not painful. All you feel is a gush of warm liquid. Be prepared for contractions to increase in intensity after this has happened. ARM can shorten labour by 30–45 minutes if the membranes have still not ruptured spontaneously by the end of the first stage, since the baby's head is pressing harder against the cervix once the cushion of fluid is gone, and this produces a rush of oxytocin in your system, which triggers the start of strong contractions.

REASONS FOR AMNIOTOMY
Besides being a part of induction, rupturing the membranes also allows the obstetrician to assess the state of the amniotic fluid. When a fetus is in distress it passes meconium, the first contents of the bowels, into the amniotic fluid, which is easily seen when the fluid is released. Many obstetricians believe that amniotomy is important in assessing the condition of the baby. Once it has been done, it is possible to insert an electrode in the baby's scalp so that its heartbeat can be recorded throughout labour (see pages 330–333).

In some countries, obstetricians prefer to use an amnioscope in order to examine the amniotic fluid while still keeping the membrane intact. A cone-shaped instrument with a fibre-optic light positioned inside it is introduced through the vagina and cervix. Although it may be very uncomfortable, this technique is less invasive than ARM.

THE RISKS OF ROUTINE AMNIOTOMY
Pressure on the cord Intact membranes protect the baby's head. The amniotic fluid equalizes pressure on the head, and amniotomy takes away the cushion of water in which the fetus lies, thus exposing its head to the direct effect of contractions. Rupture of the membranes also gives rise to the possibility of pressure on the cord, which may

hinder the flow of blood through it. It is not rare for a baby to have the cord around its neck, and without the cushion provided by the amniotic fluid, such babies are particularly vulnerable to pressure on the cord. It has also been suggested that once the amniotic fluid is gone, the fetal surface of the placenta is compressed, which may reduce the flow of blood to and from the baby.*

Pelvic infection Amniotomy increases the possibility of pelvic infection.* Infection is more likely if labour continues for more than 24 hours after amniotomy, especially if there is no restriction on vaginal exams, and operative delivery may be necessary if the baby has not been born naturally by that time.

Sometimes when the membranes are ruptured before labour is going strong, later contractions become weak or stop altogether, and it turns out that the woman was in "false" labour. Because of the risk of ascending infection if labour takes a long time following rupture of the membranes, it is often decided to stimulate the uterus with an oxytocin intravenous drip.

Deceleration of the baby's heartbeat Some studies have shown that after amniotomy there are more early decelerations of the baby's heartbeat. These early decelerations occur at the start of a contraction and the heart is back to normal by the end of the contraction. The slowing down is slight, by less than 40 beats a minute. Many obstetricians consider this innocuous and quite normal.* Because babies who are born after amniotomy are generally in good condition, with high Apgar scores (see page 356), some doctors have concluded that the procedure does not subject the fetus to any special stress during labour.

Head moulding Some obstetricians are concerned about head moulding and disalignment of the cranial bones, which may be increased after amniotomy. There is some disagreement about this, but, in any case, the moulding of the baby's head gradually disappears during the first week or two of life.

So amniotomy raises many questions that have yet to be answered. You may want to discuss it with your obstetrician or midwife. You have a right to be fully informed. You can, if you wish, request that amniotomy be done only if the baby is showing signs of distress.

THE INTRAVENOUS DRIP
In almost all hospitals in the United States, and increasingly in Britain, an intravenous drip is set up for every woman in labour. A fine catheter (hollow tube) is introduced into a vein in your arm or hand and fixed with adhesive tape so that fluids can be infused straight into your bloodstream. The argument for setting up a drip is that once a vein is open, emergency action can be taken rapidly and your strength can be kept up without you needing to eat or,

A typical hospital partogram

This is a series of graphs used to record the main events of labour. It is particularly useful for isolating problems. In the course of a normal labour it also acts as a clear record of progress, and is useful for any new staff that may come on duty.

Fetal Heart Rate (FHR)
Charted in beats per minute, with 120 to 160 beats considered normal. (Any deceleration is shown as an arrow down to the lowest level.) The condition of the amniotic fluid (waters) is also recorded. I means "intact"; C means "clear".

Cervical Dilatation
The degree of dilatation (X) is noted every 3 or 4 hours and a curve is drawn. If there is a 2-hour delay compared with the norm, the doctor stimulates the labour with an oxytocin drip. The descent of the baby's head through the pelvis (O) is also indicated.

Drugs
Any drugs given are noted on the partogram chart. In this case entonox (gas and oxygen) was given for pain relief and syntometrine to stimulate the delivery of the placenta.

Contractions
Frequency, strength (by shading) and length of contractions in seconds are shown.

Blood Pressure
The mother's blood pressure and pulse are recorded several times during labour. The upper level recorded is the systolic pressure, the lower one the diastolic (see page 40).

Temperature
The mother's temperature is also taken throughout the labour and recorded on the partogram.

Mother's Details
Facts about the mother are recorded including: her last period (LMP); the estimated date of delivery (EDD); when the membranes ruptured (2 hours before birth).

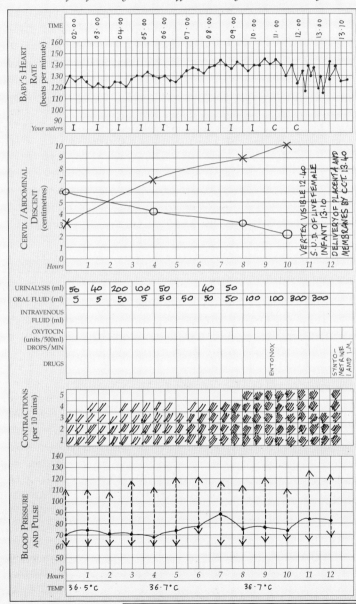

No. EP 8247	Surname PERRY	First Name CAMILLA
Parity 0+0	Age 25	Date 2-9-97
LMP 22·11·96 EDD 29-8-97		
Duration of Labour 12 HRS.	Duration of Ruptured Membranes 2HRS.	

sometimes, even drink anything. This means that if a Caesarean section is necessary (see pages 336–338) and a general anaesthetic is used, your stomach is likely to be almost empty already and there is not a great deal of risk that you will regurgitate or inhale its contents. If needs be, to lower the risk even further, you can have an antacid drink to reduce the acid of your stomach contents.

Forcing women to go through labour without food and drink is bad policy.* It medicalizes the birth experience and is unnecessary. Labour is hard work. In the early phases especially, you may get hungry, and should be allowed to eat whatever you fancy. And you will certainly be thirsty and should feel free to drink.

Dextrose, a glucose solution or "Ringer's lactate" solution, containing electrolytes and water, may be given through a drip to act as a "pick-me-up" in labour. Since it bypasses the stomach, you do not have to digest it. Dextrose may be useful if labour is long and you are becoming dehydrated, or if lactic acid builds up in the course of a difficult labour, causing acetone to appear in the urine – an indication that your body is short of glucose. But a dextrose drip can lead to hypoglycemia (low blood sugar) in your baby after birth.

If you have a drip set up it is especially important to remember to empty your bladder regularly: every hour is not too frequent. You will be accumulating fluid, and should urinate frequently to prevent urine from building up in your bladder.

Once a drip is in place, other substances can be introduced by the same route. This may be done without your consenting to or being aware of the administration of drugs. If you have an intravenous infusion and the bag or bottle is changed, ask why. Your partner will be able to get close enough to read the label. Oxytocin is introduced by this means. The label for this will probably read "Syntocinon." You can find more information about this in the section on induced labour on pages 324–329.

Other medicines and narcotics are also given via the drip. You need not consent to an intravenous drip unless you are confident that there are good reasons for it. It is yet another way in which women are sometimes made needlessly uncomfortable in labour. The drip can be very helpful when needed, but used routinely it merely makes it difficult for you to move. In most hospitals where intravenous drips are administered as a matter of course it is taken for granted that the woman in labour stays in bed.

EPISIOTOMY

An episiotomy is a surgical cut made to enlarge the birth opening. It is done with scissors, under local anaesthetic, just before the baby is born. It can be midline (down from the bottom of the vagina towards the anus) or mediolateral (sloping out to the side, away from the anus, or down and then out again in the shape of a hockey stick). In Britain the episiotomy is usually mediolateral. Mediolateral incisions are virtually never done in North America.

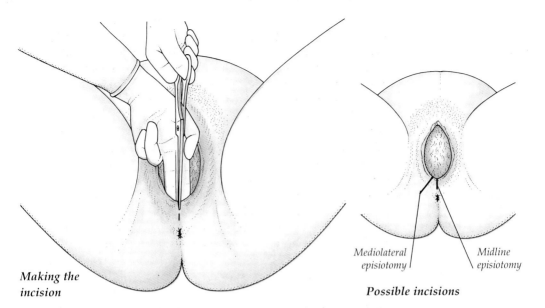

Making the incision

Mediolateral episiotomy | *Midline episiotomy*

Possible incisions

Since the incision is made through both skin and muscle, careful repair of the wound must be made afterwards. The local anaesthetic given before the episiotomy is usually enough for the repair. If not, more can be given. This requires a few minutes to take effect, and the doctor or midwife should wait until the area is fully anaesthetized before stitching the wound. The suturing is done with a curved needle and it may take as long as an hour to sew up a mediolateral episiotomy or one that has been extended by tearing. Stitching a midline episiotomy is usually quicker, because there is a natural dividing line between muscles in the midline, which makes the repair much simpler to carry out.

The stitches can be left in if they are the kind that dissolve, but you should have a look at the area in a mirror every couple of days to make sure that they have disappeared, since sometimes they do not drop out and become embedded in tissue. You may feel as if you are sitting on thorns. When this happens, the stitches should be snipped out by a midwife on or before the tenth day after the birth.

After an episiotomy your perineum is likely to be very tender, swollen and sore for days, or even weeks. Ask for a local anaesthetic spray to apply to the area. This really helps.*

REASONS FOR EPISIOTOMY

Some obstetricians believe that all first-time mothers should have an episiotomy to relieve strain on their tissues and get the baby delivered quickly. When there are signs of fetal distress an episiotomy can speed delivery and make birth easier for the baby. You may be told that it is a good idea to have an episiotomy because "a straight, clean cut is better than a nasty, jagged tear", which is more difficult to sew up. Sometimes episiotomy is done

Having an episiotomy

An episiotomy is done as the baby's head crowns and between contractions. The local anaesthetic, combined with the numbing effect of the baby's head pressing against the perineum, results in the cut being rarely felt.

321

in an attempt to prevent damage to tissues inside the vagina when there is evidence of "buttonhole" tearing (that is, a series of very tiny lacerations deep inside).

The practice of routine episiotomy is still favored by many North American obstetricians and those on the European continent, but is declining in British hospitals. In the Seventies, almost 100 per cent of women had episiotomies in certain hospitals in Britain. Now the proportion is generally below 40 per cent. As soon as a research project investigating episiotomy was begun in any hospital – that is, as soon as questions were raised about its necessity – the rate dropped by about a third, even before any results were obtained.

PROBLEMS WITH EPISIOTOMY

Trials conducted in Dublin, Montreal,* and Argentina* have revealed that women with an intact perineum, or only a superficial tear, experience less pain after childbirth than those who have undergone an episiotomy. The pain after an episiotomy is about the same as that experienced from a second-degree tear (one that affects the underlying muscle). Women are also more likely to suffer severe tears into the anus when they have had an episiotomy than when they have not had one.* Another trial, in England, as well as the Montreal trial, showed that there is no advantage to episiotomy over a natural first- or second-degree tear.*

Many women say that they feel terribly uncomfortable when making love for several months after an episiotomy, and they tend to resume intercourse later than women who have had a tear.

There are other problems with episiotomy that should be borne in mind: if done too early – before the perineum has thinned out – it can cause unnecessary bleeding; sometimes the cut is much larger than a tear would have been; and quite often the stitches get infected and antibiotics are then necessary.*

With skilled guidance at delivery and a gentle birth (see pages 343–353), more and more women are now having no injury to the perineum – and this makes an enormous difference to how they feel in the days and weeks after the baby is born.

MANAGING THE THIRD STAGE

A now widely accepted method of controlling the third stage of labour, the expulsion of the placenta, is to give an intramuscular injection of oxytocin directly after the delivery of the baby's shoulder nearest your front (the anterior shoulder). The placenta then usually separates from the lining of the uterus with the next contraction and is expelled within five minutes of the birth.

However, if the placenta does *not* separate completely after the injection, it can be trapped by the powerfully contracting uterus. So attendants clamp and cut the cord as soon as the baby is born and then press a hand on the top of the uterus, pulling on the cord at the same time in order to get the placenta out.

A healthy placenta

Controlled cord traction

Cord traction
After the birth of your baby your uterus continues to contract strongly to expel the placenta. You may be asked to push the placenta out, once it has peeled off the wall of the uterus, by pushing against the doctor's or midwife's hand placed against your lower abdomen, while he or she gently pulls on the cord with the other hand.

If the placenta is left to separate naturally, it may take half an hour or longer. Clamping of the cord immediately at delivery may make a retained placenta more likely. If the cord is not clamped until after it has stopped pulsating there is much less chance of a retained placenta. This is because when the cord is clamped blood cannot flow out of it, which would encourage the now defunct placenta to peel away from the uterine wall. A blood-packed placenta stays firm and full and is less likely to separate.

If the third stage is allowed to proceed naturally, your first physical contact with your baby produces a rush of emotion that is accompanied by the release of oxytocin. This *natural* oxytocin rush keeps the uterus firm and causes further contractions. Once the placenta has separated, the doctor or midwife gently places one flat hand over your lower tummy, just above the pubic bone, and you push against the hand, in order to deliver the placenta and membranes. It often helps to have a hand to push against like this. The alternative is to squat over a bowl or pail and to deliver the placenta with the help of gravity.

There is no reason for a cord to be clamped before the placenta has been delivered except for convenience, although sometimes the cord is so short that it is impossible for the mother to hold her baby unless it is cut first; or it is twisted in a succession of loops around the baby's neck and is cut so that the baby can slide out. If a woman is Rhesus negative with a Rhesus positive baby (see page 113), there is a case for *delayed* cord clamping. If the cord is clamped while still pulsating fetal blood is retained in the placenta, blood vessels rupture as the uterus contracts, and the chances of Rhesus positive blood being pushed back into the mother's blood stream are greatly increased.

Induced labour

Induction is the obstetric way of starting off labour that has not begun by itself. When labour begins naturally, the uterus becomes sensitive to hormones present in your bloodstream at the end of pregnancy. When labour is induced the doctor tries to obtain a similar result by flooding your system with hormones, until they reach a level much higher than that which occurs naturally. This can be done by introducing synthetic hormones into your bloodstream through a continuous intravenous drip, or by inserting prostaglandin pessaries into your vagina. Both methods are usually combined with artificial rupture of the membranes.

INDUCTION PROCEDURES

Remember that you have the right to receive full details of exactly what is going to be done and why *before* being admitted to hospital for induction, and you can then choose to accept or refuse the treatment once you know all the facts.

Stripping the membranes Some doctors strip the membranes to stimulate labour. This is done by pushing the membranes away from the cervix by hand, while leaving them intact. This is a rather uncomfortable procedure, but may successfully start things off.

Artificial rupture of the membranes (see page 317) This may be performed as the only means of induction if your cervix is already starting to dilate. Most obstetricians believe that once the membranes are ruptured the baby ought to be born within 24 hours, because there is some risk of infection if labour is long and drawn out. So you need to be aware that if your labour is started by ARM but is slow to get going, it may then have to be accelerated with hormones.

Prostaglandin pessaries One way of inducing labour that is commonly employed is to introduce prostaglandin pessaries into and around the cervix. While prostaglandin pessaries may not start labour, they help to ripen and efface a firm, thick cervix, making it more likely to dilate when oxytocin is given. If the pessaries are inserted in the evening, labour may have started by the following morning. It may be unnecessary to have amniotomy (see page 317) and an oxytocin drip as well, and pessaries have the great advantage of allowing you freedom to move about in labour.

Oxytocin drip If induction involves being connected to an oxytocin (syntocinon) drip, ask for it to be placed in the arm or hand you use less. If the connecting tube is short, you cannot easily move your arm or change position without dislodging it, but there is no need for it to be short, and you can ask for it to be securely fixed so that you can still change position. Many women have discovered that they get backache simply from lying in one position for too long, quite apart from the backache caused by contractions. A glucose solution may be passed through the drip first. The drip can be turned down or removed once contractions are effective and

"I found it so much easier to be upright and moving that I got out of the bed and walked around attached to the intravenous drip stand."

the cervix is 5 cm dilated. You can ask the obstetrician to do this. But the drip is usually kept in until after the end of the third stage, since it can control bleeding from the uterus by keeping it contracting hard.

WHEN INDUCTION MAY HELP

Induction is useful when a baby must be born without delay. Many doctors believe that between 15 and 25 per cent of labours benefit from either induction or acceleration. Some believe that these figures are too high, while others contend that 60 per cent or more of labours ought to be induced. Symptoms of pre-eclampsia (see page 139), including high blood pressure, albumin in the urine, sudden, excessive weight gain and oedema (puffiness resulting from fluid retention), are a good reason for induction, since the baby may not continue to be well nourished in your uterus if the pregnancy is allowed to go on. If you have had a previous forceps delivery because a baby was a tight fit, inducing the next baby before term may allow you to give birth more easily, but this can not be guaranteed because pain is usually more severe in induced labours.

Induction before the EDD Some babies stop growing because the placenta, through which they receive nourishment and oxygen, is not working well at the end of pregnancy, even before there is any question of being "overdue", although the mother may be feeling fit and healthy. Such babies may flourish better outside the uterus.

Induction after the EDD Between 10 and 12 per cent of women go two weeks or more "overdue" (known as "post-dates"), but in only 1 per cent of these cases is there any evidence of post-maturity (the baby's skin is dry and peeling and the fingernails require cutting). The start of pregnancy has usually been miscalculated or normal variations in the length of pregnancy ignored. Growing a baby is not a factory process.

If you are 43 weeks pregnant, there is a chance of the placenta not functioning so well because it is aging. However, *premature babies are most at risk*, so you need to be sure that the baby really is overdue before inducing. Some doctors make it a rule to induce if you are more than a week overdue. Others like all their patients to deliver at about term, and bring you into hospital even if you are just a few days past your date. Ultrasound can be used to check the flow of blood to the baby and the volume of amniotic fluid – which is reduced once a baby really is post-term – and to discover whether induction is necessary (see pages 223–226).

THE LENGTH OF INDUCED LABOURS

Although you may have a rapid labour with induction, this cannot be guaranteed. Some obstetricians prefer labours not to last longer than ten, eight or even five hours and deliver with forceps or by Caesarean section if labour is prolonged beyond that fixed point. When a policy of routine induction in birth is introduced into a hospital, there is often a large increase in the number of instrumental deliveries and Caesarean sections performed, and the proportion of babies with low Apgar scores (see page 356) goes up – evidence that a policy of routine induction is bad for babies as well as mothers.* Since there is so much variation in obstetric policy, it may be a good idea when discussing the possibility of induction with the doctor to ask what his or her practice is. Depending on whether or not you want a short, sharp labour, this may affect your decision about whether to agree to induction if it is not urgently necessary for your baby's sake.

"I declined the offer of induction at 42 weeks and asked for some tests to be done instead. The baby was fine, and I went into labour the next day."

Induction is a form of intervention that, while useful when necessary, is not without risks, and the relative risks of leaving the baby inside your uterus and of inducing labour have to be assessed.

Unripe cervix It has been stated that "the major factor governing the success of induction is the state of the cervix".* When the cervix feels soft – like your lips when you hold your mouth slack – then it is ripe and ready for labour. Unfortunately, induction is often done before the cervix is ripe, and in consequence the uterus may not respond to hormones. If the membranes have been ruptured, then the only way to get the baby born is by Caesarean section. In cases where an induction is necessary and the cervix is unripe, prostaglandin pessaries over a period of several days may be used before oxytocin is administered.

Powerful contractions If the uterus is triggered to work harder, labour is more violent than when started naturally. In a labour that has been induced there are often two "peaks" to each contraction, and each may last one minute or longer. Women who have had babies before, and whose previous labours were not induced, say that contractions start more powerfully and that there is not much lead-up to each contraction, but instead a sudden "explosion". There may be only a short interval between contractions; just time to let out one relaxing breath, and then you are into the next one! You may find you need to go straight into the breathing patterns you will have learned about for half-dilatation (see pages 201–208).

Interrupted blood flow Extremely powerful contractions are likely to interfere with the blood flow through the uterus. In one study it was discovered that fetal distress was significantly more common in women taking oxytocin, that the babies were more likely to have low Apgar scores (see page 356), and that far more of these babies than usual went to the nursery for special care.*

If labour is induced the baby's heart will be monitored continuously. If you experience a contraction that lasts longer than 90 seconds, let the midwife know immediately. Even with a small dose of oxytocin, some women have a prolonged contraction in which the uterus clamps down on itself – and on the baby. There is no test by which the sensitivity of your uterus to oxytocin can be known beforehand, so it is best to start with a small dose and gradually build up until good contractions result. The aim should be to simulate normal labour.

Measuring contractions
During an induced labour, an intrauterine pressure catheter may be used to monitor the pressure of uterine contractions, and slow down or stop the flow of oxytocin when the uterus is contracting too hard. Another machine automatically adjusts the flow according to the amount of pressure in the uterus, which is measured by a small intrauterine pressure catheter so that the woman does not have to be strapped into a tight belt to record the contractions. This technology aims to solve the problem of too strong, harsh labour, which results when more oxytocin is infiltrated into a woman's bloodstream than her particular uterus needs.

Induction with epidural anaesthesia
In some hospitals you may be offered a "package deal" of induction combined with epidural anaesthesia. (For more about epidurals see pages 309–313.) This new style of childbirth is attractive to many obstetricians and to many women, too.

As with any intravenous drip, if you are receiving a large quantity of fluid, it is important that you remember to empty your bladder regularly. If you cannot urinate (and you often cannot if you have had an epidural), the midwife will insert a catheter and draw off the urine for you. A full bladder makes contractions painful (sometimes even with an epidural) by acting as a barrier between the baby's head and the base that forms the front of your pelvic arch.

Elective induction
Sometimes called induction for convenience, elective induction is induction with no medical indication. Some doctors believe that most women should be induced. Some think it is the only way in

which all labours can be efficiently managed. They say that it is important for women to be in labour when doctors and midwives are on duty, that hospital organization is easier when it is known how many women will be in labour each day and that it is better if women are not in labour at night. There will always be those women who go into labour spontaneously at inconvenient times, but the earlier they are induced the less likely this is to happen. Because of this some obstetricians believe that induction any time after 38 or 39 weeks is right for most women. The logical development of this approach to obstetrics is that all spontaneous labours will come to be considered as "emergencies" and "normal" labours will all be induced.

After considering the findings of research, the United States Food and Drug Administration withdrew approval for the use of oxytocin for the elective induction of labour, asserting that it can expose both mother and baby to unnecessary danger.

COPING WITH INDUCTION

While there are basic questions that women need to ask about induction and acceleration of labour in terms of our increasingly technological style of childbirth in the West, these may not seem very relevant if your doctor advises you that your labour should be induced. It may come as a shock. You may even feel that all your careful preparation for the birth of your baby is pointless now.

Many women have enjoyed induced labours and coped with them well. But unfortunately many whose labours were induced say that they did not have any choice and that they were given inadequate information. Yet the British Department of Health has stated: "A mother should have learned about induction at antenatal classes and if later it appears that induction would be the safer course of action for her, she should have every opportunity of discussing it with professional advisers. Knowing what is likely to be involved, she can make a fully informed decision about it".*

The important thing is to ask questions. Do not wait and hope that someone will explain things to you. Discuss it all fully, learn about what might happen and share in the decision-making rather than feeling it is all being decided for you. When you have the facts and your obstetrician's advice, take time to weigh them and choose what seems to be the best path, always leaving your mind open to new evidence that may later point to a different course of action. Remember that it is your baby and your body and the experts are there to help you, not to take over.

ACCELERATED LABOUR

Labour is said to be augmented or accelerated when it has already started and then been speeded up by the use of an oxytocin drip. If a drip is used *before* the cervix has started to dilate progressively, even though you have felt contractions and have had a "false labour" or many Braxton Hicks contractions, your labour is being induced, not augmented. Labour may be augmented when there is uterine inertia or inco-ordination – that is, when the uterus is not working effectively (see page 276). Some of the most difficult labours are long ones, and if you are getting tired out with the stress of experiencing continued back pain, for example, augmentation may help you cope because it stimulates uterine action.

If it looks as if labour ought to be induced or accelerated, there are breathing skills you can use in order to help you deal with the challenge (see pages 201–208). You need not give up when this occurs, feeling that the doctors have now taken over.

ACTIVE MANAGEMENT OF LABOUR

This is a system of controlling and hastening labour, and ensuring rapid and efficient uterine action, by introducing the hormone oxytocin into a woman's bloodstream. It is claimed that it cuts the Caesarean section rate. It was devised by obstetricians in the National Maternity Hospital in Dublin, where 40 per cent of women have their labours stimulated in this way, and is increasingly popular with obstetricians all over the world. A woman is told that under no circumstances will her labour be allowed to last longer than 12 hours, and if her cervix does not dilate by at least one centimeter every hour, the uterus is stimulated artificially to work harder and faster.

In Dublin the administration of uterine stimulation is restricted to women giving birth for the first time. Its use is considered potentially dangerous for women who have already had babies – multigravidae.* In addition, an important part of labour management is one-to-one care from a personal midwife who usually stays with each woman until the baby is born. Her duties primarily involve continuous presence, eye contact and encouragement throughout every contraction, along with some clinical responsibilities.

"The birth was turned into a race against time, for no reason except that the obstetrician believed the best labours were the fastest."

Obstetricians outside Dublin often use active management indiscriminately. They favour active management for multigravidae, as well as for primigravidae (women having their first baby). And they neglect or forget that one-to-one care is part of the method, because it is administratively difficult. There is evidence, however, that it is not active management, but continuous one-to-one care, that reduces the need for Caesarean section.* It is having someone with you who has experience and who gives emotional support that is the single most effective element in this method of labour management. With this in mind, the decision to have a birth partner with you is probably one of the best ways of keeping your labour normal and reducing the chances of a Caesarean delivery, and you may want to ensure that you have the same midwife, or a birth companion, present with you throughout the birth.

The electronic fetal monitor is close to the the bed so you can see when the next contraction is starting even before you feel it, and can get ready to meet it with your breathing. Before you are attached to a monitor, get into an upright position so that you are not stuck lying down.

Electronic fetal monitoring

The electronic fetal monitor (EFM) is used to track the fetal heartbeat and to record the pressure of the uterus during contractions. Either a transducer is placed over your abdomen near the baby's heart (external monitoring), or a spiral wire electrode is inserted through the open cervix and fastened to the baby's scalp (internal monitoring). A printout, usually in the form of a continuous graph on a long spool of tape rather like ticker tape, shows the baby's heart rate in relation to the work being done by the uterus. The monitor is a compact box that can amplify the baby's heartbeat so that it becomes clearly audible. It incorporates a flashing light that also registers the beating of the baby's heart and the contraction intensity, but this can be turned off. If anything goes wrong, the monitor sounds an alarm. This often indicates that there is something wrong with the machine rather than with the baby.

MAKING A DECISION ABOUT ELECTRONIC FETAL MONITORING
When EFM was invented in the 1970s, it was believed that it would make birth safer for babies, allowing fetal heart rate to be monitored constantly. But nine randomized controlled trials have shown that it does not. Babies are just as safe when someone listens to the fetal heart just after a contraction has finished and in the interval between contractions with a Pinard's stethoscope or a hand-held Doppler machine. Babies who are intermittently monitored are no

more likely to have low Apgar scores or go to the special care unit.*
In fact, more babies suffer from cerebral palsy after EFM labours
than when they are monitored intermittently.*

Research has shown monitoring reduces the rate of neonatal
seizures (fits). Some people concluded that this affirmed the value of
continuous monitoring. Then it was revealed that this kind of
neonatal seizure was not the type that produced long-term health
problems, which occurred only in babies whose mothers had
received oxytocin in labour. A major disadvantage of EFM is that it
increases the Caesarean section rate by 160 per cent, without any
benefit to the baby.* This rate is reduced if fetal blood sampling is
done before the decision to proceed to operative delivery, but there is
still a 30 per cent increase in the Caesarean section rate, again without
any benefit to the baby.* Continuous monitoring also has a profound
effect on the way that labour is conducted. With the monitoring set-
up, the woman is unable to move freely. She is more likely to be left
alone at times during the labour, because the caregivers believe that
the electronic equipment is doing the job of monitoring for them. She
cannot use a birth pool or have transcutaneous electronic nerve
stimulation for pain relief. For many women the process of electronic
monitoring makes the labour much more stressful than it need be.

THE EXTERNAL MONITOR
An external monitor has two straps that are attached to your
abdomen. One strap holds the tocodynamometer (the pressure
gauge that records contractions). The other holds the ultrasound
transducer that registers the baby's heartbeats.

THE INTERNAL MONITOR
The internal monitor, which is more accurate than the external
monitor, is inserted through the vagina and cervix, and fixed to the
skin of the baby's head. It is connected to a wire leading to the
machine. An intrauterine pressure catheter is inserted into the uterus
to record the pressure of contractions; or you may wear a single
strap around your abdomen to hold the tocodynamometer. An
internal monitor cannot be used until the membranes have ruptured
and until the cervix is dilated at least 2 cm.

ADVANTAGES OF MONITORING
The electronic monitor may be useful when labour is induced or
augmented with an oxytocin drip, as the length, power and frequency
of the contractions produced by the drip, and their effect on the baby,
must be carefully observed lest they prove to be too stressful for the
baby to cope with. Until recently induction was often done "blind,"
and as a result enormous, turbulent contractions were produced that
sometimes cut off the fetal blood supply. This is much less likely
nowadays since, by monitoring these artificially aided births, it has
been discovered that small amounts of oxytocin are effective.

Another advantage of monitoring during labour is that the monitor indicates when the next contraction is beginning, so that however drowsy you are feeling during labour you can breathe out and relax, and get ready to breathe over the contraction.

PROBLEMS OF MONITORING

Many women say that the abdominal strapping of the external monitor is very uncomfortable during labour. Some even say that the pressure of the transducer on their tummies was the most painful thing about labour. Sometimes the internal electrode slips off the baby's head or, if an external monitor is being used, the baby moves and its heartbeat is then lost on the monitor. Some new external monitors have transducers that track the position of the baby's heart so that they do not lose it in this way. As in the case of an intravenous drip, an external monitor requires you to remain more or less in one position lest the transducer slip off. This immobility results in discomfort for you (page 320) and possibly problems for the baby. So monitoring may sometimes produce the failing fetal heart rate that it then records. Do not allow the monitor to keep you from moving around within the range of the wires to which you are attached. The midwife will be able to adjust the monitor when you move.

Some women in labour are wired to the monitor only to find that nothing is being recorded at all because the machine is not operating. It is very irritating to be immobilized and connected to a machine when it cannot possibly be doing anything to help. Yet staff sometimes appear shocked at a woman's request for the transducer to be detached so that she can move about and get on with her labour unhindered. If this happens to you, you are entirely justified in insisting that the monitor be disconnected. But when the monitor is working well some women are reassured to know that every heartbeat of the baby is being recorded.

TELEMETRY

Monitoring by telemetry (radio waves) is an advance on the older method, allowing you to be up and about in labour unattached to wires but continuously monitored at the same time. The equipment is not cumbersome and can be placed at some distance from you. Women prefer it, labours seem to go faster than with other methods of monitoring, and babies do better. Because you are able to stay upright, you may feel less pain, and the uterus can work more efficiently.

Even monitoring by telemetry can often be invasive, since internal monitoring methods are sometimes used with telemetry, although a method of sticking the monitor on to the baby's scalp with epoxy resin is now available. Any invasive technique (one that entails entering your body) introduces added risk of infection. This is a risk worth taking when there is reason to suspect that the baby is encountering difficulties, but not when everything seems to be straightforward.

A scalp electrode probably causes the baby some pain. It involves breaking the skin of the baby's scalp. (It is uncomfortable to prick your finger on one.) It remains on the baby's head until after delivery, when it should be removed gently and deftly, not merely yanked. In 85 per cent of newborn babies a rash appears at the site of the electrode and in 20 per cent a small abscess develops.* Sometimes the child is left with a permanent bald patch.

INTERPRETING THE DATA

Although it is estimated that the fetal monitor enables an obstetrician to save one life for every 1000 babies monitored, the interpretation of data is of first importance. The machine itself can do nothing to make childbirth safer. It is only too easy to interpret normal variations in the fetal heart rate as pathological, sometimes because of the design of the machine, or to miss clinical signs that something is wrong because the monitor indicates that everything is normal. Obstetricians and midwives experienced in auscultating the fetal heart (listening with ultrasound or a Pinard's stethoscope) have a valuable skill that is neglected as more and more confidence is placed in electronic monitors.

Interpretation of electronic monitoring data sometimes causes more harm than good. Half of all babies show some irregularities of heartbeat during labour. Usually this is of no significance. We don't know how they manage it, but babies actually sleep during labour. They change from rapid eye movement (REM) or dreaming sleep to deep, quiet sleep for a period of up to 40 minutes, and then back again. As the sleep state varies, so the heart rate changes; in deep sleep, the heartbeat stays steady, and the printout of the heart rate tends to be flat. Until the deep sleep was understood, this trace made doctors anxious; but it has now been discovered that the baby only has to be roused a little for the heartbeat to pick up. One way of doing this is to touch the top of the baby's head. Mothers have their own ways of achieving the same result – changing position, for example, or talking to the baby – and this may reassure the doctors.

"There was some concern about the baby's heart rate because it was abnormally slow. Then they found they were picking up my heartbeat, not the baby's."

The baby's heart rate is usually between 120 and 160 beats per minute. A quicker rate than this is termed tachycardia, and a slower rate, bradycardia. Incomplete understanding of the normal range of variation in the fetal heart rate during and between contractions leads to a great deal of intervention. Emergency Caesarean sections are often performed because of changes in the fetal heart rate that are judged to be signs of asphyxia. Yet more than 50 per cent of babies delivered by Caesarean section turn out to be in good condition, so operating was unnecessary. What has actually occurred is a series of complex changes in the baby's heartbeat as a result of a normal catecholamine (stress hormone) surge, and these alterations have then been misinterpreted as signs of fetal distress.

In Spain and Germany, when abnormal fetal heart patterns are recorded obstetricians stop the uterus from contracting by introducing drugs into the mother's bloodstream. In all countries, electronic fetal monitoring has led to more forceps deliveries and Caesarean sections, and the introduction of a monitor in any hospital is always associated with a sharp increase in the rate of operative deliveries – although this often drops after a while as staff become more comfortable with the normal variations in fetal heart rate. The American College of Obstetricians and Gynecologists (ACOG) and the Society of Obstetricians and Gynecologists of Canada (SOGC) now support a policy of regular, frequent listening with an ultrasound stethoscope (auscultation) as equal or superior to electronic fetal heart monitoring. Despite this reversal of support for electronic fetal heart monitoring by the leaders in obstetrics, most doctors and even many midwives have not been well trained in auscultation, and so continue to rely on EFM.

TESTING THE BABY'S BLOOD

If the fetal monitor suggests that the baby is under stress, the baby's blood should be tested in order to check the findings, since if the baby is having any difficulties this always shows up in the blood chemistry. But this testing is not always done. A biochemical test carried out in order to assess the pH level of the baby's blood cuts down the number of unnecessary Caesarean deliveries. One kind of electrode both records the baby's heart rate and also tests its blood.

It has usually been accepted that if a blood test reveals high levels of lactic acid, which builds up if the baby is short of oxygen in the second stage of labour, the baby's brain will be damaged. But it is now known that if it does become short of oxygen, a healthy baby can switch to another kind of metabolism that allows it to draw on energy reserves that have been built up over the previous weeks; in this way the baby can survive on less oxygen with no ill effects whatsoever. Indeed, babies whose blood is acid at birth often have high Apgar scores (see page 356). Moreover, neurological studies on four-year-olds whose blood was acid at birth due to oxygen shortage show that this had no harmful effects.*

Helping the baby out

In most British hospitals nowadays about one baby in every ten is delivered by forceps. The rate is higher in some hospitals.

FORCEPS DELIVERY

Forceps look like metal salad servers and dovetail into each other so that they cannot press too far in on the baby's head. If the woman has not already had an epidural, an injection to numb the birth outlet is given first. The curved blades are inserted one at a time and cradled around the baby's head, one at each temple.

Vacuum extraction

Simple forceps delivery

Vacuum
extractor

Forceps

Forceps are of different shapes for different situations: most draw your baby down the birth canal, although some are simply used to lift the baby out. If the baby's head is occipito transverse or occipito posterior (see page 263), the obstetrician may first turn the head manually, or may use curved Kiellands forceps for the delivery to rotate the head from the transverse or posterior to the anterior.

VACUUM EXTRACTION

Increasingly, a vacuum extractor is used in preference to forceps. There is evidence that vacuum extraction may be better for both mother and baby than forceps extraction. But, of course, it is a skill that needs to be learned.* A vacuum extractor works like a miniature vacuum cleaner to suck the baby out. A vacuum cup is attached to the baby's head. It may take between 10 and 20 minutes to be applied. During this time if you want to push, push. Once the cup is on, it helps if you can bear down, so that the baby is pressed down from above as well as being pulled down the birth canal by the suction that is being applied from below.

REASONS FOR FORCEPS DELIVERY OR VACUUM EXTRACTION

Forceps or vacuum extraction are used only during the second stage when delivery needs to be hastened because your blood pressure has risen dramatically, for example, or because there are signs of fetal distress, or when the baby is in an unusual position, making its journey through the pelvic outlet difficult.

The obstetrician has to use clinical judgment to decide whether your baby will pop out like a cork from a bottle given a firm, long pull, or whether it is so firmly wedged that it might harm both you and the baby to deliver vaginally. Sometimes a Caesarean section is performed after forceps or vacuum have failed. Forceps or

Help with delivery
Vacuum extraction
(left) can sometimes
avoid a difficult forceps
delivery, and the
suction cup may be
attached to the baby
before it has started to
descend the birth canal.
The forceps (right)
are the kind used
simply for lifting the
baby's head out of
the birth canal.

335

vacuum extraction may also be used if you have had an epidural (see pages 309–313), because in this case you may well feel too numb to be able to work with contractions.

A forceps delivery or vacuum extraction is frequently advised if you are having a prolonged second stage. Different obstetricians have different ideas of what a prolonged second stage is. Some would say that it is any second stage longer than half an hour in which there are no signs of progress. Many set a definite time limit on the second stage and instruct nurses to call them when it looks as if this stage is extending. Others believe that this is rather doctrinaire and that the important thing is to observe whether or not the baby is coming down the birth canal progressively, while checking its condition carefully and regularly.

Some women seem to be able to cope with long second stages without tiring, whereas others quickly become exhausted. If you have already had a long labour and then a slow second stage, it is difficult to retain enthusiasm and, unless given a great deal of encouragement, you may hope that someone would just come and take the baby out of your body one way or another.

A woman may be given encouragement to push or be persuaded to hold her breath too long, when she does not feel any spontaneous urge to bear down. This is because the midwife knows that the delivery will be by forceps unless the baby is born within the time decreed by the obstetrician, so she tries to avoid the intervention by encouraging the mother to push more strenuously in the hope that this will help the baby to be born before the deadline.

AVOIDING A FORCEPS DELIVERY OR VACUUM EXTRACTION

If you have been struggling to push the baby out and it is suggested that forceps may be necessary because the second stage is taking too long, you are becoming too tired or the fetal heart rate is slow, explore the effect of *not pushing*. You may find that you do not need to push at all for several contractions – a welcome rest for both you and the baby – and then there is an unmistakable and irresistible pushing sensation that is much more effective than pushing just because you are following instructions. It is a good idea to stand, squat or kneel so that gravity can help the baby out.

Caesarean section

If the obstetrician tells you that you need to give birth by Caesarean section, this means that you will be anaesthetized and your baby will then be delivered abdominally rather than vaginally.

The most common reason for Caesarean section is the failure of your labour to progress, due to malposition of the baby or to cephalopelvic disproportion, when the baby's head is too large to pass through the pelvis. Some obstetricians prefer to deliver all breech babies abdominally, or all breech babies of first-time mothers, because they believe that it is safer for the baby. But the size of the baby in relation to the maternal pelvis and the way the baby is lying are factors to take into account. If fetal distress is picked up by an electronic monitor and the obstetrician becomes anxious about the state of the baby, he or she may decide to perform an emergency Caesarean section. A biochemical test of the baby's scalp blood should be done first to check whether the baby is finding birth hard going.

Abdominal delivery may also be performed for twins, when amniocentesis has revealed that a baby is damaged, for very low-weight babies, and also for women suffering from active herpes or diseases such as diabetes, renal disease and severe hypertension. Research has been carried out on the outcomes of automatic Caesarean sections for multiple births and when women have diabetes, and it has been shown that this practice is unlikely to be of benefit.* Delivering all twins by Caesarean section does not save babies' lives or produce babies in better condition. A study compared birth outcomes in two parts of Denmark, one where the rate of Caesarean section was about twice as high as the other, and found no differences in perinatal mortality or morbidity.*

THE RISE IN CAESAREAN BIRTHS

Caesarean rates vary. In Britain, they make up about 15 per cent of all births. In some cities in Latin America, a staggering 85 per cent of babies are delivered abdominally, whereas in the Netherlands the overall rate is less than 10 per cent. In South Africa the rate varies from 14 to 17 per cent in state teaching hospitals to 33 per cent in private hospitals. Private obstetricians there, as in other countries, are much more likely to opt for Caesarean sections than those in a national health service. South African obstetricians themselves report that they do Caesarean section for convenience in 75 per cent of cases.* The Caesarean rate in the United States is approximately 24 per cent. In some hospitals it is 50 per cent or more. But there has not been a corresponding rise in the fetal survival rate. And Caesarean section imposes on women extra risk, as well as unnecessary pain and, often, postoperative infection. The World Health Organization recommends that Caesarean section rates should never be allowed to go higher than 10 to 12 per cent.

"It was a shock to have a Caesarean section, as I'd looked forward to a natural birth. I felt cheated and as if I weren't a normal woman."

In the past the obstetrician would have corrected a breech baby's position by external version through the mother's abdominal wall (see page 234). This practice declined for a generation and it became the tendency to deliver by section rather than attempting to turn the baby first. As a result, doctors no longer knew *how* to perform external version. Now doctors are starting to learn this technique again.

More and more women are now included in the category of "high risk". The age at which a woman is considered obstetrically high risk went down from 40 to 35, then to 30. If you are over 35 and it seems likely that there may be problems with your labour, you may find that you are advised to deliver by Caesarean section. Some obstetricians like to do a Caesarean section just because a baby looks as if it is going to be big. This is not a good reason for Caesarean section.* Throughout North America it is also the practice to do *repeat* Caesarean sections, even when the conditions that resulted in the first section are not present: "Once a Caesarean, always a Caesarean." Many repeat Caesareans are unnecessary. Only about one woman in four who had a Caesarean with one birth even tries for a VBAC (vaginal birth after Caesarean) with her next. Women often ask to have a Caesarean in order to avoid the pain of labour and because they can be conveniently scheduled. American doctors argue that the uterine scar might possibly break open during VBAC, but British obstetricians differ. They normally prefer a "trial" of labour but are ready to do a Caesarean if necessary. One professor of obstetrics says that problems of scar separation are "much less than the one per cent that is often quoted" and that even if the scar is pulled open by strong contractions, "careful monitoring of the fetus and mother usually means that any harm to either is rare."*

Planned Caesarean section

The decision to perform a Caesarean section is often made days or weeks in advance. As one woman said, "I got out my diary and wrote 'BABY' in a square several months ahead."A section will usually be planned if it is known that the baby is in a difficult position to be delivered vaginally. You may also be advised to have a Caesarean if there is evidence of cephalopelvic disproportion – although you can be certain that there is genuine CPD only when you are actually in labour. The baby must be delivered abdominally if the placenta is lying at the bottom of the uterus and over the os (the mouth of the cervix), in front of the baby's presenting part (placenta previa). You usually have a scan at 32 weeks to confirm that the placenta is still in this position. If your placenta is low lying, surgery is arranged either for the 39th week or as soon as the baby's lungs are known to be mature, which can be tested by amniocentesis.

Unplanned (just-in-case) Caesarean section

During a long labour in which there is little progress, the obstetrician may make the decision to perform a Caesarean section for no other reason than that dilatation is slow. It is important that you share in the decision-making about this. It is up to you.

Emergency Caesarean section

Some of the different reasons for a planned Caesarean section (such as cephalopelvic disproportion) may also apply to an emergency section, when the condition has not been obvious until labour. An emergency section may also be decided on during a long labour in which the baby is in obvious difficulties and is short of oxygen; if the placenta is failing to service the baby sufficiently or is becoming detached from the lining of the uterus, causing the mother to haemorrhage; or if there is a prolapsed umbilical cord.

ANAESTHESIA FOR CAESAREAN SECTION

Caesarean section in the past was always performed with the patient having first been given general anaesthesia, but now epidural or spinal anaesthesia (see below) is preferred for this operation. Although general anaesthesia still has to be used when a very quick decision has to be made to do a Caesarean section, those women who have epidural or spinal anaesthesia have usually liked being awake, aware of what is going on and ready to welcome the baby as soon as he or she is lifted out.

General anaesthesia If general anaesthesia is used, you are given as small a dose as possible for the baby's sake, and you may be unconscious for only a few minutes. All the preparation for the operation is done while you are awake and you are often given pure oxygen to breathe in during this time. It should also be possible to arrange for the baby who is in good condition to be held by the father while you are still unconscious.

Epidural anaesthesia You are given the epidural after being taken to the operating theatre or an existing epidural will be increased – the dosage is larger for surgery than it would be if an epidural were being given just for pain relief. An anaesthetist checks carefully to see that the anaesthesia is sufficient for the operation, and is ready with general anaesthesia if the epidural does not take effectively enough. With epidural anaesthesia you may possibly have some postoperative nausea and vomiting, as is often the case with general anaesthesia. An epidural is safer for you because there is no danger of inhaling your stomach contents, and safer for the baby, who does not receive a knock-out dose of anaesthesia. Another advantage of the epidural is that you can hold your baby and put it to the breast immediately after the operation.

Spinal anaethesia If you have had no anaesthetic prior to the decision to do a Caesarean, a spinal anaesthetic may be preferred to an epidural because it can be done more quickly and achieves good anaesthesia more simply than an epidural.

HORIZONTAL OR VERTICAL UTERINE INCISION

Incisions for Caesarean section are either horizontal or vertical. The classical incision is vertical but this is rarely done now unless there is no time to spare. The main advantages of the horizontal incision are that it is made low down near the line of the pubic hair, in the area that would be covered by a bikini, and that a horizontal scar is less likely to break down than a vertical scar.

Caesarean incisions
The classic Caesarean incision is vertical. Although this is still used in emergencies, horizontal incision is now more common, because it reduces the risk of rupture in another pregnancy. The positioning of a vertical and a horizontal incision is shown below.

WHAT HAPPENS DURING A CAESAREAN SECTION

Before you have a Caesarean section, you should be given antibiotics because one very frequent problem is pelvic infection afterwards.* A midwife will shave off your pubic hair and slip a catheter into your bladder so that it is kept empty. In the operating room sterile drapes are put around your tummy, and if you are going to be awake, a screen is erected at about chest level so that you do not see the surgery. Your tummy is washed in antiseptic solution. If there is anything you want to know, ask.

You will be given an epidural, spinal or, rarely, a general anaesthetic. When your whole tummy is numb, or you have become unconscious, a series of small cuts is made through the layers in your lower abdominal wall until the lower uterine segment is revealed. Packs of surgical gauze are pressed in to keep other organs out of the way. A horizontal slit is made through the uterus and the bag of waters then bulges through it. The obstetrician pops the bag and sucks out the amniotic fluid – if you have had an epidural or spinal you may hear the glug-glug-swoosh sound – and uses a forceps blade or a hand under the baby's presenting part to ease it out of the small opening, at the same time pushing with one hand on the upper part of the uterus so that the baby is pressed down through the incision.

If you have had an epidural or spinal it may be possible for you to watch the birth at this stage. Ask the doctor to put the screen down for a few moments. You will see your baby emerging and, from your horizontal position, will not see anything gruesome. In fact you will have eyes only for your baby. The baby is lifted out, suctioned with a mucus catheter and, once it is breathing well, can be handed to you or your partner. The process from the beginning of surgery to the birth need take only about four minutes in an emergency, but usually takes approximately 10 to 15 minutes.

As the baby is delivered, you may be given an injection of oxytocin to make the placenta peel away from the wall of the uterus. It will then be lifted out through the abdominal opening that has been made. The obstetrician stitches the cut in the uterus, layer by layer, with absorbable sutures. Suction instruments are used to draw out blood and amniotic fluid, and then the obstetrician repairs the abdominal wall. This takes much longer than the birth – up to an hour – and entails repairing the skin with non-absorbable sutures, staples or metal clips, which are removed the next day.

HAVING YOUR PARTNER WITH YOU

Not all couples want to be together during surgery. You may worry that perhaps it will be too much for your partner to cope with, or he may expect the experience to be so distressing that he will be unable to give you any support. Those couples who do want to be together feel that the birth of a baby, by whatever route, is something they want to share, and that if the mother is not able to cuddle the newborn baby the father should be there to do so. A father who is present sits by your head, supporting you emotionally; there is no necessity to watch the operation since the screen restricts his view.

AFTER THE DELIVERY

When the operation is over, say that you want to hold your baby if he or she is not already beside you. An intravenous drip is left in for some hours so that you can be given plenty of fluids straight into your bloodstream if this is necessary. If you had general anaesthesia, you may feel sick and weak for the first day or so. As soon as you feel that you can move about in bed a little, do so. Even small actions such as wiggling your toes and rotating your ankles are good for you and prevent pooling of blood in your legs.

Whatever anaesthesia you have had, the nurses will help you to get up later the same day. Although it hurts, moving around is important in order to avoid thrombosis. To move off the bed, first work your way to the side of it, roll on to your side, and push yourself to a sitting position with your hands. As you get up you may have a lot of bleeding from the vagina. This also tends to happen after a vaginal delivery and is simply the blood that has pooled in your pelvic region. Stroll around the room to encourage good circulation and, as you do so, use the slow, complete breathing that you learned in antenatal classes.

If you feel that you need drugs for pain relief, ask for them. Although you probably want to be awake to enjoy your baby, you cannot do this if you are in discomfort. The more your partner can be with you, even while you doze, the more you can relax, feeling that the baby is being looked after by someone who loves her. You will probably go home between 72 hours and five days after surgery, with instructions on self-care. Ring the hospital or your doctor if you have problems or questions. Dressings will be removed three or four days later. Because the obstetrician has had to cut through muscle, your tummy will look very big and soggy. The stitches inside your body dissolve naturally, but the external stitches or staples will be removed before you go home. Do not worry about stitches bursting – with every layer stitched separately there is very little chance of this.

After general anaesthesia, fluid collects in the lungs and then has to be coughed up. A midwife or physiotherapist will teach you the way to do this that causes least discomfort. The breathing techniques you learned in pregnancy can help too. It is natural to feel a flood of conflicting emotions after a Caesarean. Some women say that they are grateful to have the baby, but at the same time they feel "cheated". A Caesarean birth is a surgical operation and you need time to recover from it as from any abdominal surgery. For the first six weeks after the birth you should avoid any heavy lifting. If it is possible to arrange for extra help at home, especially if you already have a toddler who expects to be lifted, it is an enormous benefit for someone else to do the more strenuous work.

The passage is narrow but yielding, and the baby's body is massaged vigorously with each new contraction as she gradually descends. Beneath the stretched abdominal skin and the thinned, translucent wall of the uterus itself the baby has been aware in the last weeks of pregnancy of glowing light whenever bright sun or artificial light shone on your body. It must be rather like firelight or the light cast by a red-shaded lamp. When the journey to birth begins the baby is pressed deeper into the cavity of the pelvis, under arches of bone and a canopy of thick, supportive ligaments and muscles. Perhaps it is a sensation rather like travelling through a long, dark avenue of overhanging trees.

The baby is not just a hunk of flesh or a life-sized doll. She is a human being fully equipped to feel pain and pleasure, a person coming to birth. The baby cannot remember or anticipate in the same way that we can, but nevertheless feels keenly and is a fully sentient being. The uterus holds and presses tightly in on the child not yet born, with steadily escalating power. By the end of the first stage of labour it is embracing the baby tightly for one or two minutes each time. Each hug begins gently and grows tighter and tighter until at the height of the contractions the baby is being gripped fast for 20 to 30 seconds. Then the wave of pressure recedes again and the baby floats once more in her inner sea: she is in labour along with you.

NEWBORN REFLEXES IN LABOUR

In some obstetric textbooks the baby is described simply as "a passenger", and purely in mechanical terms as two ovoids, the head and the trunk, the long axes of which are at right angles to each other and which can take the curve of the pelvic axis independently. While this is accurate as a description of the mechanics of fetal descent, it omits any mention of what the baby might be doing during this process and how the reflexes with which she is born are also already functioning during labour.

The baby changes position in response to the power unleashed in your body, and does this not only because of mechanical forces which act on her but probably also because she is making active movements. Your baby is working *with* you towards birth, a partner in the struggle, not just a passenger, and can do this because of built-in reflexes (see page 357). A newborn baby turns her head in the direction of a touch, moves her head up and down against a firm surface, curls her toes down when pressure is applied to the ball of the foot, lifts her foot up and puts it down at a higher level when pressure is applied over the top of the foot, and makes forward stepping movements when tilted forwards with her feet against a firm surface. Two of these actions probably operate to help the baby onwards in her journey. One is the reflex to move her head up and down against firm resistance, which means that she actually wriggles her way forwards

"I expected a baby, of course, something I would hold. But he was born with eyes wide open, and as he looked at me I realized, 'this is a person!'"

through the cervix and the fanned-out tissues of the vagina, with much the same action that we make when putting on a new sweater with a rather tight neck. The other is the stepping movement when resistance is offered to the feet, so that in effect the baby pushes away from the solid wall of the uterus as it tightens around her.

THE IMPACT OF THE OUTSIDE WORLD

In the second stage the head has to take a nearly right-angled bend. The pressure builds up until it swivels the neck around so that the baby is facing downwards and ready to slide out. You can imagine that this provides a very sharp stimulus to the baby, a message that says unmistakably, "Things are changing. Wake up! It's all systems go!" At last the crown of the head oozes through the vagina and remains there. Perhaps you reach down with eager hands to stroke the damp, warm top of your baby's head. This is the first greeting.

The head slips out and suddenly the baby encounters space and air. The shoulders and chest slide forwards, followed by the whole body. There is a gasp and air rushes into the lungs, inflating them for the first time. The damp inner surfaces of the lungs, previously clinging together like wet plastic bags, open up with the first cry with which the baby meets life.

Air, space, the baby's own limbs moving in an unfamiliar medium, weight, strange sounds, glaring lights, cold hands picking the baby up and turning her over – all at once a myriad of new sensations assail the newborn. Not only must the lungs fill with air and start to function rhythmically, but the circulation must find new pathways.

LABOUR AS A STIMULUS

In his book *Birth Without Violence,** Dr Frederick Leboyer calls the mother "a monster" because of the pain he believes she cannot help but inflict on the baby as she passes through the throes of birth. But the process of being born can also be seen to involve stimulation and awakening for which the baby is ready and that prepares her for life. Looked at from this point of view, muscles hold and embrace the baby, triggering powerful sensations, then soften again in a rhythmic pattern. The space between contractions is like the trough between two waves. Inevitably the next wave comes and again the muscles tighten firmly around the child.

Although labour is undoubtedly traumatic for some babies, others look extraordinarily peaceful and contented after their journey. It may feel to you as if you are swimming in a stormy sea when you reach the end of the first stage of labour. You may be anxious that these massive squeezings of the great muscle of the uterus are causing your baby suffering. Yet in spite of the relentless onslaught of contractions as full dilatation approaches, the baby who is pressed through the cervix and down the 23-cm (9-inch) birth canal responds more vigorously to life than do most babies who are merely lifted out through an abdominal incision. The baby born vaginally has less mucus in her respiratory tract than one delivered by Caesarean section (especially an elective Caesarean) and is better prepared for the great new activity of breathing. The baby can also maintain her own body temperature better after a vaginal birth than after a Caesarean with little or no labour.

CATECHOLAMINES: THE AMAZING "STRESS" HORMONES

Stress is often talked about as if it were invariably harmful. But stress is part of active living. Labour is exciting, challenging – and stressful, for both you and the baby. As a result, hormones pour into your bloodstream and give you a "buzz." They are the same hormones that come with the triumph and satisfaction of at last climbing to the top of a mountain, or of drawing on all your reserves of strength and persistence in a race, the same hormones that flood through you when the curtain rises and you stand

"My labour was long and hard and I felt sorry for the baby. But he came out alert, peaceful, and soon started to search for my breast."

floodlit in front of an audience. There is striving, longing concern to give your utmost, and the thrill of the unknown. It is like that, too, when labour begins. These hormones are produced by the baby as well as by you, and the baby produces them in vast quantities.

All hormones are chemical messengers. Catecholamines give the baby the message of life. A surge of the stress hormones – adrenaline and noradrenaline – courses through the baby's bloodstream before labour starts. They protect the baby from shortage of oxygen, shunt blood away from non-essential organs – the skin, for example, – ensure a rich supply of blood to the heart, brain and muscles, slow down the heart rate so that the heart does not have to work so hard or need so much oxygen, prepare the lungs for breathing by dilating the bronchioles, cause fat and glycogen to be broken down and available for quick energy and in all these ways prepare the baby for the demands of life outside the uterus.

A scientist who researches the function of catecholamines at birth writes, "Nearly every newborn has an oxygen debt akin to that of a sprinter after a run".* This catecholamine surge is the reason why babies can cope so well with oxygen deprivation at birth. They handle it much better than adults, who develop heart rate irregularities after just a few minutes.

Catecholamine levels in the baby build up even in early labour, when the cervix is still only 2 or 3 cm dilated, and are about five times the concentration of those in a resting adult. These hormones surge still higher in the second stage of labour, and after the birth are double or triple the level of the early first stage, dropping to a resting level after about two hours.

Pressure on the head of the fetus causes increased secretion of catecholamines. Babies who have not experienced labour and been delivered by elective Caesarean section have much lower levels. This is why whenever possible the mother should experience some labour. A baby who is simply removed through an abdominal incision is likely to have breathing difficulties because liquid in the lungs has not been absorbed during the process of birth and because the lungs have not produced much surfactant – the substance like soap bubbles that prevents the lung surfaces from sticking together. Both absorption of lung liquid and release of surfactant are dependent on catecholamines in the hours immediately before the baby is born. Some drugs used to treat hypertension in the mother also interfere with the action of catecholamines.

A newborn baby loses heat rapidly because of her high surface-to-volume ratio. If a baby gets cold after birth, catecholamines also activate special heat-producing tissue called "brown fat". Another effect of catecholamines is to dilate the pupils of the baby's eyes and increase alertness. Mother and baby fix their gaze on each other. Each is for the other the most interesting person in the world. The baby is not only cuddly and warm, but also alert and responsive. In this way catecholamines are an element in the process of bonding between mother and baby.

WELCOMING YOUR BABY

Have you thought about how you want to welcome your baby into the world? This is not just a matter of safe or speedy delivery, of making sure that the baby has enough oxygen or is not traumatized by delivery, but also one of greeting the baby with gentleness.

Most babies cry at the shock of birth and this first cry ensures that a rush of air enters the lungs. But if they *go on* crying there is something wrong. The crying of abandonment and distress is quite different from the healthy crying of the newborn. Yet people often take persistent crying for granted and even smile indulgently and say, "She's got a fine pair of lungs!" The newborn baby continues to scream because of insensitivity to her needs and the lack of a sufficiently caring environment. If the setting for birth is changed and, above all, if the attitudes of those assisting are different, so that the baby is treated with respect, the child will become quiet, open her eyes, reach out her hands and start to discover herself. But if this is to happen the birth room must be calm and hushed, the lights dimmed and those handling the baby must do so slowly, carefully and lovingly. This is *gentle birth*.

Creating a caring environment

Gentle birth need not start only as the baby is born. In the way that labour is conducted, and in the whole atmosphere of the birth room, an environment of peace and serenity can be created. As a mother you are in such a subtle and yet intense relationship with your baby that everything done to you during labour must affect the way in which you are able to respond to your newborn baby. If you are treated as if your body is merely the container from which a baby is removed, or as an irresponsible child who has to be given orders, you will find it very difficult to be in harmony with the forces that are bringing the baby to birth, with your own body in its work of creation, and also with the baby. The caring environment for the newborn starts with a caring environment for you, a respect for your rhythms, patience to wait and watch and loving support.

Dimming the lights

It is irritating for you to labour under bright lights, just as it is for the baby to confront brilliant fluorescent light at delivery. For a gentle birth all unnecessary lighting is switched off so that the room is softly illuminated, with a clear light only on the perineum. Instead of lying flat on your back or with your legs suspended in lithotomy stirrups you need to be in a position you find comfortable and in which you can be an active birthgiver. Many women like to be sitting up, crouching or kneeling so that they can catch the first glimpse of the baby's head and can touch it even before it has started to emerge through the vagina. We have already seen (on page 246) that an upright position has many advantages for the mother in terms of mechanical function. If you are well raised you are also in a splendid position for greeting your baby.

When the head crowns some women put their hands down to caress the top of the baby's head. The head feels warm and firm and as it eases forwards you touch more and more warm, damp, silky hair. This very first contact between mother and child is beyond excitement; it is a moment of awe.

Then the head slides out and turns to align with the shoulders still inside and you can see your baby's profile; with a rush the shoulders and whole body are born. As the baby slips out and starts to breathe the lights can be dimmed further so that the baby can take her time to open her eyes in the half-light. Many years ago Maria Montessori, the educationalist, stressed that babies are assaulted by bright light. She said that they should be able to begin the gradual exploration of the world with their senses in a soft glow and shadows, similar to the uterine environment they have just left. Yet we have subjected newborns to harsh hospital lights and acted as if they were unable to see or hear.

Reducing the noise level

In non-violent birth there is no unnecessary conversation and those attendants who speak do so in hushed voices. Dr Frederick Leboyer believed that the mother should be quiet, too, and that excited voices can startle the baby. When he wrote his book, it was not known that the intrauterine environment was full of sound, particularly the mother's heartbeat and voice and the voices of others. Dr Michel Odent thinks that there is too much emphasis nowadays on the father's presence in childbirth and that fathers sometimes get too emotional. Couples who value sharing birth together would not

In a tranquil setting, the midwife lifts the baby into the mother's arms, with her finger resting on the baby's chest to feel the heartbeat (opposite).

348

agree. I feel myself and know many women who also feel that it would not have been possible to go through labour and birth without the child's father there. In fact, couples often do cry out with astonishment and wonder when they see their baby leap into life and this is a spontaneous outpouring of emotion, of joy, an integral part of childbirth, which *in itself* is a life-enhancing experience for both parents. We do not carefully work out exactly what we are going to do when we are caught up in other sorts of peak experience; we do not weigh the different factors and come up with a formula. To do so would diminish the experience. Life is exultant and we are borne along with it. Birth is that kind of climactic process. It is also an act of love, the culmination of the passion that first started the development of that baby.

PHYSICAL CONTACT

It is because birth is a peak experience that arms reach out to take and hold the baby and draw her close. It is not just that this small, wrinkled, vulnerable baby is yours and that therefore you decide to take her in your arms (although unfortunately this is just how it is for some women in a loveless, uncaring environment); if the right atmosphere exists you are totally enveloped in a rush of intense feeling. This does not mean that the baby is neglected in an orgy of self-indulgent emotion. The baby is drawn into the warm circle of love between the parents and becomes part of it. This is what it means for not only a baby to be born but also a *family*. In non-violent birth the baby is handled gently and slowly, without haste. There are no rough, quick movements. He or she is delivered up on to your tummy or over your thigh. If you ask beforehand it is often possible to do this yourself and the midwife or doctor will remind you to reach out and draw the baby on to your body.

"I lifted her out and up on to my tummy and held and stroked her. It suddenly burst on me that this incredible little creature had come out of my body! She had been a part of me. Now we were separate but we needed each other."

Leboyer believed that the baby should be lovingly and gently massaged until she stops crying and gradually becomes calm. Only then does Leboyer think the baby is ready to go to the mother's arms. In his own obstetric practice he used to do this massaging. But many women think that this is yet one more way in which professionals, however caring, attempt to take over childbirth and to intrude on the mother's natural role.

Where gentle birth is practised today it is usually the mother who holds and caresses her baby. You do not have to learn how to massage your newborn. The way you explore and stroke her is spontaneous and right. But this is only possible if the baby is naked and in skin contact with you. Babies are often bundled up in wrappings in case they lose heat. It is true that new babies quickly become chilled unless they are in a warm atmosphere and are held close. Research has shown that the baby, even the low-birthweight baby, keeps warmer when in flesh-to-flesh contact with her mother and nestling against her breast than when wrapped up and put in a cot. So ask a helper to slip your gown down over your shoulders or even to take it right off before delivery.

A blanket can easily be thrown over you and your baby or a heater can be placed over you both. Mothers often feel chilled and shaky after giving birth and appreciate the warmth. Covering the baby's head also helps to avoid heat loss.

If your baby is handed to you bundled up in a cloth, unwrap the covers and cuddle her close. Do not be afraid to talk to your baby. He or she will respond to the sound of your voice and be especially sensitive to the higher-pitched tone of a woman's voice. The baby is also getting to know your unique scent and by the time she is a few days old will already prefer a cloth that has been against your body to one that has been close to another new mother's body.

DELAYING THE CLAMPING OF THE CORD

Ask your midwife or doctor to wait to clamp the cord until it has stopped pulsating. Midwives always used to wait, but nowadays the whole birth is often so rushed that the cord is sometimes clamped and cut immediately while blood is still flowing back and forth between placenta and baby. Even though this blood is not particularly well oxygenated – because the placenta begins to peel off the wall of the uterus as soon as delivery takes place – it is important that the correct balance between blood supply in baby and placenta be reached. The way to ensure that is to hold the baby at approximately the same level as the placenta and wait for the cord to become flaccid, indicating no further flow of blood in either direction (to or from the baby). There are occasionally reasons for early cord clamping, such as a Rhesus negative mother who has already produced antibodies against her Rhesus positive baby (see pages 113–114), or a cord wrapped tightly around the baby's neck. Otherwise there is no reason why the cord has to be cut until after the placenta is delivered; it is separated only for convenience.

You can rest your fingers on the cord and feel the blood throbbing through it and wait for the moment when it stops completely. Cutting the cord between two clamps is a very simple procedure and something that a father may enjoy doing. If you would like him to do this, ask in advance.

Some obstetricians are concerned that blood could drain back into the placenta if the baby is placed above the placenta with the cord still unclamped. This is not a sufficient reason for early clamping or not placing the baby against your body. The baby can be rested over your thigh at the level of the placenta, where you can hold him. Mucus usually drains out naturally and there is therefore no need to use a mucus extractor, although the baby should be carefully observed and a mucus extractor used if his or her airways are blocked, followed by a few puffs of oxygen.

WAITING FOR THE ROOTING REFLEX

Your baby may emerge from your body already wanting to suck. But many babies need time to feel secure before they reach out to find the nipple. The rooting reflex (see page 357) is a sure sign that the baby is ready to be put to the breast. Wait until the baby shows interest rather than stuffing your breast into her mouth. Women often try to breastfeed before the baby is ready. Then even breastfeeding is another assault on the newborn. Many women are anxious to put the baby to the breast immediately after delivery and their anxiety to do this in an alien environment, and one which they may feel is hostile, makes them rush things. Be patient if you can. Let the baby rest against your bare breast and in her own time she will start to explore with mouth, hands and eyes. This time is precious for you and your baby. It cannot be speeded up without interfering with spontaneous, natural rhythms. The baby begins to lick your nipple, then seeks it and, with just a little help as you lift your breast into her searching mouth, latches on and begins to suck.

BATHING THE BABY

An important part of the Leboyer style of birth was the warm water bath in which the baby is supported shortly after delivery, and in his film illustrating gentle birth the bath is given even before the mother holds her baby. Leboyer believed that the baby needs time to feel safe in the medium which she has just left in the uterus – water – and that suspended in a bath the baby becomes peaceful and sometimes positively beatific, discovers herself, and starts to open her eyes and explore the world around her. It is true that some babies seem to enjoy the bath very much, but only if it is given slowly and calmly and if the water is deep enough for the baby to float. The ideal way to give a bath is in a container with a thermal lining and an air heater over the bath or, alternatively, the mother may prefer a water birth.

You may find that the hospital where you are having your baby does not allow a bath because of the risk of hypothermia (chilling). Unfortunately, cold air ventilation ducts have been incorporated into the design of many modern maternity units and the baby in water or exposed to this air is likely to get chilled. Many hospital paediatricians are concerned that the baby can lose a great deal of body heat while wet through evaporation or in a bath that is too cool; they say that if a bath is given at all it should be done speedily, which defeats its purpose. You obviously cannot add hot water to a bath when the baby is in it, and you know yourself how shivery you feel when you get out of a hot bath into a relatively cold atmosphere. It is much harder for a newborn baby, who cannot shiver yet and whose largest area of heat loss is her big head, to keep warm. The baby can maintain heat through brown fat that creates warmth, just as a bear or any

"She looked at me very critically at first as if to say, 'Do you know what you are doing?' Then she relaxed and it was like watching a flower open in water."

cold-adapted hibernating animal does. A low-birthweight baby does not have enough brown fat to do this. Muscular activity and crying also help the baby to keep warm; a baby in a cool room will hyperventilate, although one with respiratory depression cannot do this. Heat loss is also reduced when blood vessels near the surface of the skin tighten up. But babies who have received drugs from their mothers' bloodstreams, including narcotics, are not only sedated but also unable to prevent heat loss efficiently. So if you want the bath to be given, bear in mind that you should not have had narcotics in the last five hours; that your baby should be full term, weigh more than 2.5 kg (5 lb) and not have had breathing difficulties at delivery; and that the room should be warm.

Parents are sometimes very doubtful about the advantages of the bath, preferring to be in skin contact with their baby and to let him or her suck at the breast indefinitely instead. If a baby is happy lying against her mother and ready to go to the breast after a little while, it seems purely ritualistic to insist on putting her in a bath because of preconceived ideas about how babies *ought* to behave.

Dr Michel Odent* uses the bath in a different way. The baby goes first to the mother's arms and sucks if she is rooting; only then is she immersed in a bath, and instead of the doctor bathing the baby the father takes over this responsibility, but close enough to the mother so that she can see and touch, too. It can be moving to watch a father doing this first service for his newborn child.

A midwife described what happened in one case when a father bathed his baby in this way: "The baby, who had been resting quietly with its mother, gradually opening its eyes, now seemed to wake to its surroundings and gaze serenely around. It is this serenity which is so remarkable and such a joy to watch. The baby's body was totally immersed in the water, which kept it warm, and gave it total relaxation. After five to ten minutes a midwife took over and gently lifted the baby on to the warmed towel below the overhead heater. There was not one cry and all handling was done with an awareness that the baby had never been handled before and that its skin was acutely sensitive. There were no sudden jerks, movements or pulling while the baby was being dressed. I now realize that the crying which so often accompanies these tasks is the result of sheer fright."*

AFTER THE DELIVERY

Gentle birth does not end with the minutes after delivery. It is part of a continuum, a flow of interaction between you and your baby, beginning in pregnancy and going on following childbirth. It is a question not just of how the delivery is conducted or even whether you are able to hold your baby right away, but also of creating an environment in which throughout the 24 hours you have access to your baby, feel she is yours, and can act spontaneously. You need to know that everyone around you understands what you are feeling, and to be confident of emotional support as you learn to be parents.

You and your newborn

The first hours of life **356**

The baby who needs special care **366**

Losing a baby **372**

The first ten days **381**

The challenge of new parenthood **396**

The first hours of life

The hours immediately following birth are for many women some of the most intense of their lives. A peak experience like that of giving birth does not suddenly subside after you have spent half an hour holding the baby or end when the lights are turned out. After such a dramatic time it is not surprising that some women cannot sleep, and that many remain in a party spirit for hours or even days after.

Unfortunately, many hospitals treat the period after birth as a time for quiet rest, once you are clean and tidy; if you are too excited to sleep you may be offered some sleeping pills or tranquillizers. Most hospitals do not make provision for the continuity of passionate feeling which ensures that motherhood becomes part of you as a person and is not just something that you are straining to learn. These overpowering emotions propel you through the interim phase between knowing nothing about your baby, who is like a stranger, and realizing you know everything about her and have become centred in this tiny new existence as much as you are in yourself.

YOUR FIRST MEETING WITH YOUR NEWBORN

You look down at this new little person, and feel the weight of the body as he or she begins to relax after the struggle to birth. The head is the biggest part, the hair silken and perhaps still wet and curled in damp fronds or streaked back as if after a swim. The ears are tiny and carved like convoluted shells and the fingernails, too, are like

THE APGAR SCALE

Immediately after birth your baby's vitality is tested; it is tested again after about five minutes. Babies who get low marks the first time usually score nine or ten when tested the second time; but a baby does not have to cry to be vigorous and healthy.

What is Tested	0 Points	1 Point	2 Points
Heart rate	Absent	Below 100 beats per minute	100 beats per minute or more
Breathing	Absent	Slow or irregular	Regular
Skin colour	Blue	Body pink, extremities blue	Pink all over
Muscle tone	Limp	Some movements	Active movements
Reflex response	Absent	Grimace only	Cry

Newborn reflexes

Babies are born with reflexes to help them adjust to life outside the uterus. Breathing, sucking, and swallowing are the most important reflexes in a newborn baby. Some others are illustrated below.

Rooting
The baby opens her mouth, often screws up one eye, and turns her head. This is known as "rooting" for the nipple.

The startle reflex
If the baby is handled abruptly or roughly the Moro or startle reflex will be seen. The baby throws up her arms and trembles.

Hand gripping
The baby is born with a strong grasp reflex and will usually grip your finger tightly.

About to crawl
When you place a newborn baby on her tummy she will automatically assume what appears to be a crawling position.

Stepping
When you stand a newborn baby up she will make "stepping" movements.

the little pink shells you picked up from the sand when you were a child. If the baby is still crying the mouth looks huge, a most efficient organ capable of reaching out to and grasping the breast for essential nourishment. And the cry itself, a high-pitched, almost animal wail, is well adapted to summon immediate attention, to drive you to find out what is wrong and how you can answer the baby's needs, and to be intensely anxious until you have stilled the crying. It is a biological mechanism of vital importance for survival.

As you hold the baby, the hands start to scan the air, encountering space, meeting the face, perhaps brushing against your body or hand. The fingers move and undulate like sea anemones, embarking on the important task of finding out about this new world.

If lights have been dimmed the baby will open wide eyes and look straight at you some time during this process of unfolding. It has been discovered that newborn babies find the human face the most attractive thing to look at, far more so than woolly bunnies or painted ducks – and the moving, speaking human face is best of all.

THE EXPERIENCE OF BONDING

The environment into which the baby is born and the attitude of all those handling the baby are important not only for the baby's sake but for yours, too, and for the relationship between you. It is far more difficult for a mother to feel that her baby belongs to her and she to him – to bond – if she does not have time immediately following birth to begin to get to know her baby.* An important element in this is naked skin contact. The baby should not be wrapped up and turned into a solid little package which you are allowed to hold but not to explore. He should be delivered on to your body and you should be able to put the baby to the breast as soon as he is ready to suck.

Marshall Klaus and John Kennel,* working at a hospital in Cleveland, recommended that mothers be able to hold their babies naked on the delivery bed and have undisturbed time to get to know them, and then be encouraged to look after them themselves, with help available if they needed it. They should have their babies with them and be responsible for them at least five hours a day, and be given ample emotional support from hospital staff. They found that when mothers and infants remained together undisturbed for the first hour after birth, and had extended contact with their babies in the first 48 hours, the attachment between mother and baby was stronger than when minimal contact (for feeds only) was allowed.

Still, in many hospitals the hours after birth are used mainly for medically processing you and your baby; and you must pass tests of fitness before being pronounced not "at risk" and discharged.

WHAT TESTS ARE CARRIED OUT?

As soon as the baby is born the midwife or doctor assesses the baby's condition and rates it at one and five minutes of age, according to the Apgar scale (see page 356). This is done by simple

Testing the newborn

These are some of the standard tests that are given routinely to all new babies. You can ask that they be done right beside you so that you can discuss the results.

The baby's mouth is checked for cleft palate ...

... the diameter of the head is measured ...

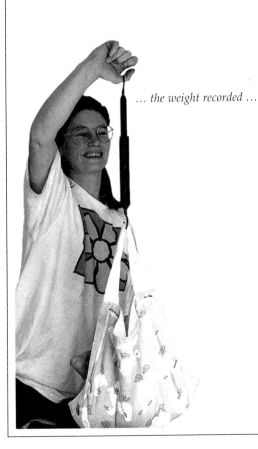

... the weight recorded ...

... jaw and hips tested for dislocation ...

... length measured from head to foot.

observation of the baby's breathing, skin colour, muscle tone, heart rate and reflexes. The important measurement is the one done at five minutes when a baby has had time to adjust to life and has received any help necessary, such as a whiff of oxygen. The highest score is ten and most babies get seven or higher. Once you have had a cuddle a further check is made on the baby. Many women say they like this check-up to be done close beside them so that they can see what is happening and can discuss with the paediatrician anything that they find worrying. If the baby stays by your side and never leaves you this will happen as a matter of course.

The baby's weight and the length of the body are recorded. The depth of breathing is assessed and noted, whether the extremities are still blue, and whether he or she responds vigorously to stimuli and seems to be strong and healthy.

Certain specific things are looked for, too. These include the size of the head, the genitals and – in a boy – whether both testes are descended. If the baby has not already passed meconium the anus is checked to ensure that it is formed normally. And the baby's heart is listened to (auscultated). The upper part of the mouth is examined to ensure that the palate is complete, and the legs are gently bent up and circled outwards to make sure that there is no dislocation of the hips. Gentle feeling of the baby's tummy discloses whether the liver and spleen are the right size, and feeling around the top of the baby's head reveals the state of the skull bones. It is usual practice to give an injection or oral dose of Vitamin K. This vitamin is necessary for formation of the enzyme thrombin, without which blood cannot clot.

"I never thought I could create something so beautiful. He is perfect, and I just lie and stare at him in wonder. And when he opens his eyes and looks at me, I am bowled over."

RELATING TO YOUR BABY

The adjustment of mother and baby to each other is sometimes treated as of secondary importance to the process of medical screening. As a result many new mothers lack confidence in handling and relating to their babies. Much of what is called "postnatal depression" is connected with a mother's inability to relate to her baby; it feels to her as if the baby belongs not to her, but to the hospital. It can be even more difficult for a man to feel that his baby belongs to him. In one Stockholm hospital, men were shown how to handle, change, bathe and weigh their babies and were helped to understand the emotional and physical stresses of pregnancy and birth on their partners. This was done on two separate occasions while the women were in the postpartum ward. These fathers became more involved in baby care later on and it seemed that they were more understanding than another group of fathers who had not been given the chance to become involved with their babies in this way. Research shows that *both* parents need an unhurried and peaceful time with their baby in the hour following birth.

How your baby may look

Your new baby may have a low, sloping forehead, a receding chin, hair in sideburns (low on the brow, in the nape of the neck and sometimes down the back as well), an odd, bumpy head that has been moulded like a ripe grapefruit in its passage down the birth canal, a squashed boxer's nose and blotchy skin. Yet to most new parents their baby looks beautiful! You respond in a protective way to the wonder of this new human being who has come out of the inner depths of your body, having been pressed and squeezed out of the uterus and down the vagina to the outside world.

Even if you are unaware of feeling anything remarkable at the time, you will probably look back at those moments as being special, as you piece together the fragments of the birth experience and place it in its setting of life lived. This kind of reflection and thinking back is especially important after a difficult labour. It probably comes spontaneously to the majority of women if they allow themselves time and do not try to forget about what happened to them.

HOW THE BABY HAS HAD TO ADJUST

Enormous changes occur as the baby adjusts to the challenges of an extra-uterine existence. One of the most dramatic things that happens, although unseen, is the change from fetal to newborn circulation, with the blood flowing along different pathways. When the baby is inside you all the blood flows in and out through the umbilical cord and bypasses the lungs, which do not need to function (see page 70–71). Since the placenta is doing much of the work that will later be performed by the baby's liver and kidneys, little blood needs to be carried to these organs in the intrauterine state.

At birth the first great gasp of air causes pressure changes in the whole circulatory system so that the baby's blood enters the lungs, liver and kidneys. The increased pressure in these organs brings about the collapse of the umbilical blood vessels and of the bypasses around lungs, liver and kidneys. Once these pressure changes have taken place the system is all set to work for a lifetime and the blood vessels that are no longer used waste away.

WHY YOUR BABY MAY LOOK STRANGE

Many things you notice about your baby may worry you. It helps to understand the wide range of the normal and to realize that the baby may look very different once she has uncrumpled after a few days.

Lanugo The dark hair that may cover large parts of the newborn's body, especially if it is premature, is called lanugo and drops out over the next week or so. The hair on the head is often a different shade from that which will grow in a few weeks' time to replace the original hair. One of my babies was born with almost black hair and in a few months was a flaxen blond.

Vernix The creamy substance that may coat the baby's skin, sometimes quite thickly, is vernix. It is produced by skin cells as they drop off into the amniotic fluid and forms a protective coating. Vernix is gradually absorbed, so it is not necessary to wipe it off, except on the head, where it tends to stick to the hair, and in the folds and creases under the arms, in the neck and in the groin.

Caput Some babies are born with a peculiar bump like a large blister on their heads, often just off centre. This is where the head was pressing down through the inadequately dilated cervix before the second stage of labour; the swelling does not affect the baby's brain, and will gradually go away. The bump is known as a caput.

Moulding Usually the brow is sloped back and rather low in a newborn baby, but some babies who were in a posterior position during labour have, when they are born, high, domed heads like figures in an Egyptian hieroglyph.

A baby who was presenting by the face is usually very swollen, bruised and puffy but, again, this gradually goes away.

Mongolian spots Some babies have patches of slate-blue skin on their tummies or backs. These are called "Mongolian spots". They have nothing to do with mental handicap or Down's syndrome, and are completely harmless. They occur most often in families of African, Asian, Mediterranean or Native American and Canadian origin.

Sexual characteristics A newborn baby's genitals can look very large, especially if the baby is premature. Sometimes there is milk in the breasts of both girl and boy babies. It is harmless and disappears without treatment. This is a result of the withdrawal of oestrogen received from the mother's bloodstream and the action of prolactin released by the baby's pituitary. Some baby girls even experience pseudo-menstruation as the result of the withdrawal of maternal oestrogen. It is nothing to worry about, and stops within a few days.

BONDING AS A GRADUAL PROCESS

Some of the reactions that you have to your newborn baby are instinctive. You respond to the sight of the baby's plumpness, the rounded head, the large forehead, the smell of the skin, the bright gaze of her eyes (which look as if they say "So that is who you are!"), your baby's cry, her exploring hands and mouth, her vigorous movement and the extraordinary compactness of her neat little body. But even instinctive behaviour needs the right setting if it is to be triggered and to unfold into appropriate nurturing. Then you can go on to learn from the baby how to respond to her signals.

Bonding is often talked about as if it were instant glue that sticks a mother and baby together the minute after delivery, and some women who do not spend the time immediately after the birth with

Meeting a new brother or sister, encountering the amazing reality of a newborn person, is a very important event in a child's life (opposite).

their babies worry that they have failed a test in motherhood and are anxious that this will have lasting effects. In fact, bonding is a gradually unfolding process that only *starts* then and develops each hour you and your baby are together. During all this time you are both learning about each other, and further physical changes in you are set off by stimuli provided by the baby. The most obvious of these is the milk ejection reflex (let-down response), which is stimulated by the baby's crying and searching for the nipple, the touch of his mouth against the breast and his sucking.

One aspect of hospital care that Klaus and Kennel stress is the way in which caregivers can support the family – not just the mother, father and baby, but also other children. Older brothers and sisters should be allowed to have close contact with the baby, too, and be made welcome in the hospital. In practice, some hospitals are still restrictive about sibling visits.*

THE IMPORTANCE OF THE TIME AFTER BIRTH
Wherever you are having a baby, and even if you are "high risk" and need obstetric help, provision should be made for a quiet, intimate time together after birth. This can be done in a big teaching hospital just as it can in a small birth centre, *and it is part of the job of the hospital to create that environment for each mother, each father and each baby*. It is only when doctors, nurses and midwives know what women want that they will be sufficiently enlightened to offer the loving environment which is every baby's birthright.

The minutes, hours and days after birth are a time for emotional "work" that may be no less significant in the lives of the newborn baby and of both parents than the sheer physical work of labour. The hospital should provide an environment that supports these unfolding emotional processes. New parents do not need to be shown how to develop a relationship with their babies. They do need, however, to feel that they are among friends, to be handed the baby at birth and to be left in peace and privacy together.

The question of circumcision

Circumcision is an unnecessary operation. It can be dangerous, too. It may result in excessive bleeding or infection. Sometimes the penis is damaged irreparably. Some babies have to be rushed to a hospital intensive care unit because of complications following circumcision. Occasionally a baby dies.

Newborn babies feel pain. In fact, they may feel it more acutely than adults. At least an adult knows that the pain caused by an operation will end. A baby cannot know this. If you are considering circumcising your son, bear in mind that amputation of the foreskin, even when a local anaesthetic is injected into the penis, is an intensely painful and traumatic procedure. It is true that some babies do not cry during circumcision. They are too deeply shocked to do so; instead, they withdraw. Whether a baby cries inconsolably or is overwhelmed by shock, he has a raw and painful scar afterwards. He is often so distressed that there are feeding problems, and a woman who longed to breastfeed may be unable to do so. Sometimes a mother observes that her baby's personality seems to have changed. Perhaps it is not only the pain. Trust has been destroyed. The rhythms of love and intimacy between a mother and her newborn are disrupted. We can only guess the possible long-term emotional effects of this mutilating surgery.

Although few doctors still defend circumcision as medically necessary, they are often slow to criticize the practice because they believe that babies cannot really feel very much, and perhaps also because they are concerned that to challenge circumcision may appear to be anti-Semitic. Men who were circumcised may believe that it never did them any harm. Some want a son circumcised so that he can be the same as "everyone else" – an argument that is also used to support the practice of female clitoridectomy and infibulation in Egypt and Somalia.

"We were under pressure from our parents to circumcise him. We did research and decided that we could not do this to our child."

The foreskin protects the tip – the glans – of a baby's penis. You do not need to retract it or work it loose. Trying to do so may tear delicate structures and hurt the baby. By the time a boy reaches adolescence it will have become more flexible.

If you are Jewish you may want to welcome your baby into Judaism in a ceremony of blessing and thanksgiving that does not entail mutilation. Do not expect grandparents to find this an easy adjustment. You may need to acknowledge the pain that your decision causes them. But ultimately it is a choice that *you* make.

The baby who needs special care

About 6 per cent of all babies weigh 5 lb (2.27 kg) or less (the internationally agreed definition of a low-birthweight baby). Such babies can be divided into two categories – pre-term and small-for-dates – and they generally require special care.

Half or more of low-birthweight babies are born too soon – pre-term or premature babies. There seems to be no obvious reason why such babies should be expelled from the uterus so early, and research is still being carried out into the causes of pre-term delivery. Maternal illness, smoking, poor nutrition, a high-stress lifestyle and poverty are all associated with pre-term delivery, but sometimes none of these factors is present in pre-term births.

Small-for-dates babies are born at the right time but have not flourished in the uterus in the last months of pregnancy for a variety of reasons. Sometimes this happens because of malnutrition in the mother, because of her smoking, pre-eclampsia or high blood pressure, because the placenta has not been working well (placental insufficiency), or because she was carrying twins or more. These undernourished babies often have difficulty during labour, are short of oxygen and have problems with breathing after delivery. They may suffer from hypoglycaemia (low blood sugar) or have convulsions. A few small-for-dates babies, however, are small right through pregnancy for genetic, chromosomal, or other reasons.

THE BABY WITH POOR TEMPERATURE CONTROL

Low-birthweight babies may have problems during labour and are also more likely to have poor temperature control, because there is very little fat under the skin. They may be jaundiced, difficult to feed and susceptible to infection. Their skin is usually red because the blood vessels are visible through the thin layer of fat. Such babies are kept in a nursery that is warmer than the wards and may be cared for in incubators. A thermostat may be strapped to a baby's tummy so that the temperature can be regulated according to his or her needs. Sometimes a baby is placed under a plastic heat shield and wears a hat. Tiny babies who are kept warm grow faster.*

THE BABY WITH BREATHING DIFFICULTIES

Premature and low-birthweight babies may have interrupted breathing (apnoea) in the early days after the birth. This is why a very tiny baby is kept on a special mattress which sets off an alarm should breathing stop. All that is usually needed to start the baby's breathing is a little stimulation of the baby by touch. One in every ten premature babies has insufficient surfactant in its lungs.

care unit rather than merely visiting. When a woman can start to look after her baby herself, she begins to feel that her baby belongs to her. One model intensive care unit has rooms where babies are cared for by their mothers, with a glass wall at the side of the babies' cubicles so that nurses can keep a constant eye on them. A nurse in this unit said: "One thing the nurses must not do is to take away responsibility for the baby. We always try to make a mother feel that it is her baby, even when it is very small and sick".

THE BABY WITH A DISABILITY

The moment when someone tells you, or when you yourself recognize, that your baby is not "normal" is engraved on your mind forever. This happens to 3 in every 100 women. The most common handicaps are cerebral palsy, which can affect both brain and body, and Down's syndrome, which has a genetic cause. For many disabilities no cause is known. It used to be thought that cerebral palsy was always caused by lack of oxygen during labour and birth, but it is now known that it is more likely to be a result of oxygen deprivation during pregnancy. There is no way a mother could have known about this or taken steps to avoid it.

Your first reaction to being told that an abnormality is suspected may be simple denial. It cannot possibly be, or if there really is something wrong they will discover that it is minor. As tests are done and information trickles in, you may start to feel cheated. You see other mothers with their perfect babies and ask, "Why me?" Having a baby with a disability sets you apart from other mothers and may make you feel not only different but stigmatized. There may be an overwhelming sense of guilt: "What did I do wrong?" Although you are assured that nothing you did or did not do brought about this outcome, you probably continue to blame yourself even when your rational mind acknowledges that bad things

"We couldn't believe it. We hoped that they'd say, 'There has been a mistake. The baby is going to be fine.'"

happen in life that you cannot possibly control. Other peoples' attitudes are often very difficult to cope with, whether it be their careful avoidance of the topic, their pity or the ways in which they try to be positive and reassuring. Feelings of shame and resentment jostle with anger. You want to blame someone but there is no one to blame and, of course, you feel a realistic anxiety about the future. Since one of the most painful things about having a child who is different is the isolation that often results, it is a good idea to contact one of the organizations that enable you to meet other parents who have children with the same disability, in order to learn more, share experiences and develop coping strategies. Addresses of these organizations are given on pages 413–414.

Losing a baby

Many women know what it is like to have an interrupted pregnancy, although the distress caused by even an early miscarriage is often underestimated. Stillbirth, on the other hand, is now rare. But still today, for a small number of women, the birth is also a death.

Women who make the painful decision to have a termination, because of fetal handicap or for any other reason, may grieve deeply, too. This is so even though they know that they have made the best possible choice under the circumstances and have behaved sensibly. A termination should never be dismissed as a simple expedient to get rid of an unwanted pregnancy. Yet it is still largely a taboo subject, and women often have to go through the experience alone, without any help, socially isolated and deprived of the emotional support they need.

Most people might find it easier to sympathize with a woman whose baby dies at birth. Yet often they do not know how to help and they withdraw from her grief in embarrassment. After all the woman's preparations and her happy expectations, she goes through a labour that culminates in the delivery of a stillborn baby, or of a frail or handicapped baby who dies a week or so after birth. Her arms are empty and she is left alone. The more medical advances reduce perinatal mortality, the more isolated is the woman whose baby dies.

Miscarriage

A miscarriage usually comes as a terrible shock, and yet one in every five pregnancies probably ends in miscarriage or "spontaneous abortion". In three out of four cases this occurs before the tenth week and sometimes even before the woman realizes she is pregnant.

THREATENED MISCARRIAGE
In the first three months of pregnancy, you may notice a heavy feeling around your pelvis and in the pit of your tummy and have period-like twinges and aches.

Sometimes you may have bleeding that is really a suppressed period. This happens when there is insufficient pregnancy hormone to stop your period, even though it will be scanty. Such bleeding is not a miscarriage and the blood comes from the endometrium, not from the placenta or the baby. Sometimes this also occurs at the time when each period would have been due, and right through the early months of pregnancy each would-be period is marked by slight bleeding. Some doctors may advise injections of progesterone to stop this bleeding. Bleeding in pregnancy is not the baby's blood but yours, and comes from the maternal side of the placenta where it is not adhering to the uterus, or from around the cervix. It used to be thought that the best thing was to go to bed and stay there until the bleeding stopped. There is, however, no evidence that this is of any help at all.* So do whatever makes you feel more comfortable.

INEVITABLE ABORTION
An "inevitable abortion" is a miscarriage that occurs because the baby is no longer alive and, whatever you do, the bleeding is bound to continue. If the fetal heart cannot be detected by ultrasound (see pages 223–226), the abortion is inevitable and you might just as well be up and about and let it run its course. If ultrasound picks up the baby's heartbeat, there is only a 10 per cent chance that you will miscarry, even though you may go on bleeding for a while.

POSSIBLE CAUSES OF EARLY MISCARRIAGE
The cause of early miscarriage is often not known. Defective embryos with abnormalities that would not allow them to survive after birth are usually miscarried, and a large proportion of miscarriages are probably the natural way of getting rid of imperfect babies. Sometimes there has been no development beyond the very early stages of segmentation and what is termed a blighted ovum is passed. It is estimated that one in six miscarriages may result from fertilized eggs that do not develop properly.

After it had been noted that more women than usual miscarry in early pregnancy during influenza epidemics, it was discovered that a high fever can result in miscarriage. There is more about this on page 111. Sometimes the presence of uterine fibroids (common in older mothers) or an oddly formed uterus results in there not being enough space for the pregnancy to develop.

Cleaning out the uterus Some doctors take it for granted that a woman who has had a miscarriage should go to hospital for a D & C (dilatation and curettage) to scrape out surgically any remaining contents of the uterus, in order to avoid infection. This is a traumatic experience. Research using ultrasound shows that it is rarely necessary.*

There may be a hormonal factor in some miscarriages, since one third of women who have repeated miscarriages have also found it difficult to get pregnant. (Insulin-dependent diabetic women with poor glucose control have up to three times more miscarriages than other women.) Occasionally, recurrent miscarriage is a sign of an auto-immune condition. The mother produces antibodies that cause blood clots in the placenta. Low doses of aspirin throughout pregnancy may help these women.

LATE MISCARRIAGE
Miscarriage after the 12th week of pregnancy is approximately three times less common than in early pregnancy. Miscarriage is more likely as you grow older (over 35), if you have had difficulty in conceiving (if it has taken longer than six months), and if you have

had two or more previous miscarriages. If you have had only one miscarriage before, there is no obvious reason why the next pregnancy should not be straightforward. After three miscarriages there is a 50/50 chance of miscarrying again, so talk to your doctor *before* you become pregnant again and plan your time to include extra rest from the first days after possible conception.

"Incompetent" cervix Late miscarriage is often the result of a weak or "incompetent" cervix which starts to dilate long before it should. The bag of waters is wedged between the baby and the cervix and ruptures as the cervix starts to dilate, so the first sign may be the breaking of the waters. This type of miscarriage is particularly likely if a woman has already miscarried repeatedly in mid-pregnancy. An incompetent cervix may be the result of a previous abortion if it was done after the 12th week, or of a previous difficult labour. There is more information about this on page 115.

Placental insufficiency Miscarriage after the 20th week may occur because the placenta has failed to function in servicing the baby. (After 21 weeks the loss of the baby is termed a stillbirth.) If there is evidence of poor placental function and inadequate growth of the baby in the uterus, bedrest will allow a better flow of blood through the placenta to the baby. One way you can improve the efficiency of the placenta is by making sure that you have a good diet during pregnancy. If you have had a miscarriage, it is recommended that you start a high-standard diet before you become pregnant again (see pages 93–100). If you have had a series of miscarriages, keep any large blood clots from the latest one (a vacuum-sealed jar is suitable) for the doctor to see and perhaps have tested in a laboratory.

GUILT ABOUT A MISCARRIAGE

Every woman who has had a miscarriage wonders if anything she did or failed to do caused it. A miscarriage can happen at any time, so most women will be able to think of some event that might have triggered it. You had a fight with someone in the office, your mother-in-law came to stay, you slipped in the street, had just had intercourse or were overtired from a party the night before.

"I miscarried late in pregnancy, so I started to lactate. It felt as if my breasts were weeping milk for my lost baby and it was all being wasted."

Whatever your guilty suspicions, none of these things has been shown to cause miscarriage. However, it can be difficult to convince yourself that you are in no way responsible.

GRIEVING FOR THE LOST BABY

Miscarriage, however early it occurs, is for most women equivalent to the loss of a baby. If it was to be your first child it is also the loss of yourself as a mother, and when you have had repeated miscarriages you have experienced this loss over and over again. It may be the loss of your partner as a father, too, and of your parents as grandparents. It may be a child's loss of an expected brother or sister. So it is a time for grieving. But women often feel ashamed about this and fear that they are being "over-emotional" or "silly".

Talk with your partner about what you are feeling. Even if you have not yet felt fetal movements, the loss of your baby is sometimes emotionally shattering. If you have had miscarriage after miscarriage or are slow to conceive, you may experience every single period as the loss of a baby and may grieve as a result. This grieving is necessary for you to be able to look forward to the future with confidence in yourself as a "real woman". Suppressed grief always causes trouble later.

Your partner, however, may not have accepted the reality of the pregnancy by the time you miscarry, so that it can be difficult for him to understand why you need to mourn, but it will help you if he can take time to listen. Or you may find you can talk more easily with another woman who has been through a miscarriage herself.

After it is all over, the longing to start another pregnancy can interfere with relaxed and spontaneous sex. If you feel that you are getting anxious and that this is spoiling your sexual relationship, try having a holiday from each other and coming together again at the time when you expect to be ovulating (see pages 62 and 405).

Stillbirth

"I'm so sorry. Your baby has died." Almost every expectant mother has thought at some time that someone might say these words to her. For some women it is a nagging fear that haunts them as they punish themselves for negative feelings they have about the baby and about becoming a mother, or for daring to expect too much of the birth and the baby. Sometimes, not as often as in the past, but nonetheless in about eight out of every thousand births, it really happens and the baby dies before, during or shortly after birth.

THE EXPERIENCE OF LOSS
Despite everything that anyone can do you are suddenly confronted with the experience of loss. This is a loss not only of the baby, but of all the expectations of yourselves as parents and the new images of the self and the family that have been built up through pregnancy.

Nothing can take away the suffering that accompanies stillbirth. This is so even when the care that is given to you is loving and sympathetic, although such emotional support can help you deal gradually with the experience and eventually come to terms with it. Unfortunately some members of hospital staff cannot cope with their own feelings of guilt and distress when a baby dies, and you may be left alone in your room, avoided as much as possible by nurses and doctors who do not want to "upset" you by referring to what has happened. When they do talk to you, they may urge you to put it behind you, say that you will forget when you have another baby or tell you to think of your partner. The more such advice is given the longer it may take to live through the experience.

You will be offered bereavement counselling, and although you may not feel like it at the time, it helps to have someone to talk to who is not a friend or relation. The task of grieving is a personal and intimate one. It consists of slowly and painfully integrating the experience into the total pattern of your life and finding a place for it in which it has meaning. (Sometimes you may feel that you will never succeed in doing it.) Once you have done this you will be able to stand back from it a little and will no longer be overwhelmed by it. This process cannot be hurried and if an attempt is made to force the pace grieving will be delayed and you may be overpowered by grief at a later stage of your life.

Stillbirth in Third World societies

A hundred years ago everyone expected a certain proportion of babies to die. A woman bore ten and reared six if she was lucky. In many Third World countries even today, babies are not named or spoken of publicly for the first few weeks because the chances are that they will not survive. It has been suggested that the mothers themselves are able to remain slightly emotionally detached from a new baby whose life may be transitory.*

In these societies death is incorporated into the web of life and there are supportive rituals to deal with it, whereas we are ill-prepared in Western society for facing death. We each struggle to find our own way and often feel that we are the only people who have ever faced such emotional upheavals. Death is a shocking intrusion into the normality of existence.

Facing up to the loss

If professional helpers know that something is going wrong with your birth, you have a right to expect them to give you clear information, discuss the difficulties openly and honestly and stand by you as you try to cope emotionally with what is happening. Women who have been through this ordeal say that it helped to be told the truth and to be fully involved rather than shielded from the event by the mystique of medical practice. If your baby dies while still inside the uterus, you know that you are carrying a dead baby. It is then as if your uterus, a place of life, has become a grave. The obstetrician may advise that it is safer to wait to go into labour naturally, which often happens within a couple of weeks, but may offer you induction if you wish. Many women feel an urgent need to "get it over with"; others feel that they want to spend the last remaining days possible with the baby inside them.

When something so distressing happens, there is no easy "solution", no one course of action that can wipe out the anguish. Sometimes a man asks what he can say or do to help his partner and to make the suffering less, or other family members or friends want to help but do not know how. People are so different in their responses to loss that the most helpers can do is to make themselves available, reach out and be ready to receive whatever the bereaved person wants to tell them, without holding back for fear of intruding or feeling embarrassment at her grief. The most valuable thing they can offer is a *waiting silence*, without tension or unnecessary words, so that the sufferer's pain can flow into them.

MOURNING FOR THE BABY

This may sound simple, but it can be very difficult, because grieving is a matter not just of tears and sadness, but also of numb shock and guilt and anger, all of which are felt at different phases of the experience. It is not easy to acknowledge destructive guilt, and even harder to cope with anger that involves hostility towards people, including doctors, and midwives who tried to help.

For you the time immediately following the death of a baby may be a time of frozen half-awareness of what has happened, and frequently it is not until at least three weeks afterwards that you begin to live through these other phases of grieving.

It is sometimes difficult for a mother to mourn her stillborn baby because she never really knew this person for whom she is grieving. It can be still more difficult if you have not *seen* the dead baby and realized that your bulging tummy held a living creature that has since died. This is why some grief counsellors and paediatricians think it is a good idea for a mother to touch her stillborn child, and encourage her to do so. You can ask to hold your baby and to be left alone to say goodbye to her. Take as long as you need.

"I needed to be held and cuddled, but it was hard for my husband to do this, as he was trying to be strong and hide his emotions."

THE BABY'S BURIAL

You and your partner may wish to discuss together arrangements for the baby's burial. Some women do not wish to know where the baby is buried, but others do. It is up to you to learn as much or as little as you wish to know. Some women feel afterwards that perhaps the baby was a figment of their imagination and never actually existed at all. It was removed from them like a tooth that was causing trouble and was then extracted. You may think of your baby's body being handled with indifference and lie awake wondering what "they" did with it.

THE EFFECT ON YOUR RELATIONSHIPS

Being depressed affects all our relationships with other people, including those we love and need the most. Although the death of a baby may draw you and your partner closer together, it introduces stresses into the relationship that may be too severe for you to be able to cope with effectively. You both may need help from other people. Your partner has to grieve, too, and yet may feel that it is "unmanly" for him to show any emotional weakness and that he must be strong to support you. The result may be that he simulates a matter-of-fact acceptance of the inevitable and leaves you feeling isolated because he seems not to understand.

If the baby lived for a time and went to the special care nursery, your partner probably had a chance to go there and see and touch the baby while you may have stayed on the maternity floor. So you rely on his descriptions and the details he can give you to be able to build up a complete picture. Yet a man who is himself depressed and grieving may find it difficult to talk about such things without showing his own distress and may resist it, thus giving you the impression that he is holding back on vital information.

Losing a baby almost invariably causes a deterioration in the couple's sexual relationship. It is difficult to feel sexually excited when you are depressed. Even when you are beginning to "function" again, feelings of pleasure can be followed by a rush of grief. When you start to enjoy life again, or start to feel sexually aroused, you may both feel at times that you are betraying your dead child.* So both of you need to give understanding to each other.

If you have lost your baby and want to be in touch with other people who have undergone this experience, contact one of the organizations that are listed on page 413–414.

The next pregnancy

If you have had a termination or have lost a previous baby as a result of miscarriage or stillbirth, or if your baby died after birth, the previous experience tends to cast its shadow forwards. Strangely, this tends to happen even if you really did not want that particular pregnancy to continue.

A woman who has lost a baby through accident, who has had miscarriages, for example, or a cot death, may feel angry that the emotions of one who has had a termination should be discussed in the same context as her own ordeal and even that the woman who got rid of a baby deserves whatever happens to her. Yet the experience of loss may be equally haunting and the sense of guilt even greater.

We tend to compare and contrast the progress of the present pregnancy with past pregnancies. If a previous pregnancy had an unhappy outcome, it colours our view of the whole experience and it is natural to become acutely conscious of risks and dangers. We do not always realize that this is what we are doing, since a common way of trying to deal with fear and anxiety about repeating a traumatic experience is to attempt to shut out thoughts of it, to protect ourselves from the pain of yet another failure.

A woman who feels guilty about aborting a previous baby or who feels somehow responsible for a miscarriage may transfer this guilt to the present pregnancy and be anxious that she is going to have a terrible labour, bear an abnormal baby or lose the baby as a kind of retribution or punishment. This is not a rational or even necessarily a conscious thinking-through of the risks, but a kind of primitive expectation that automatic punishment comes from the gods.

If you try to forget what happened or to put it to the back of your mind, you will be unprepared for the emotions that may assail you in stressful situations, when you have a vaginal examination for example, or when you go into hospital. When labour starts you may find that you cannot help thinking back to the loss of the other baby.

You may tell yourself to be sensible and not to dwell on negative thoughts. Although understandable, this is rarely successful. You are right to acknowledge your feelings and also justified in getting those who care for you to take them seriously. But do not leave this process until the end of pregnancy and certainly not until you go into labour. Try to find the kind of preparation for birth that includes frank and open acceptance of any previous unhappy experience.

"It was as if I were betraying my dead baby when I became pregnant again. I couldn't help feeling guilty."

In a pregnancy following the loss of the baby, women often experience painful, disturbing dreams about bearing a damaged child or losing the baby and feel that in some awful way this is their own fault. The dreams may be clearly about birth and babies or may be heavily disguised. The baby is often represented in such dreams as a doll or small animal or one's own tooth or limb, and death as the irretrievable loss of something that is treasured.

You may feel that you are carrying a baby of the same sex as the previous one or even that you are pregnant with the child you lost before. That is one way of trying to cope with the painful experience. In fact, some people even say, "Have another baby and you'll forget about it". But of course you cannot really substitute one baby for another or replace a lost baby by getting pregnant again. It is vital for both you and the baby you are bearing that you work towards an acknowledgment that this baby is its own unique self.

The first ten days

It is recognized that a woman with a child who is handicapped or ill, or who has a baby who dies, needs to pass through a period of grieving. It is less well understood that for *any* woman the time immediately after birth may be experienced as a loss which she needs to grieve over, however perfect the baby. As a new mother you are on the threshold of a new beginning that entails the death of some aspects of your self and, with the birth of a first baby, also the relinquishing of the self as child and adolescent.

Emotions after birth

UNSUSPECTED EMOTIONS
Many women need time to part with the fantasy baby they carried inside them before they can come to terms with the real baby who has been born. The real baby is often astonishingly different from the one they imagined they were bearing. The death of a fantasy that has been cherished can be painful. It is especially threatening if the baby is premature and needs to have special care, or suffers from any form of handicap. But even a healthy, mature baby may be so unlike what you expected that you cannot come to terms with the reality or with the fact that you have been turned into a mother with different responsibilities from those you had before, who is emotionally committed to that baby for every minute of every day.

CHANGES IN MOOD
All the intense feelings you have during the hours and days after having given birth have biological survival value for the baby. Without them you would be just a caretaker. Sometimes your emotions are mind-altering and if you had not just had a baby would rightly be thought pathological. But during the first week after birth they are perfectly normal and experienced by many more women than ever openly admit to them.

It is not just a matter of depression. In fact, you may feel on a permanent high. But it is likely that at some time during the first five days after the birth you will experience an abrupt drop in mood and a sudden feeling of depression. Your stitches are uncomfortable, the first days at home are like a thick fog, you start to worry about the baby or whether you will be a good mother, or you simply feel flat because the party is over and it is now "the morning after the night before". Then again, you may experience violent mood swings and feel you are on an emotional roller coaster in the days immediately after the birth. You are more likely to feel like this if you usually have pronounced mood swings anyway. Our society often has a very romanticized stereotype of the new mother in a frothy pink negligée

A mother gives her newborn his first taste of one of the great pleasures of the first year of life (opposite).

381

with a cherubic baby in her arms. The violent mood swings that you may experience can come as a shock because they are so different from the way you think you *ought* to feel.

NEEDING TO BEHAVE SPONTANEOUSLY

You do not become a different person once you have a baby, but all the colours of your personality become more vivid. You want to cry and then a short while later laugh helplessly at something that is not really very funny. And this is why indignation you may feel about something or someone in the hospital – and above all, longing for your baby if he or she is in a nursery – seems to have a physical impact, knotting your stomach, drying your throat, burning you up.

Some women who have their babies in hospital are emotionally unstable until they get home. For these women an institutional setting is unsettling and confusing. They have a great need to be *in their own place*. On the other hand, if you are sent home within 24 or 48 hours of the birth, you may not feel ready. You may not have successfully breastfed your baby; you may have painful stitches; there may be no one there to help you. You may feel frightened and helpless at the prospect of taking on all that responsibility so soon. There is nothing at all abnormal about you if you feel like this. The most important thing is to acknowledge the kind of person you are and for your partner to accept it, too. Then you can make arrangements as decisively and speedily as possible.

"I was very depressed but told no one, as no one asked and I felt too terrible about it to bring up the problem."

If all is going well with you and the baby, and you have help at home, it works well to leave hospital as soon as possible. A midwife will visit you at home for ten days following the birth, and longer if necessary. There is a strong case to be made for being in contact with her before you have your baby and to have her telephone number. You will then avoid the occasional breakdown in liaison between hospitals and community health services, or the times when the whole machinery suddenly grinds to a halt, such as during public holidays as well as weekends.

COMPLICATED EMOTIONS

Your partner may be experiencing violent emotions at this time; he too may be torn between laughter and tears. Our society tends to stress that men ought to be strong and offer broad shoulders for a new mother to lean on, but some men are so deeply touched by the experience of birth that they undergo much the same emotional turmoil as the new mother. A father may suffer as he goes back home after the birth, because he is surrendering you and his newborn baby to the care of strangers. In spite of rejoicing and excitement, there may be an undercurrent of grief. The intimate bond linking him to the woman who has borne his child is cut by enforced separation. When he returns to the hospital it is as a visitor.

Your changed body

After you have had a baby you encounter your body in a dramatically changed state. Whereas before you enjoyed your smooth body heavy with fruit, the curve of your abdomen like an enormous melon still awaiting the harvest of birth, after birth you may feel astonishingly alone, bereft and empty. If you are in the hospital without people you love near you, in the care of people who treat you as just another "mum" or, worse still, as an involuting uterus, a sutured perineum and a couple of lactating breasts, you need time to come to terms with your changed body and to rediscover yourself as a person.

For many women the euphoria of having given birth and of having produced a real baby, which comes as a delightful surprise at first, gives way to this confrontation with the body. Changes in the breasts associated with breastfeeding can be an ordeal for some women. Many set their sights on the birth, seeing labour and delivery as the challenge, and are ill-prepared for the new challenges that follow immediately afterwards. One mother who felt a revulsion at her much-changed body exclaimed: "But it was all supposed to be *over!*" Once the baby had arrived she wanted her self back again.

WEIGHT LOSS

Immediately following delivery you probably feel beautifully slim and lightweight. You have lost the combined weight of the baby, the placenta, the amniotic fluid and membranes. It is only when you first put your hand down on your tummy that you become aware of the folds of skin, like a soft and soggy cream puff. When you first catch sight of yourself naked in a full-length mirror you may be horrified at the amount of weight you have put on: the thickened waist, the heavy thighs and (if you are breastfeeding) the ballooning breasts – which you and your partner may enjoy if you were small and flat before, but which can be too much of a good thing if you were top-heavy anyway.

Water loss During the week after childbirth most women sweat out the excess fluid they no longer need, and any puffiness you may have noticed in your legs and ankles will disappear; so will the plumped-out facial features and the fluid that might have been retained in your fingers, making them fatter than usual.

Restoring muscle tone If you use your abdominal muscles your tummy will flatten after a few weeks, but you cannot achieve this if you go without exercise. Some exercises suitable for the early postpartum period are illustrated on pages 398–401. Brisk walking is good for the abdominal muscles: if the weather is suitable, put the baby in a carrier against your body and walk, in the country if possible. At first your pelvic floor muscles may feel as if they are sagging like a heavy hammock, but their tone will be gradually restored over the next three months and, if you use them regularly, without straining them, rehabilitation will be complete.

Breasts and breastfeeding

The sooner you put your baby to the breast the sooner her stomach will be lined with colostrum, a substance that forms a protective "paint" and a barrier to invading bacteria. Colostrum also provides the baby with antibodies to diseases to which you yourself are resistant. Ready in your breasts at the end of pregnancy, it is the earliest form of milk, rich in protein, and an ideal first concentrated food for your baby. Do not wash your nipples before breastfeeding. Babies are attracted to the breast partly by their sense of smell, and prefer an unwashed to a washed breast.*

THE MILK EJECTION REFLEX

When your baby sucks, the sucking action stimulates an area in your brain (the hypothalamus), which in turn activates the pituitary gland at the base of your brain to release oxytocin into your bloodstream. Oxytocin flows into the blood vessels in your breasts and causes specific cells around the milk glands deep inside your breasts to contract. This has the effect of squeezing the milk out through the tiny holes in your nipples.

The shape of the baby's face is perfectly adapted to sucking at the breast: a snubnose, receding chin, and a mouth that opens wide and latches on.

Oxytocin also makes your uterus contract, so you can have the odd feeling of milk being pushed down into your baby's mouth at the same time as your uterus is squeezing tight. After about a week you can no longer feel uterine contractions when you breastfeed. You will probably feel the warm, tingling glow of the milk ejection reflex immediately preceding the flow of milk. This occurs as the oxytocin-carrying blood rushes into the breasts and you feel them getting warmer. Infrared photographs of lactating breasts show that they really do grow hotter in response to the baby's cry.

The first feeds Notice what happens when you put the baby to the breast. He should have the nipple deep in his mouth and as much of the areola as will make a good mouthful. Cuddle the baby close and wait. Drop your shoulders: if they feel really stiff *pull* them down and then let them go. Sometimes it may take a few minutes for the sensation to come and then suddenly it is there: deep inside both breasts, not just the one the baby is sucking, there is a prickling, buzzing feeling as if champagne were flowing through your veins, while a wave of heat flows towards your nipples. And then you see the baby's jaws beginning to work, and the strong, steady movement of the bone at the top of the baby's jawbone, just by his ear, as he begins to swallow as well as suck.

The milk ejection reflex can happen spontaneously when you just think about feeding the baby or when you hear his crying. If he is not in your arms you can press the palm of a hand firmly against your breast and the milk flow – a slow but steady dripping from the nipple – will then come to a stop.

THE DIFFERENCE BETWEEN SUCKING AND FEEDING

Having milk in your breasts is just the beginning. Obviously the important thing is to *release* it so that it flows into your baby. For nutritional purposes it is not enough to have a baby sucking at your breasts, although he will enjoy this anyway. He needs to *swallow,* and until this happens he is not feeding.

Hospitals are more relaxed than they used to be about the time babies spend at the breast, but if you are in one where feeding time is still restricted, you should count the time from the moment the baby is actually feeding, not from when he is just sucking.

Even before the reflex occurs the baby gets some milk, because it collects in the ducts just behind the nipple. This is called "foremilk" and is rich in protein. It usually keeps the baby happy until the rush of milk comes with the reflex. But if you give a baby foremilk only, because he is not sucking long enough to stimulate the reflex, your milk supply will dwindle or never build up.

If you feel embarrassed or self-conscious or experience strong emotions of anxiety, fear or anger, the milk ejection reflex will probably be slower in coming, and sometimes may not occur at all. This is why the setting for breastfeeding in the first days after birth is so important and why emotional support from your partner or someone else who understands how you feel is helpful. Even though you may think you have emptied a breast, a fresh reflex can occur when you put the baby back to it again. A breast is not like a jug of milk, but produces a constant supply, provided that the baby gives the right stimulus.

LITTLE AND OFTEN

If you can, keep your baby with you all 24 hours of the day, and feed whenever the baby wants. If you are concerned that the baby is taking too little milk, bear in mind that the frequency of feeds is more important than their length. Look at your baby's little clenched fist: that is about the size of her stomach. Although some babies, especially in the first four to six weeks of life, enjoy sucking more or less continuously at certain times of the day, the main nutritional content of the milk is obtained during the first five to seven minutes. This is why many short feeds, with the baby dropping off to sleep in between, is for many mothers and babies the perfect style of feeding in these first weeks. You may be able to unplug the baby's mouth gently from your nipple by depressing the breast with a finger, or by slipping a finger just inside the baby's mouth to break the vacuum – but do not, whatever you do, just pull the nipple out.

BABIES LIKE SUCKING FOR COMFORT

You may feel very "drained" when nursing is long and drawn out: if you are tired and the baby is constantly demanding to be fed, it is easy to think that you cannot be providing enough milk. Although this is sometimes the case, many babies want to go on feeding nonstop because they like it so much, not because they are starving. So after about ten minutes' sucking it is sensible to put the baby down or hand him or her over to a friend or your partner for a cuddle. Relax a bit; offer some more breast milk on whichever side feels more generously supplied; then have another break, and so on.

EACH BABY'S FEEDING PATTERN IS DIFFERENT

Breastfed babies do not suck continuously through a feeding. They enjoy bursts of sucking, stopping for a while, then starting again. This is normal. If you think about meals you enjoy you will realize that you do not chomp away non-stop, either. Nor do you want an equal quantity of food at each meal. Babies are the same.

Think of each feeding as divided into different courses. Some will be seven- or eight-course banquets, but others will be only two courses. You will gradually be able to work out when the baby likes the banquets, and then you may be able to cater for them by arranging your day to fit this pattern. Somehow, anticipating and preparing for feeding sessions of this kind make them much easier to cope with, and you are less likely to feel exhausted by them.

IS BREAST MILK ENOUGH?

You may wonder if and when your baby needs any food other than your breast milk, especially if you secretly feel that your baby is not getting enough milk from you.

Water Some hospitals still give water or sugar water. The baby needs milk, not water. If your baby is producing six or more wet nappies in the course of 24 hours and frequent bowel movements and is having no other fluid, and if the urine is pale amber or colourless, this is an indication that she is indeed getting enough milk from you. You will probably find that *you* are thirstier than usual. Drink as much as you like, although there is no point in having more than you want, since it will not produce more milk. Giving a newborn baby any fluid other than breast milk may be harmful.

Supplementary bottles If you think your baby is not getting enough milk and you start to give bottle feeds, the amount of milk you are producing will diminish, since demand stimulates supply.

Solid foods When you introduce solid foods, be prepared for your milk supply to be reduced. This is one reason why introducing solid foods early is counterproductive. It replaces food the baby needs, human milk, with food she does not need until she is about six months old. A baby's appetite cannot cope with human milk *plus* all the other foods that are on the market. Manufacturers of so-called "baby foods" are often responsible for breastfeeding difficulties that start at three to four months, a common time for mothers to discover that they are failing to produce enough milk.

Test weighing Weighing the baby before and after a feed (test weighing) is a method of finding out exactly how much breast milk he or she has taken. It is a pointless exercise unless done over a 24-hour period, since the baby takes different quantities of milk at different times; even then it tends to increase your anxiety and make you feel inadequate. A much better guide to your baby's wellbeing is good muscle tone and alert responses.

Breastfeeding
For the breastfeeding to go well the baby needs to suck at the breast, not just the nipple. The nipple is drawn back into the baby's mouth and the jaws press on the areola to pump the milk.

More frequent breastfeeding When you want to increase the quantity of milk you are making, put the baby to the breast more often. If the baby has not gained weight, or has lost weight, breastfeed every time he stirs over a 24-hour period. If the baby is very sleepy, rouse him every two and a half hours if you can, except at night. Unwrap him, talk to him and "woo" him with the breast. I call this my *"Twenty-Four-Hour Peak Production Plan"*. It works in the first weeks after birth and is also useful at about six weeks.

BREASTFEEDING DIFFICULTIES
Engorged breasts Many new mothers find that they are engorged on the third or fourth day after birth, when the milk really floods in. The longer you go between feeds the more likely you are to be painfully

Funnel

Inner cylinder

Outer cylinder

Using a breast pump　　　　　**Giving expressed milk**

Expressing milk
A small breast pump is a useful accessory. Sometimes breasts become so full of milk that the baby cannot latch on. You can either hand express or express a little with a breast pump.

engorged. A cold compress, such as a cloth with some ice inside, resting against your breast, will ease the pain of engorgement, and the baby's frequent sucking will help you through this difficult transitional phase. The hospital will have a breast pump that you can use if it is important to draw off some milk and you find it difficult to express by hand, but make sure to draw off only enough for comfort.

Sore nipples Nipple soreness, especially when the baby is a vigorous sucker, is common in the first few weeks after birth and does not mean that you will fail at breastfeeding. Studies show that those mothers who go on to enjoy breastfeeding include many women who have had initial trouble with sores and cracks, and that the only difference between these and others who give up is that they persevere. Ensure that your baby is well latched on the breast and has a good mouthful.

Go topless whenever you can; avoid using soap on your nipples or using breast pads against them; and let them dry off after a feed, exposed to warm air. It is best not to use a towel and to avoid cotton wool, which tends to disintegrate and stick to your skin.

Cracked nipples Sometimes a crack appears at the point where the nipple joins the areola. This is almost invariably because the baby has not fixed well on the surrounding tissue and has not obtained a really good mouthful. If a baby drags on the nipple stem and does not draw the nipple into the back of the mouth, not only will you have problems with sores and cracks but also the baby will not be able to take enough milk after the first spurts at the beginning of a feeding. A soft, flexible nipple shield made of rubber, with a wide brim like a Mexican sombrero, can sometimes help to relieve the soreness that is caused by cracks and make nursing tolerable until the nipple has had time in which to heal. Avoid using plastic-lined breast pads, since if there is any leaking your nipples will be sitting in dampness.

Breast tenderness If you develop a red area on a breast, feeding more frequently can help. Ensure that the baby is well latched on. Exercise your arms to increase the circulation to your breasts (see page 401). If an infection develops and you run a temperature while you have a red area, cold compresses and oral antibiotics prescribed by the doctor will quickly treat it. Continue breastfeeding the baby, since this makes it far less likely that you will develop an abscess.

Excitable babies Some babies nurse with great bluster and excitement, spluttering and coughing and really making a meal out of it. In the first weeks they suddenly draw back as they start to choke, pulling on the nipple at the same time. Or they may let go for a second and then grab on again, but because they have jerked their heads back they now have only the nipple stem in their mouths so that they are dragging on the place where the stem joins the areola. These babies need a calm environment in which to feed. Talk to yours soothingly and reassuringly, and reposition her firmly and securely. If your milk comes with a sudden rush after the ejection reflex has occurred, you can see if a little boiled water or mint tea, which can be given by spoon or in a bottle, encourages her to be more relaxed at the breast. If your milk streams out fast you may need to express a little before each feed.

Sore abdomen After a Caesarean section, breastfeeding may be difficult because you find it almost impossible to settle with the baby in a position where she is not pressing on the wound. Try placing a pillow on the wound and lie on your side, or sit up and prop the baby's legs under the arm on the same side as the breast you are using.

Giving breast milk in a bottle
When you desperately need sleep and your partner wants to give the baby some feeds, it can be a good idea to express some breast milk after each feed and store it in the refrigerator. (This is perfectly safe for 2 or 3 days.) Use a sterile plastic container. If you want to keep your milk longer than that, freeze it. Express the milk after each feeding, either immediately or about 30 minutes later. If you find that milk shoots out of one breast when you put the baby to the other, you can collect this milk, too. If you do not find it easy to express milk by hand, you can buy a small breast pump. There are several different varieties on the market.

A woman who meets obstacles to breastfeeding – who discovers, perhaps, that her husband does not like her feeding in front of other men, or who sees disgust on peoples' faces when she is breastfeeding in a public place – is coming up against a social system in which breasts are considered exclusively as playthings for sexually aroused men, and in which the life-giving milk with which she sustains her baby is treated like an unclean physical discharge. Breastfeeding is an intimate personal experience and a way of loving. Once it is going well it often brings sensual feelings of closeness to and pleasure in your baby. When women fail to breastfeed it may have less to do with failing to get the techniques right than with the fact that breastfeeding can be a lonely struggle in a culture that disapproves of it being visible.

It helps to get together with other women who are breastfeeding so that you can discuss your experiences, including any problems and the strategies you have worked out to deal with them. Organizations that can put you in touch with other breastfeeding mothers are listed on page 413.

Bottlefeeding

If you decide to bottlefeed, avoid taking lactation suppressants. Bromocriptine, the generic name of the drug that was once used widely to suppress breast milk, has not been proved safe. Some women who took it have had strokes or seizures. If you want to bottlefeed or to give occasional bottles because it is more convenient, the formula you choose for your baby should be as much like your own milk as possible.

No manufacturer has yet been able to invent anything better than an *approximation* of human milk, because your own milk adapts to your baby's individual needs. Substitute milks are a great improvement over unmodified cow's milk, however, and those that are "humanized" have the proportions of fats, sugars and trace elements changed to be more like the real thing.

DIFFERENT KINDS OF FORMULA

If there are allergies in your or your partner's family, breastfeeding is the easiest way to help protect your baby against eczema, asthma and other allergies, although it is no guarantee that a child will never develop such conditions. Some babies are allergic to the protein in cow's milk. With this in mind, formula companies promote milk containing hydrolyzed protein, although it does not always solve the problem and there are reports of babies becoming ill from it. Another alternative is to use soya milk, but this may not be a good idea. Babies fed on soya milk receive the equivalent of up to five contraceptive pills a day, because soya milk contains 100 times more oestrogen than breast milk. Such an oestrogen overdose may have toxic effects.

Human milk also contains long-chain fatty acids which help brain development.* Some formula companies are now adding long-chain lipids derived from egg yolk or bio-engineered yeasts. But some babies are allergic to these lipids. Discuss with your doctor or midwife the choices that are available.

MAKING UP BOTTLE FEEDS

You do need to be scrupulously hygienic when preparing formula. It is vital that your kitchen and all utensils be clean and that you sterilize both bottles and teats carefully, and follow the instructions on the can. You can make up enough feeds for 24 hours, put caps on the bottles, and store them in the refrigerator. It is then easy to feed your baby whenever he or she shows signs of hunger, just as you would if you were breastfeeding.

Never leave warm formula out for more than a few minutes, as harmful bacteria may multiply. After the feed, always throw away any leftover milk, clean out the bottle immediately and sterilize it. Keep teats in sterilized, covered containers. When you go out, do not take warm milk with you. Take it cold, straight from the refrigerator, and reheat it in a pan of hot water or an electric bottle warmer. It is tempting to tuck the bottle under the baby's covers to keep it snug and ready as soon as the baby wants it. But if you do this you are running the risk of harbouring bacteria that is capable of causing your baby gastrointestinal illness.

Although it seems pleasanter for a baby to have warm milk, this is not strictly necessary; if the baby is impatient for a feed and you are in a hurry, it is quite all right to give a cold bottle. Powdered formula must be thoroughly mixed. Some brands dissolve more easily than others. Even the tiniest lumps can block the hole in the

When giving milk in a bottle, hold the baby close. Never feed a baby who is lying in a cot or leave a baby with a propped-up bottle.

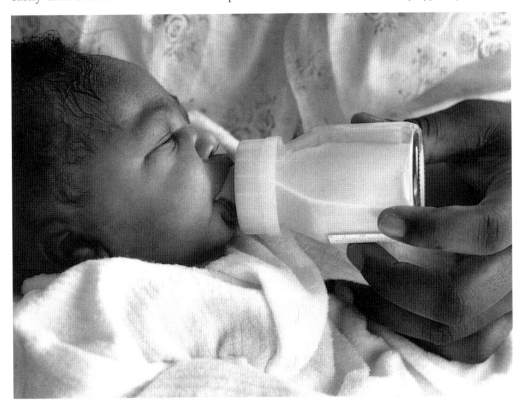

nipple and, if your baby splutters or vomits, can be inhaled and cause trouble with breathing. When you are making up dried milk, measure it very carefully and never be tempted to put in an extra scoop to make it richer, since this overloads the baby with minerals that his system can absorb only with difficulty.

The baby who is fed on formula may go longer between feeds since the milk takes longer to digest. Avoid trying to make the baby finish the bottle just because there is milk in it. In hot weather give drinks of water, too, and introduce sips of fruit juice for vitamin C at any time from 6 weeks. Formulas do contain some extra vitamins, so do not give vitamin supplements unless you are advised to do so by your doctor, and then take care that you do not exceed the prescribed dose.

FEEDING FOR PLEASURE

When bottlefeeding, remember to hold the baby close, cheek against your breast, just as if you were breastfeeding. Although it may produce a less comfortable cushion for the baby's head, a man can also do this. The baby may sometimes like to lie nestled against your partner's bare skin, and fathers who give a feed like this in the middle of the night say how much they enjoy it.

Never prop a baby up to feed on its own in a cot, however rushed you are. It can be dangerous, and it means that the baby misses out on one of the most important experiences of early life.

Sleep and crying

After being awake and alert, eyes wide open, for an hour or so after birth, the baby often sinks into a deep sleep for about 24 hours, waking only to suck and then dropping off to sleep again while still at the breast. This period is often followed by another lasting about 24 hours in which the baby may be sucking almost continuously. This is a normal pattern. It is the frequent sucking that stimulates your milk supply. Some babies suck in short bursts, get drowsy, then suck again. Others sleep for two to three hours between prolonged sucking sessions. Some babies start a pattern of evening fussing when they are one or two weeks old, which may then continue for three months or longer. Although this behaviour is tiring for you, it is completely normal. It may be a sign that the baby is over-stimulated and therefore needs to discharge tension.

SLEEP PATTERNS OF NEWBORN BABIES

When your baby is asleep you will sometimes notice that the eyelids flicker and the eyeballs are moving behind them. This is rapid eye movement (REM) sleep similar to that which adults have – the dreaming time. It has been discovered that REM sleep is essential for mental wellbeing and to prevent exhaustion.* These little eye movements also stimulate the flow of blood to the brain. Even if the baby seems to be stirring and is making little jerking movements or fussing noises, this is not a time to wake her. This kind of sleep is probably just as important for babies as it is for adults.

THE MEANING OF YOUR BABY'S CRY
Another innate biological mechanism is your baby's cry on waking, which alerts you to care for her. Your baby may also cry whenever you undress her and seem to hate being without clothes. This is nerve wracking for the new mother and father, especially if they are about to bath her. But remember that the baby was held firmly inside your uterus, hugged by its tightly enclosing walls. If your baby startles and cries when you change a nappy or when you start taking off her clothes, keep your movements slow and firm. With one hand hold the baby's arms over her chest, as they would have been folded inside the uterus at the end of pregnancy, and speak soothingly.

You will soon discover that the baby has different cries to express different needs. But in the first weeks the cry nearly always means hunger and the right thing to do is to let the baby suck. At this age a wet or dirty nappy does not really concern most babies.

Practical care
There is a great gap between studying something in a book and doing it in practice. Experiment and see what works best for you.

BATHING YOUR BABY
It does not matter how you bath your baby, so long as he is head-above-water, keeps warm and has a chance to enjoy it. Many babies hate being undressed and abhor being bathed in the first weeks of life, and make you feel that you must be a tyrant for ever doing either of these things to them. And because they cry you are convinced that you must be utterly incompetent and hopeless as a mother. The single most important thing to remember is to talk to your baby while dressing, undressing and bathing him.

If you do not want a very hot bath yourself, you can take the baby with you into your own bath. This provides the baby with a personal swimming pool. Start by placing him facing you on your knee and have a conversation. Then you will discover that you can work out little games together and the baby will find out what fun it is to splash. Have ready the biggest bath towel you can find and make the patting-dry fun, too, so that the whole process is enjoyable.

NAPPIES
The main choice is between cloth nappies and disposables. Cloth nappies really are more ecologically sound, and many women find that with a bit of extra organization washing becomes routine and they do not mind the extra laundry. Although they entail high initial expense, you can often get them secondhand, and they do work out

more cheaply in the long run if you have a washing machine. Even so, you would be wise to buy a packet of disposables before the baby is born. You are bound to resort to them occasionally when you go out for the day. Babies often soil or wet their nappies before, during and after a feed. Since many like to suck every two or three hours at first, you may need as many as 24 nappies to see you through the 24 hours, especially if you do not have an efficient tumble dryer. You can save some washing by buying disposable nappy liners and plastic pants. A nappy service may solve all the problems.

On the other hand you will be busy with a baby, and disposable nappies save time and work. There will be no pails of dirty nappies soaking, no frantic hunt for clean ones on days when you have not been able to catch up with yourself and no waiting for nappies to dry. Mothers tend to change their babies more often when it is simply a matter of taking another nappy out of a packet, rather than estimating how many clean ones are left, and that must be more comfortable for their babies. But disposables end up being more expensive, and there are none that are completely biodegradable.

MOTHERS WITH DISABILITIES
If you have a disability that makes caring for your baby difficult, you will want special equipment to help you. A woman in a wheelchair, for example, welcomes a cot and a bath on a stand the height of which can be adjusted, and with space underneath so that she can get up close to the baby. If you have back pain you will want equipment that reduces the need to bend and lift. (For organizations, see page 413–414.)

THE BABY'S CLOTHING
Newborn babies lose heat rapidly, so they need to be warm and cozy. You can achieve this any way you like, but several fine layers are usually warmer than one thick one. Choose clothes that do not have to be pulled over the head, since most babies hate narrow neck holes. In cold weather the baby's head ought to be covered outdoors.

Avoid strings and ribbons near the baby's mouth and hands, and lacy knitted jackets and shawls in which the baby will catch fingers and toes. You are bound to be given bootees and mittens; these can be wriggled off or lost, get dirty and germ-ridden. Stretchy one-piece suits are better for keeping feet covered; babies should be able to get at their hands and explore with them when they are awake.

A baby carrier is not strictly clothing but is important for your mobility. And the most useful item of clothing in cold weather is something for you, not the baby. It is a big, wrap-around overcoat, cape or other voluminous top garment. Then you can tuck the baby underneath it in a baby carrier against your body with just her face peeping out; your own body heat will provide warmth and the outer garment will hold the warmth around the baby. The baby carrier you use to begin with should be one of those where the baby is held in front of you and the head is supported.

Most babies love to be bathed when handled gently and reassuringly, although they might not take to it the first few times (opposite).

The challenge of new parenthood

Although most women look forwards to the time after the birth when they will have their new baby under their own roof, taking an important part in family life, the first days at home alone with a new baby can be filled with unexpected worry and even a sense of panic. You may suddenly feel like a stranger in your own home as you try to both understand and cope with the various needs of this demanding new person. However, you will soon learn to be able to interpret the different cries of your baby and understand exactly what it is that he or she is trying to tell you.

POSTNATAL CHECKUP

Your postnatal checkup will take place between five and seven weeks after the birth. This checkup is important in ensuring that you have complete physical rehabilitation after childbirth. The doctor or midwife will give you an internal examination to see if your pelvic floor muscles are well toned and that the uterus and bladder are correctly positioned, and will also check on the state of any scar tissue. If you have been finding that sexual intercourse is difficult and uncomfortable or if you are feeling depressed and unhappy, it is a good idea to tell the doctor at this visit. If you are dissatisfied with any aspect of the care you have received or seek further explanation of things that happened to you in labour, take the opportunity to discuss these things, too.

Sex after childbirth

For many women the full flood of passion is slow to return after childbirth. This is not really surprising, considering that so much has happened in your body and to your emotions; you may need time to find yourself again and to get in touch with your feelings. If your labour was unpleasant or the delivery traumatic then you may need additional time, too, in order to like yourself again and to gain back trust in your body.

If you have had stitches after the birth you may feel at first as if you will never want to make love again. If you are one of the minority of women who do not have stitches then you may not be able to wait to make love. So there is a great difference in attitude to making love after giving birth, depending very much on the state of your perineum. The initial healing of the tear or episiotomy wound (and it is a wound) often takes two weeks or sometimes longer, and even then you may be very conscious of having scar tissue at the lower end of your vagina.

REDISCOVERING EACH OTHERS' BODIES

Make sure that your partner knows which areas are likely to feel sore and help him to discover what feels good and where. Do not attempt to have intercourse at first and certainly do not try to prove anything to yourselves. Choose a quiet time when you need not be rushed, perhaps after a feeding when you know the baby is most likely to settle and sleep soundly. Squeeze a little lubricant jelly on to your partner's fingers and, taking his hands in yours, guide him, showing him where you like to be touched. Many couples need two or three exploratory sessions like this before they feel sufficiently confident and passionate to have complete intercourse. If you rush it, you may have unexpected discomfort and will then tense up in anticipation of pain next time, and because your pelvic floor muscles have contracted you will experience more pain.

"I was sore, and a bit scared. The baby had an uncanny knack of knowing when we were making love and wanting a feed."

When you feel that you are ready for intercourse, adopt a position in which your partner's weight is not going to pull and drag on the lower part of your vagina or, if you are breastfeeding, on your breasts. For example, if you lie or sit with your legs over the side of a low bed, feet on the floor, your partner will be able to penetrate you gently without pressing against or pulling on any tender areas. You will probably feel extraordinarily full up. Release your *throat* and this will help to release muscles around your vagina. It is best if you do not aim for simultaneous orgasm. It is usually very much more comfortable and pleasurable for you in the weeks immediately after birth if your partner comes to orgasm first and then stays still inside until you have an orgasm too.

ADJUSTING TO YOUR CHANGED BODY

You and your partner will learn a lot more about each other after the birth and, as a result, sex will sometimes be funny, sometimes tender and occasionally passionate. Even if you do not feel that you are making a wild success of your sex life in the first few months after birth, lovemaking helps both you and your baby by releasing oxytocin into your bloodstream. This helps the uterus to contract so that it returns to its previous size and shape, and it also encourages the flow of breast milk. When you do have an orgasm, milk may actually shoot out of your nipples.

You will probably find that the shape of your body has changed after giving birth to a first baby. The labia, like the outside petals of a flower, are now softer and fleshier, and away from the site of the episiotomy you may find the entrance to the vagina also more yielding. If your uterus is still involuting, you will also feel after-contractions following lovemaking. This is a good sign. If they are uncomfortable, then it is a good idea to use a hot-water bottle against your lower tummy or against your back. Even if you thoroughly enjoyed lovemaking, you may feel slightly sore

Postnatal exercises

Many of the exercises recommended during pregnancy are also good for getting your figure back after birth. It is important to remember, though, that postnatal exercises should be progressive. Do only the gentlest exercises for the first day or two. Then move on to the more strenuous ones. Never do an exercise that hurts.

Pelvic rock

Lie on your back on the floor, knees bent, soles of feet flat and your baby lying between your legs and along your tummy. Breathe out and push against the floor with your feet. Allow your pelvis to roll and your lower back to press against the floor. Then release your feet and rock your pelvis so that the pressure of your lower back is lifted away from the floor. Notice the movement all along your spine to your head, and how your back flattens as your chin rolls up from your chest and arches as it rolls down on to your chest.

The leg slide

1 *Lie on your back, knees bent, feet flat on the floor. Place one hand under the small of your back. Release your chest, press against the floor with your feet, and notice how your back also presses against your hand.*

2 *Keeping up this pressure against your hand, slowly allow both feet to slide forwards so that you extend your legs and feel the pull of your abdominal muscles. Let your toes come up off the floor. Continue to breathe.*

Feel how your back pushes against your hand

Unfolding

1 *Sit on the floor, knees bent and together, soles flat, with your hands crossed on your chest. Relax your chest and let your back drop slowly backwards with your legs sliding forwards. Feel how vertebrae in your lower back press on the floor one after the other like a string of pearls unfolding.*

Fold and unfold yourself in a rhythmic way

2 *Fold yourself together by moving your knees and nose towards each other. Then lean back and unfold again, continuing this folding and unfolding movement rhythmically.*

Sideways curl-up

1 *Lie on your back on the floor, knees bent, with your left hand tucked behind your head. Breathe in, breathe out, let your chest become soft, lift your head and shoulders and lift your left knee.*

2 *Continue to lift your knee until it touches the elbow. Stay in the position for a few seconds, breathing gently. Then slowly return to the starting position. Continue the movement on your right side, then repeat the left side again, and so on.*

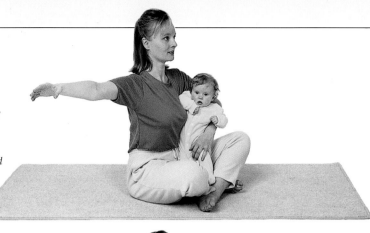

The twist

1 *Sit on the floor, legs crossed, holding your baby in your lap. Extend one arm behind you at shoulder level, allowing your body to turn with it and turning your head to look at your hand.*

2 *Lower your hands to the floor behind you and continue to look over your shoulder. Hold this position for ten seconds. Return to the starting position. Repeat the movement with the other arm.*

Make sure you are holding the baby firmly with the other hand

The hammock

Lie on your back on the floor, knees bent, feet flat, holding your baby sitting on your tummy. Soften your chest and press your feet and head against the floor, allowing your bottom to lift up off it. Rock your baby by swinging from side to side in this position. Then relax your body and let your bottom drop back to the floor.

Rocking the baby

Lie on your back, knees bent, feet up off the floor so that your lower legs are parallel with it and your baby is resting on your lower legs, face down and supported under the arms. Tuck your chin in and, slowly lifting your head and shoulders, rock forwards and back, alternately lifting and lowering to and from the floor.

Complete rock

1 *Lie on your back, knees bent, feet lifted off the floor, your hands behind your knees. Rock backwards and forwards, keeping your back rounded and an equal distance between your nose and your knees.*

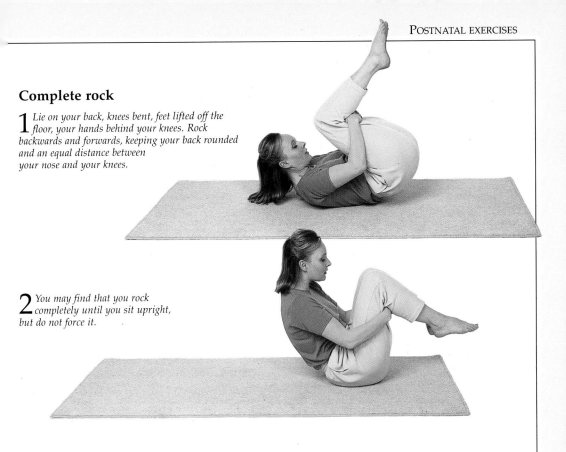

2 *You may find that you rock completely until you sit upright, but do not force it.*

Roll up

Lie on your back, knees bent, your hands holding your lower legs, elbows forwards. Let your head and knees roll towards each other, then apart, then together again and continue this rocking movement. You may find that you roll right up until you are sitting. Do not force this. You can also do this movement with your hands behind your head.

Up, up and away

Lie on your back, knees bent, feet flat on the floor, your baby lying on your chest and your hands supporting her under the arms. Gently lift the baby up above your face, noticing the pressure of your lower back against the floor as you do so. Hold the baby in this position for a few seconds. Then slowly lower her on to your chest and rock her gently.

afterwards, once the sexual intensity has faded. Again, this is quite normal. A cold witch-hazel compress held against the area may feel soothing and help to bring relief.

PAINFUL INTERCOURSE

For some women intercourse is acutely painful after childbirth and no amount of trying to relax does away with the pain. This is called "dyspareunia". It can occur when stitches have been inserted too tightly and the surrounding flesh has become puffy and swollen (oedematous) and is perhaps infected. Ask your doctor or midwife to look at the sore area as soon as possible. Sometimes it is just a question of nicking a few stitches, sometimes a matter of taking antibiotics. If you have pain up near your cervix, it may be that the transverse cervical ligaments have been torn and it takes time for them to repair themselves. Make sure that your doctor knows that you are having this sort of pain.

Many women worry that they have become "frigid" after childbirth. Often a lack of interest in sex is directly caused by tiredness. Try to rest regularly with your feet up and, if it is possible, sleep at some time during the day when your baby sleeps. Even the most active baby sleeps sometimes, and you could try to discover your baby's pattern and then take advantage of it yourself. This is more difficult if you also have a toddler, but many toddlers enjoy a cuddle in bed or on the sofa.

Although you may not feel like making love for some time after childbirth, it is sensible to have explored sensations and had intercourse before your postnatal checkup. Most women with new babies are so busy that it is not easy to fit in another appointment in order to discuss sexual difficulties, and they may hope that if they take no notice then the problems will disappear gradually of their own accord. Make a note of where and when you feel pain during intercourse and let the doctor know that you are experiencing dyspareunia and that you want help.

Sex after childbirth takes you on a new journey with your partner. It involves discovery, change, for many women a fresh awareness of the depth and drama of their own sexual feelings, and for both of you a new kind of closeness and tenderness as parents of the baby who has been born of your love.

Contraception after childbirth

There is no easy answer to contraception and what pleases one couple may be completely unsuitable for another. Many couples consider the matter in advance, so that they can have intercourse safely whenever they feel ready. Barrier methods also protect against sexually transmitted diseases, which the IUD and hormonal contraceptives cannot do. You may find that a combination of methods works best for you but, whatever kind(s) you select, study

To be a parent is all about learning. A child with a younger sibling has new opportunities for development, too (opposite).

them carefully and never deviate from the correct routine. It is not worth being worried about another pregnancy when you are only just beginning to enjoy the results of the last!*

BREASTFEEDING

If you are breastfeeding, your periods may not come back until you wean the baby or introduce some form of solid food. Ovulation, and hence the possibility of conception, can occur a couple of weeks or so *before* you have this first period. Breastfeeding tends to reduce fertility but is not an effective contraceptive unless you are suckling the baby intermittently right through the 24 hours and are giving her no other food or fluid at all. A fully breastfeeding woman may not have a period for a year. In many Third World cultures, lactating women rarely conceive. Since children are breastfed for three years or longer, this is an effective method of family planning. But bear in mind that in these societies intercourse is often prohibited during lactation, too.

COITUS INTERRUPTUS

Hoping that your partner will withdraw before ejaculation, and deposit semen outside your vagina, is not a reliable method, although it is very common throughout the world. In spite of working well for some couples, it demands great control on the man's part and may lead to dissatisfaction for you both. Sperm can flow from the penis *before* ejaculation and if you have intercourse again within a short time live sperm may already be present in your partner's urethra and be introduced into your vagina before ejaculation. Sperm do not have to be deposited right inside your vagina for you to become pregnant, and even a drop or two of semen leaking against the labia may contain a million sperm or more.

NATURAL FAMILY PLANNING

Natural methods of birth control entail identifying the period of ovulation, the phase of the menstrual cycle at which you are most fertile, and abstaining from intercourse during that time. It is impossible to calculate ovulation accurately using a calendar alone. The only methods of birth control officially approved by the Roman Catholic Church are the rhythm method and the symptothermal method. They both require that you keep an accurate record of your menstrual cycle and also a daily chart of body temperature, using a special thermometer. By doing this you can identify when ovulation occurs and avoid intercourse at that time. With the symptothermal method you also observe changes in the cervical mucus, which gets thinner during your fertile period. There are drawbacks, however: in the first year or so after childbirth a woman may not have a regular menstrual cycle, and it can be difficult to work out the significance of the changes she observes; natural methods require instruction from someone who is really skilled in using them, and a firm commitment from both partners.

Ovulation prediction There are kits on the market that can tell you if and when you are ovulating, although they are expensive. They work in a way similar to chemical pregnancy tests (see page 19), and they signal, by a colour change, the presence of luteinizing hormone in your urine, which increases a couple of days before ovulation. You start testing the urine several days after the beginning of a period and go on testing, at the same time each day, noting exactly when the equipment records a surge in luteinizing hormone. You should not empty your bladder for four hours beforehand. Two to three days after you have observed a colour change you are at your most fertile.

THE CONDOM

Made of latex or polyurethane (for those allergic to latex), the condom (rubber) is the most widely used of the barrier methods. If it is employed carefully, it is reasonably effective (12 per cent failure rate without spermicide, 1 per cent with). It has no harmful side effects. The one big disadvantage of using condoms during intercourse after childbirth is that your vagina may not be well lubricated and may be tender following an episiotomy. Unless you use a lubricant cream the latex sticks and drags, interfering with pleasure and reducing confidence. So have some artificial lubrication ready – preferably a spermicidal cream or jelly, or mineral oil, but avoid Vaseline, since this causes rubber to disintegrate. Do not use old condoms; the shelf life of condoms is about two years.

THE DIAPHRAGM

If you used a diaphragm before you became pregnant you will probably need to use a larger size after you have had a baby, and it must be fitted by a doctor or midwife, who cannot do it accurately until about six weeks after childbirth. The diaphragm should always be left in place for at least six hours after intercourse; do not, however, leave it for longer than eight hours if you have had any kind of bladder infection during pregnancy or following the birth, since the pressure of the rubber rim on your bladder could cause irritation and perhaps exacerbate an existing infection. Use about one teaspoonful of spermicidal cream on the diaphragm; never use Vaseline. It is probably best not to dust the diaphragm with powder as some manufacturers advise, since some kinds of powder can contain carcinogenic substances. Cornflour is a better substitute. Using a diaphragm will not affect your breastfeeding and the spermicidal cream or jelly cannot harm your unborn baby if you should conceive accidentally. The failure rate ranges from only 4 per cent (4 pregnancies per 100 women per year) to as high as 29 per cent, but the efficiency of the diaphragm depends very much on the motivation and care of the user.

"After the baby came, I switched to a barrier method – a condom or a diaphragm, depending on how we were feeling at the time – I didn't want to introduce chemicals into my body while breastfeeding in case it would harm her."

Sometimes ligaments running across the cervix are slack after childbirth and the diaphragm cannot be wedged snugly up under the pubic bone but slips, especially when you bear down.

THE CERVICAL CAP

This is a rigid, thimble-shaped rubber dome, into which you have placed some spermicide, which fits by suction right over the cervix itself, and which you have to place in position very carefully. It can remain in place for two to three days. It is about as safe as the diaphragm. The cervical cap is not always easy to obtain, and some doctors have not even been trained to fit it. The failure rate in women who have given birth is about 26 per cent. The cap is more effective (18 per cent failure rate) in women who have never given birth (about as effective as a diaphragm).

THE SPONGE

This is a soft, round, absorbent sponge made of polyurethane foam, looking something like a doughnut, which is impregnated with spermicide. It is inserted deep into the vagina and positioned over the cervix. Each sponge is used only once. It must be left in position for at least six hours after intercourse.

SPERMICIDES

Foaming spermicides are more effective than creams or gels because they effervesce into every crevice, but you may find that this interferes with your pleasure in intercourse. Spermicides in the form of foaming tablets or suppositories are not as reliable, because women often do not place them sufficiently high up in the vagina. You must give the tablets time to dissolve thoroughly in your vagina before ejaculation.

If you notice vaginal irritation, try changing to another brand. Some spermicides come in prefilled applicators; others have to be measured out into an applicator. One problem with spermicides is that you are supposed to lie on your back so that the spermicide does not drip out before you have finished intercourse, and this may not be the position that you would like.

Spermicides are safest when they are used in combination with other contraceptives, for instance a diaphragm, cap or condom. The failure rate when used alone is anything between 5 and 30 per cent (5 to 30 pregnancies per 100 women per year). Most spermicides contain nonoxynol-9, which also provides protection against some sexually transmitted diseases.

THE INTRAUTERINE DEVICE

It is usually easier for an intrauterine device (IUD) to be inserted and retained without cramping once you have had a baby. The failure rate is less than 1 per cent, depending on the skill of the doctor who inserts it. Copper IUDs need to be replaced every few years, and after each insertion you may feel faint and sick. Progesterone-releasing

Types of contraception

There is a wide range of birth control choices on the market, from spermicides to pills, so explore your options and discover which might be the best for you and your partner. It need not be the same method as you used before you became pregnant.

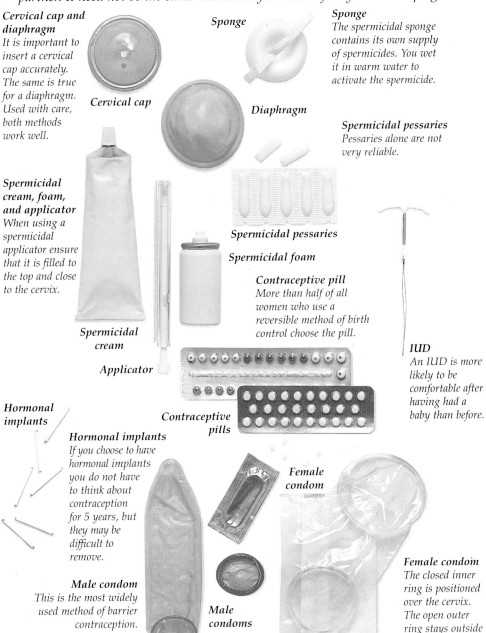

Cervical cap and diaphragm
It is important to insert a cervical cap accurately. The same is true for a diaphragm. Used with care, both methods work well.

Cervical cap

Sponge

Diaphragm

Sponge
The spermicidal sponge contains its own supply of spermicides. You wet it in warm water to activate the spermicide.

Spermicidal pessaries
Pessaries alone are not very reliable.

Spermicidal cream, foam, and applicator
When using a spermicidal applicator ensure that it is filled to the top and close to the cervix.

Spermicidal cream

Applicator

Spermicidal pessaries

Spermicidal foam

Contraceptive pill
More than half of all women who use a reversible method of birth control choose the pill.

Contraceptive pills

IUD
An IUD is more likely to be comfortable after having had a baby than before.

Hormonal implants

Hormonal implants
If you choose to have hormonal implants you do not have to think about contraception for 5 years, but they may be difficult to remove.

Male condom
This is the most widely used method of barrier contraception.

Male condoms

Female condom

Female condom
The closed inner ring is positioned over the cervix. The open outer ring stays outside the vagina.

IUDs must be replaced yearly. Avoid intercourse for the first few days. You may notice some bleeding after intercourse for the first month or so. Plastic IUDs can be left in longer; some need to be changed only every seven years. Many problems associated with IUDs are related to the way they are inserted, so the longer you can go without changing your IUD, the safer it will be.

Pelvic infection within three weeks to three months after insertion is common, but after that is unlikely in a woman who has only one partner. Infection should be treated with antibiotics, all of which pass through into your milk, although the only obvious effect on the baby may be that his or her stools become loose. In some way the thread is reassuring: occasionally an IUD is expelled or buries itself in the uterine lining and many women like to have some means of knowing whether or not their IUD is still there.

Rarely an IUD actually perforates the uterus, and this is most likely to happen if it is inserted within a short time after delivery, when the uterine wall is thin and soft. An IUD with a rounded rather than a spiky edge is less apt to do this.

There is also an IUD that works by releasing 20 micrograms of levenorgestrel, the hormone used in the progestogen pill. It is an effective contraceptive and has fewer side effects than many other kinds of IUD that are commonly available.

ORAL CONTRACEPTIVES

Although the pill is the most reliable method of contraception so far invented, there are certain conditions, some of which are not evident until pregnancy, which indicate that you should not choose the pill as your postnatal contraceptive. If you have high blood pressure that continues after the birth or if it has been discovered during pregnancy that you have diabetes, you should *probably* not go on the pill. If you are suffering from severe postnatal depression, it may also be wiser to avoid taking the pill. If you developed varicose veins during your pregnancy, you should watch for any pain that appears in your legs that could be a sign of a blood clot. If you have had a blood clot in a vein (thrombo-phlebitis), you should *not* take the pill. Progestogen changes the bacterial flora of the vagina and some women develop thrush (yeast infection) for the first time when they are taking the minipill (see opposite). If you have already had thrush this may not be the contraceptive you should choose.

The pill also needs reassessment as you get older. If you are over 35 the risk of cardiovascular disorder is increased. If you smoke you should not take the pill, since you are running grave risks.

The combined oestrogen-progestogen pill This is almost 100 per cent effective in preventing pregnancy, but is definitely *out* if you are breastfeeding. It affects your metabolism and therefore indirectly the baby's. It may alter both the quantity and the quality of milk, and there may possibly be long-term effects on the child.

The progestogen-only pill Many women who breastfeed are prescribed the progestogen-only pill, the "minipill". Since it contains no oestrogen, it probably does not prevent ovulation but works by thickening the cervical mucus, making it difficult for sperm to travel beyond the cervix. It also prevents the normal cyclical changes in the endometrium (the lining of the uterus) that allow a fertilized egg to implant. It is a less effective contraceptive than the combined pill, but has fewer side effects. There is a 1 to 4 per cent failure rate. In order to be effective it has to be taken at about the same time every day without a break.

Many women say that although their milk supply was diminished for a few days after they initially started taking the minipill, feeding their babies on demand, more or less continuously, for a day or two brought the supply back up to normal again. On the other hand, we do not really know what effects these powerful, synthetic hormones may have on the baby.

The morning-after pill (emergency contraception) A series of high-strength contraceptive pills is taken within three days of unprotected intercourse. Two pills should be taken as soon as possible after intercourse, and another two twelve hours later. This morning-after pill is useful in an emergency but, because of the strength of the hormones taken, it is not a wise form of regular contraception and often makes a woman feel nauseated. The contraceptive used is available by prescription. Your doctor can help you with this emergency contraception.

THE CONTRACEPTIVE IMPLANT

Norplant consists of six rods, the size of paper matches, which are inserted under local anaesthetic under the skin of an arm, and which release progestogen into the bloodstream for five years. As with its predecessor, Depo-Provera, approximately half of all women using this contraceptive method stop ovulating. The other half ovulate, but the hormone makes the cervix and uterus a hostile environment for sperm and discourages the implantation of a fertilized ovum. Up to 80 per cent of users have longer periods, irregular bleeding or no periods at all. The rods can be surgically removed, but sometimes there are problems with this because they have not been inserted correctly and a woman may be left with scar tissue afterwards. After successful removal, fertility returns in just two or three days. The failure rate is a tiny 0.04 per cent.

Gaining confidence as parents

Many women in our society have no experience of babies and some have never held a newborn baby in their arms. They are anxious that they will not know when the baby is hungry, that they will drop or drown him in the bath, that they will never be able to stop him

crying, or that the baby who is not crying has ceased breathing. New mothers are often too ashamed to talk about such feelings and may even repress recognition of them. Talk with other mothers and you will find that you are not alone with anxieties such as these. Talk about good feelings, too – when the baby falls asleep and lies in your arms in perfect contentment, the soft, downy head resting against your skin, when he opens his eyes wide and gazes at you with excited attention, or when you watch and feel him contentedly sucking at your breast.

You are not just a caretaker of the baby but a partner in a unique and evolving relationship. You learn more about each other every day, synchronizing with each other as dancers do. You respond to facial expression, eye movement, muscle tension – even breathing – quite spontaneously. When you act on these impulses *you are invariably doing the right thing*. When you are self-conscious you miss steps in the dance and confidence drains away.

The developing relationship between a mother and her baby is a process that needs time to unfold and blossom, patterned, just as a hyacinth bulb or a crocus is patterned, by the laws of its own inner energy. Yet this is only part of the dance. The baby's father has his own special kind of interaction with his child, as well as with you. When a man is fully involved with his baby, enjoying him, responding to his needs and getting to know him as intimately as you do, the pattern becomes even more intricate and exciting.

SHARING IN PARENTHOOD

Parenthood is a shared task. In the past fathers missed out on the baby's early months and were supposed to be interested in their children only when they started to play games and talk. But babies have astonishingly strong personalities and are different from each other even in the early weeks. It is worth getting to know the person who is your child from the outset. The man who turns his back on this opportunity to establish a relationship with the newborn baby may be denying a whole aspect of himself.

Being a parent is not just an endless series of repetitive tasks or a heavy responsibility, although all parents see it like that at times. It is a journey of discovery – discovery of the baby's personality, of who you are, who your partner is and who you are *becoming* together.

You need time to fall in love with your baby, being together in a relaxed, peaceful atmosphere.

Useful reading

Balaskas, J.
New Active Birth.
London: Thorsons. 1991.

Balaskas, J. and Y. Gordon.
Water Birth.
London: Thorsons. 1992

Bradford, N. and G. Chamberlain.
Pain Relief in Childbirth.
London: Harper Collins. 1995

Bryan, E.
Twins, Triplets and More.
London: Penguin. 1992.

Campbell, R and A. Macfarlane.
Where to be Born?
Oxford: National Perinatal Epidemiology Unit. 1994.

Clement, S.
The Caesarean Experience.
London: Pandora. 1991.

Flint, C.
Sensitive Midwifery.
London: Heinemann. 1986.

Inch, S.
Birthrights.
London: Merlin Press. 1989.

Katz Rothman, B.
The Tentative Pregnancy.
London: Pandora. 1988.

Kitzinger, S.
Birth Over Thirty-Five.
Sheldon Press. 1994.

Kitzinger, S.
Breastfeeding Your Baby.
London: Dorling Kindersley. 1989.

Kitzinger, S.
The Experience of Breastfeeding.
London: Penguin. 1987.

Kitzinger, S.
The Experience of Childbirth.
London: Penguin. 1990.

Kitzinger, S.
Freedom and Choice in Childbirth.
London: Penguin. 1988.

Kitzinger, S.
Giving Birth: How It Really Feels.
Gollancz. 1992.

Kitzinger, S.
Home Birth.
London: Dorling Kindersley. 1991.

Kitzinger, S.
Ourselves As Mothers.
Doubleday. 1992.

Kitzinger, S.
Woman's Experience of Sex.
London: Penguin. 1986.

Kitzinger, S.
The Year After Childbirth.
Oxford: Oxford University Press. 1994.

Kitzinger, S. and V. Bailey.
Pregnancy Day by Day.
London: Dorling Kindersley. 1991.

Kitzinger, S., and L. Nilsson.
Being Born.
London: Dorling Kindersley. 1990.

Lawrence Beech, B.
Water Birth Unplugged.
Hale, Cheshire: Books for Midwives Press. 1996.

Lawrence Beech, B.
Who's having your baby?
London: Camden Press. 1987.

Maxwell-Hudson, C.
Aromatherapy Massage.
London: Dorling Kindersley. 1994.

MIDIRS (Midwives Information and Resource Service)
Informed choice leaflets, often available from your Health Authority or hospital, or write with a large SAE to:
MIDIRS, Informed Choice, PO Box 669, Bristol, BS99 5FG (ask for these 'for professionals', they contain more information).

National Childbirth Trust
The National Childbirth Trust Book of Pregnancy Birth & Parenthood.
Oxford: Oxford University Press. 1992.

Odent, M.
Entering the World.
London: Marion Boyars Ltd. 1984.

Palmer, G.
The Politics of Breastfeeding.
London: Pandora. 1988.

Smale, M.
The National Childbirth Trust Book of Breastfeeding.
London: Vermilion. 1992.

Thorn, G.
Pregnancy and Birth.
London: Hamlyn. 1995.

Wagner, M.
Pursuing the Birth Machine.
ACE Graphics. 1994.
(PO Box 173, Sevenoaks, Kent, TN14 7EZ)

Mail order, massage and aromatherapy courses

Mail Order Supply of essential & carrier oils:
Clare Maxwell-Hudson
PO Box 457
London
NW2 4BR

Neal's Yard Remedies
0161 831 7875

Or visit Neal's Yard Remedies
15 Neal's Yard
London
WC2H 9DP

Massage & Aromatherapy courses:
Clare Maxwell-Hudson School
PO Box 457
London
NW2 4BR
0181 450 6494

Useful addresses

Action for Victims of Medical Accidents
Bank Chambers
1 London Road
Forest Hill
London
SE23 3PP
0181 291 2793

Active Birth Centre
25 Bickerton Road
London
N19 5JT
0171 561 9006

Association for Improvements in Maternity Services (AIMS)
40 Kingswood Avenue
London
NW6 6LS
0181 960 5585

Association for Spina Bifida and Hydrocephalus
42 Park Road
Peterborough
PE1 2UQ
01733 555988

Association of Qualified Curative Hypnotherapists
10 Balaclava Road
King's Heath
Birmingham
B14 7SG
0121 444 5435

Association of Radical Midwives
62 Greetby Hill
Ormskirk
Lancs
L39 2DT
01695 572776
This association may be able to help if you want a home birth.

BLISS (Baby Life Support System)
17–21 Emerald Street
London
WC1N 3QW
0171 831 9393
National Charity whose work includes giving support and supplying information to parents whose babies have received special care.

Bach Flower Remedies
Mount Vernon
Sotwell
Wallingford
Oxon
OX10 0PZ
Enquiries: 01491 834678
Orders: 0171 495 2404

Birth Crisis Helpline
01865 300266
Helpline for women who have been disempowered in childbirth.

Birth Works
3F Brent Mill Estate
South Brent
Devon
TQ10 9YT
01346 72802

British Acupuncture Association
34 Alderney Street
London
SW1V 4EU
0171 834 1012

British Acupuncture Council
Park House
206–208 Latimer Road
London
W10 6RE
0181 964 0222

British Chiropractic Association
29 Whiteley Street
Reading
Berks
RG2 0EG
01734 757557 Fax 01734 757257

British Homeopathic Association
27a Devonshire Street
London
W1N 1RJ
0171 935 2163

British Naturopathic & Osteopathic Association BNOA
Goswell House
2 Goswell Road
Street
Somerset
BA16 0JG
01458 840072

British Pregnancy Advisory Service
Lo-Call: 0345 304030

Community Health Council (CHC)
Association of CHC's Tel:
0171 609 8405
General advice on health services. Local numbers in phone book.

Compassionate Friends
6 Denmark Street
Bristol
BS1 5DQ
0117 953 9639
If you have suffered bereavment, will help by putting you in touch with others with a similar experience.

Contact A Family
170 Tottenham Court Road
London
W1P 0HA
0171 383 3555
This organization can put families in touch with each other whose children have disability, physical or mental.

Down's Syndrome Association
155 Mitcham Road
London
SW17 9PG
0181 682 4001

'Eating for Pregnancy' Helpline
01142 424084

Family Planning Association
St Andrew's House
27–35 Mortimer Street
London
W1N 7RJ
0171 636 7866

Gingerbread
16–17 Clerkenwell Close
London
EC1R 0AA
0171 336 8183
Local self-help groups for single parents and their children.

Incontinence Foundation
2 Doughty Street
London
WC1N 2PH
0191 213 0050 (weekdays 9am–6pm)
Information and confidential help.

Useful addresses *continued*

Independent Midwives Association
Nightingale Cottage
Shamblehurst Lane
Botley
Hampshire
SO32 2BY
Mostly home births.

International Institute of Reflexology
15 Hartfield Close
Tonbridge
TN10 4JP
01732 350629

Kith and Kids
The Irish Centre
Pretoria Road
London
N17 8DX
0181 801 7432
For parents of handicapped children.

La Leche League (Great Britain)
Box 3424
London
WC1N 3XX
0171 242 1278
Help with breastfeeding.

Maternity Alliance
45 Beech Street
London
EC2P 2LX
0171 588 8582

McTimoney College of Chiropractic
14 Park End street
Oxford
OX1 1HH
01865 246786

Meet-a-Mum Association
14 Willis Road
Croydon
Surrey
CR0 2XX
0181 665 0357

Miscarriage Association
Clayton Hospital
Northgate
Wakefield
WF1 3JS
01924 200799
Information and support during and after miscarriage.

National Childbirth Trust
Alexandra House

Oldham Terrace
Acton
London
W3 6NH
0181 922 8637
For information about antenatal classes, breastfeeding, doulas and postnatal support.

National Council for One-Parent Families
255 Kentish Town Road
London
NW5 2LX
0171 267 1361

National Drugs Helpline
Freephone: 0800 776600 (24 hours)

National Health Information Service
Freephone: 0800 665544
Information about health services and support groups.

Parentability
(See NCT above)
Mothers with disabilities

Parentline OPUS
Endway House
The Endway
Hadleigh
Essex
SS7 2AN
01702 559900
National network of support groups and day centres for parents under stress.

Parents at Work
45 Beech Street
Barbican
London
EC2Y 8AD
0171 628 3578

Patients' Association
8 Guilford Street
London WC1N 1DT
0171 242 3460
Campaingning group for NHS patients. Information and advice on how to make complaints.

PCOG (Positive Care in Obstsetrics and Gynaecology)
7 Princes Street
Oxford
OX4 1DD
01865 726755

Multi-disciplinary group of feminists working in professions concerned with midwifery, psychology and sociology.

PIPPIN (Parents in Partnership – Parent Infant Network)
Derwood
Todds Green
Stevenage
Herts
SG1 2JE

Society of Teachers of the Alexander Technique
10 London House
266 Fulham Road
London
SW10 9EL
0171 351 0828
Posture and movement in pregnancy.

Splashdown Birth Pools
No. 17 Wellington Terrace
Harrow-on-the-Hill
Middlesex
HA1 3EP
0181 422 9308

Stillbirth and Neonatal Death Society
28 Portland Place
London
W1N 3DE
0171 436 5881

Support Around Termination for Abnormality (SATFA)
73 Charlotte Street
London
W1P 1LB
0171 631 0285

TAMBA (Twins and Multiple Birth Association)
PO Box 30
Little Sutton
South Wirral
L66 1TH
0151 348 0020 Fax 0151 200 5309

Toxoplasmosis Trust
61 Collier Street London
N1 9BE
0171 713 0663

Women's Health Information Centre
52–54 Featherstone Street
London
EC1Y 8RT
0171 251 6580

Research references

These research references relate to the asterisks in the text. Where there is more than one asterisk on a page, the references appear in order. A bold dot indicates where a new reference begins.

p.22 Quoted by Pamela Nowicka, Independent, November 23, 1987.

p.24 *Pregnancy and Childbirth*, Cochrane Database, Cochrane Institute, Oxford, *available from* BMJ Publishing Group, P.O. Box 295, London WC1H 9TE.

p.36 R. Melzack, E. Bélanger and R. Lacroix, "Labor pain: effect of maternal position on front and back pain", *Journal of Pain Symptom Management*, 6, 8, 476–480, 1991.
• S-Z. Chen, K. Aisaka, H. Mori, et al., "Effects of sitting position on uterine activity during labor", *Obstetrics and Gynecology*, 69, 1, 67–73, 1987.
• *Pregnancy and Childbirth*, Cochrane Database, op. cit.
• U. Waldenström and K. Gottvall, "A randomized trial of birthing stool or conventional semirecumbent position for second-stage labor", *Birth*, 18, 1, 5–10, 1991.

p.42 "Changing Childbirth, Part 1: Report of the Expert Maternity Group", Department of Health, London, 1993.
• Christine McCourt and Lesley Page, "The Evaluation of One to One Midwifery Practice", Centre for Midwifery Practice, Thames Valley University, 1996.
• "Position Statement on Waterbirths", UKCC, London, 1994.

p.43 M. Enkin and I. Chalmers (eds.), *Effectiveness and Satisfaction in Antenatal Care*, Spastics International Medical Publications, London, 1982. Ann Oakley, *The Captured Womb*, Blackwell, Oxford, 1984.

p.45 "Routine iron supplements in pregnancy are unnecessary", *Drug and Therapeutics Bulletin*, 32, 4, 30–31, 1994.
• Jon F. R. Barrett et al.,

"Absorption of non-hem iron from food during normal pregnancy", *British Medical Journal*, 309, 79–81, 1994.

p.47 Sheila Kitzinger, *The New Good Birth Guide*, Penguin, London, 1983.
• Sheila Kitzinger, *Homebirth and Other Alternatives to the Hospital*, Dorling Kindersley, New York, 1991. Sheila Kitzinger, *Some Women's Experience of Induced Labour*, National Childbirth Trust, London, 1978.

p.52 J. G. Thornton and R. J. Lilford, "Active management of labour: current knowledge and research issues", *British Medical Journal*, 309, 366–369, 1994.

p.53 Royal College of Obstetricians and Gynaecologists. Annual statistical return; report taken from the 1993 statistics. London.

p.74 Marion H. Hall et al., "Is routine antenatal care worthwhile?", *Lancet*, 2, 78–80, 1980.

p.75 A. Saari-Kemppainen, O. Karjalainen, P. Ylöstalo, et al., "Ultrasound screening and perinatal mortality: controlled trial of systematic one-stage screening in pregnancy: the Helsinki ultrasound trial", *Lancet*, 336, 8712, 387–391, 1990. J. P. Newnham, S. F. Evans, C. A. Michael, et al., "Effects of frequent ultrasound during pregnancy: a randomized controlled trial", *Lancet*, 342, 8876, 887–891, 1993.

p.88 *Pregnancy and Childbirth*, Cochrane Database, op. cit.

p.93 Sir Dugald Baird, *Journal of Biosocial Science*, 1, 113, 1974.
• R. W. Smithells et al., "Maternal nutrition in early pregnancy", *British Journal of Nutrition*, 38, 3, 497–506, 1977. *Nutrition and Fetal Development* (ed. M. Winick), John Wiley & Sons, 1974. H. A. Kaminetzky and H. Baker, "Micronutrients in pregnancy", *Clinical Obstetrics and Gynecology*, 20, 2, 363–380, 1977. R. M. Pitkin, "Nutritional support in obstetrics

and gynecology", *Clinical Obstetrics and Gynecology*, 19, 3, 489–513, 1976.
• P. J. Illingworth, R. T. Jung, P. W. Howie and T. E. Isles, "Reduction in postprandial energy expenditure during pregnancy", *British Medical Journal*, 294, 1573–1576, 1987.

p.94 Gary K. Oakes and Ronald A. Chez, "Nutrition in pregnancy", *Contemporary Obstetrics and Gynecology*, 4, 147–150, 1974.
• M. D. G. Gillmer, "Obesity in pregnancy – physical and metabolic effects", in *Nutrition in Pregnancy: Proceedings of the Tenth Study Group of the Royal College of Obstetricians and Gynaecologists*, 213–230, RCOG, London, 1983.

p.95 Anni Somerville, *Field of Greens*, Bantam, New York, 1993.

p.97 The MRC Vitamin Study Group, "Prevention of neural tube defects: results of the Medical Research Council vitamin study", *Lancet*, 238, 131–137, 1991. Nicholas J. Wald and Carol Bower, "Folic acid and the prevention of neural tube defects", *British Medical Journal*, 310, 1019–1020, 1995.

p.98 A. Malhotri and R. S. Sawers, *British Medical Journal*, 293, 465–466, 1986.
• M. Puig-Abuli et al., "Zinc and uterine muscle contractivity", Paper given at European Congress of Perinatal Medicine, Dublin, 1984.

p.99 M. Robinson, "Salt in pregnancy", *Lancet*, 1, 178–181, 1958.
• B. S. Worthington, J. Vermeersch and S. R. Williams, *Nutrition in Pregnancy and Lactation*, Mosby, 1977.
• Ibid.

p.100 Peter C. Rubin, "Prescribing in pregnancy: general principles", *British Medical Journal*, 293, 1415–1417, 1986. Martin J. Whittle and Kevin P. Hanretty, "Identifying abnormalities", *British Medical Journal*, 293, 1485–1486, 1986.

• Jonathan Scher and Carol Dix, *Pregnancy*, Penguin, London, 1983.

p.101 G. M. Stirrat, *Obstetrics*, Grant McIntyre Ltd., 1981.

p.102 *Federal Register*, 43, 114, U.S. Department of Health, Education and Welfare, 1978.

p.103 *Perinatal Problems* (eds. N. R. Butler and E. D. Alberman), Livingstone, 1969.
• M. B. Meyer, "How does maternal smoking affect birth weight and maternal weight gain?", *American Journal of Obstetrics and Gynecology*, 131, 888–893, 1978.
• F. D. Martinez et al., "The effect of paternal smoking on the birth weight of newborns whose mothers did not smoke", *American Journal of Public Health*, 84, 9, 1489–1491, 1994.
• J. Kline et al., "Smoking: a risk factor for spontaneous abortion", *New England Journal of Medicine*, 297, 793–795, 1977. R. L. Naeye, "Relationship of cigarette smoking to congenital anomalies and perinatal death", *American Journal of Pathology*, 90, 289–297, 1978. M. B. Meyer and J. A. Tonascia, "Maternal smoking, pregnancy complications and perinatal mortality", *American Journal of Obstetrics and Gynecology*, 128, 494–502, 1977.

p.105 I. J. Chasnoff et al., "Cocaine use in pregnancy", *New England Journal of Medicine*, 313, 666–669, 1985.

p.106 Cree et al., *British Medical Journal*, 4, 251, 1973.

p.107 Peter Parish, *Medicines: a Guide for Everybody*, Penguin, London, 1976.

p.108 *Federal Register*, 41, 115, 1976.
• J. Moore-Gillon, "Asthma in pregnancy", *British Journal of Obstetrics and Gynaecology*, 1018, 658–660, 1994.

p.110 Roger Hoag, "Perinatal psychology", *Birth and the Family Journal*, 113, 1974.
• Parish, op. cit.
• Studies of babies born in England and Wales between 1943 and 1965 revealed that the children of mothers who had had pelvic X-rays in pregnancy were almost twice as likely to develop leukemia before they were 10 years old as those whose mothers had had no X-rays. The greatest risk is in the earliest weeks, when the mother may not know she is pregnant. The risk of cancer was increased 15 times when X-rays were done in the first three months of pregnancy. *See* A. Stewart and G. W. Kneale, "Radiation dose effects in relation to obstetric X-rays and childhood cancers", *Lancet*, 1, 1495, 1970.

p.111 David W. Smith, Sterling K. Clarren and Mary Ann Sedgwick Harvey, "Hyperthermia as a possible teratogenic agent", *Journal of Pediatrics*, 92, 6, 878–883, June 1978. Peter Miller, David W. Smith and Thomas H. Shepard, "Maternal hyperthermia as a possible cause of anencephaly", *Lancet*, 1, 8063, 519–521, 1978.

p.115 *British Journal of Obstetrics and Gynaecology*, 91, 724–730, 1984.
• *Pregnancy and Childbirth*, Cochrane Database, op. cit.
• Ibid.

p.119 Sarah Key, *Body in Action*, Penguin, London, 1995. I am grateful to Sarah Key for the information and imagery about the spine included in this section.

p.127 Aidan MacFarlane, *The Psychology of Childbirth*, Fontana, London, 1977.

p.130 E. Noble, *Essential Exercises for the Childbearing Year*, 3rd ed., Houghton Mifflin, Boston, 1988.

p.132 *Pregnancy and Childbirth*, Cochrane Database, op. cit.

p.135 Ibid.

p.137 Fraser R. Watson, "Bleeding during the later half of pregnancy", in I. Chalmers, M. Enkin and M. J. N. C. Keirse (eds.), *Effective Care in Pregnancy and Childbirth, Vol. 1*, Oxford University Press, Oxford, 594–611, 1989.

p.139 Baha M. Sibai et al., "Prevention of preeclampsia with low-dose aspirin in healthy, nulliparous pregnant women", *New England Journal of Medicine*, 329, 17, 1213–1218, 1993.

p.140 Christopher Redman, "Old-fashioned alertness is the key", *General Practitioner*, 1979.
• *Pregnancy and Childbirth*, Cochrane Database, op. cit.

p.143 Henci Goer, *Obstetric Myths versus Research Realities: A Guide to the Medical Literature*, Bergin and Garvey, Westport Connecticut, 1995, 157–178. R. J. Jarrett, "Gestational diabetes: a non-entity?", *British Medical Journal*, 306, 37–38, 1993.
• P. Steer, M. A. Alam, J. Wadsworth, et al., "Relation between maternal hemoglobin concentration and birth weight in different ethnic groups", *British Medical Journal*, 310, 489–491, 1995.
• Pregnant women often have "physiological" anaemia. There is a greater volume of blood circulating in their bodies; hence the red blood cells are dilated. This is normal – they are not suffering from anaemia. Unnecessary iron supplements may do more harm than good; excess iron makes the red blood cells too big to pass through some of the capillaries in the mother's and the baby's circulatory systems (macrocytosis). This deprives the baby of essential nutrients and can cause its growth to be retarded. *See* T. Lind, *British Journal of Obstetrics and Gynaecology*, 83, 760, 1976.

p.172 Sherry L. Jimenez, Linda C. Jones and Ruth G. Jungman, "Prenatal classes for repeat parents", *MCN*, 4, 305–308, Sept./Oct., 1979.

p.173 Sheila Kitzinger and Lennart Nilsson, *Being Born*, Dorling Kindersley, New York, 1989.

p.176 Penny Simkin, "Just another day in a woman's life? Part I: Women's long-term preconceptions of their first birth experiences", *Birth*, 18, 4, 203–210, 1991. Penny Simkin, "Just another day in a woman's life? Part II: Nature and consistency of women's long-term memories of their first birth experiences", *Birth*, 19, 2, 64–81, 1992.

p.179 Grantly Dick-Read, *Childbirth Without Fear*, Pan, London, 1969.
• Erna Wright, *The New Childbirth*, Tandem, London, 1969.

p.180 Janet Balaskas, *Active Birth*, Harvard Common Press, Harvard and Boston, 1992.

p.184 Marshall H. Klaus, John H. Kennel and Phyllis H. Klaus, *Mothering the Mother – How a Doula Can Help You Have a Shorter, Easier and Healthier Birth*, Addison Wesley, New York, 1993.
• *Pregnancy and Childbirth*, Cochrane Database, op. cit.

p.200 Both poems quoted in Rosemary Palmeira (ed.), in *The Gold of Flesh: Poems of Birth and Motherhood*, The Women's Press, London, 1990.

p.202 Sheila Kitzinger, *Ourselves As Mothers*, Addison Wesley, New York, 1995.

p.220 Christine Gosden, Kypros Nicolaides and Vanessa Whitting, *Is My Baby All Right?: A Guide for Expectant Parents*, Oxford University Press, Oxford, 1994.

p.225 CMO's Update 4: A communication to all doctors from the Chief Medical Officer, Department of Health, London, November 1994.

p.227 *Pregnancy and Childbirth*, Cochrane Database, op. cit.

p.229 Medical Research Council Working Party on the evaluation of chorionic villus sampling, Medical Research Council European trial of chorionic villus sampling, *Lancet*, 3, 37, 1491–1499, 1991.
• G. Kolata, "Fetuses treated through umbilical cords", *The New York Times*, March 29, 1988.

p.234 F. Chenia, Ch. B. and C. A. Crowther, "Does advice to assume knee-chest position reduce the incidence of breech presentation at delivery? A randomized clinical trial", *Birth*, 14, 2, 75–78, June 1987.
• *Pregnancy and Childbirth*, Cochrane Database, op. cit.
• J. P. VanDorsten, B. S. Schifrin and R. L. Wallace, "Randomized controlled trial of external cephalic version with tocolysis in late pregnancy", *American Journal of Obstetrics and Gynecology*, 141, 417, 1981.

p.236 *Pregnancy and Childbirth*, Cochrane Database, op. cit.

p.243 S. L. B. Duncan and S. Beckley, "Prelabour rupture of membranes – why hurry?", *British Journal of Obstetrics and Gynaecology*, 99, 543–545, 1992.
• J. Grant and M. J. N. C. Keirse, "Prelabour rupture of membranes at term", in I. Chalmers, M. Enkin and M. J. N. C. Keirse (eds.), *Effective Care in Pregnancy and Childbirth*, Oxford University Press, Oxford, 1112–1117, 1989.

p.247 Professor Mendez-Bauer found that dilatation of the cervix and the efficiency of contractions is far greater when a woman stands up than when she lies on her back. The uterus works nearly twice as well. [1]

Professor Caldeyro-Barcia discovered that contractions were just as frequent when a woman was standing as when she was lying on her back, but that the contractions were stronger when she stood. He concluded that for the uterus to work really effectively, the woman should be standing. [2, 3]

Eleven hospitals in seven Latin-American countries joined in a study of the effects of the mother's position in labour. Half the mothers were told to lie in bed during the first stage and the other half to get up or sit or lie in bed as they liked. Some 95 per cent of the women did not want to lie down. First-time mothers who stayed upright had shorter first stages than those who were lying down. The majority were more comfortable when upright.

To find out whether an upright position could produce traumatic pressure on the baby's head the researchers studied the incidence of caput and also the effect on the baby's heart rate. They found that, when the membranes had not ruptured, there was no increased rate of caput if the mother was upright, nor was there an increase in deceleration of the fetal heart as recorded by an electronic monitor. They concluded that in normal labour an upright position is fine for the baby, shortens labour and reduces pain. [4]

Further research conducted at the Queen Elizabeth Hospital, Birmingham, England, came up with the same results. [5]

See 1 Peter M. Dunn, "Obstetric delivery today", *Lancet*, 1, 7963, 790–793, 1976.
2 R. Caldeyro-Barcia et al., "Effects of position changes on the intensity and frequency of uterine contractions during labor", *American Journal of Obstetric Gynecology*, 80, 284, 1960.
3 Yuen Chou-liu, "Effects of an upright position during labor", *American Journal of Nursing*, December 1974.
4 R. L. Schwarcz et al., "Fetal heart rate patterns in labors with intact and with ruptured membranes", *Journal of Perinatal Medicine*, 1, 153, 1973.
5 A. M. Flynn, J. Kelly, G. Hollins and P. F. Lynch, "Ambulation in labour", *British Medical Journal*, 11, 591–593, 26 August 1978.

p.252 *Pregnancy and Childbirth*, Cochrane Database, op. cit.

p.253 Ibid.

p.264 C. M. Andrews and E. C. Andrews, "Nursing, maternal postures and foetal position", *Nursing Research*, 32, 336–341, 1983.

p.272 S. A. Huchcroft, M. P. Wearing and C. W. Buck, "Late results of cesarean and vaginal deliveries in cases of breech presentation", *Canadian Medical Association Journal*, 125, 726, 1982.

p.274 J. G. B. Russell, "Moulding of the pelvic outlet", *Journal of Obstetrics and Gynaecology, British Commonwealth*, 76, 817, 1967.
• Michel Odent, *Birth Reborn*, Fontana, London, 1986.

p.275 Emanuel A. Friedman, *Labor: Clinical Evaluation and Management*, Meredith Publishing Co., 1967.

p.276 K. S. Olah and J. P. Neilson, "Failure to progress in the management of labour", *British Journal of Obstetrics and Gynaecology*, 101.1, 1–3, 1994.

p.277 Marshall H. Klaus, John H. Kennel, Steven S. Robertson and Roberto Sósa, "Effects of social support during parturition and infant morbidity", *British Medical Journal*, 293, 585–587, 1986.

p.295 Ronald Melzack, *The Puzzle of Pain*, Penguin, London, 1973.

p.296 Melzack, op. cit.
• Ibid.
• Ibid.

p.300 Josephine A. Williamson, "Hypnosis in obstetrics", *Nursing Mirror*, November 27, 1975.

p.301 Sharon Yellard, "Using acupuncture in midwifery care", *Modern Midwife*, 5, 1, 8–11, 1995.
• Song Meiyu, "Acupuncture anaesthesia for caesarean section", *Midwives' Chronicle*, April 1985.
• I. F. Skelton, "Acupuncture in labor", *Society of Bio-physical Medicine*, June 1985.

p.303 Peter Webb, *Homoeopathy for Midwives*, British Homoeopathic Association, London, 1992, 30–31.

p.304 Christine Brown, "Therapeutic effects of bathing during labor", *Journal of Nurse-Midwifery*, 27, 1, 1982.

p.305 F. Alderdice et al., "Labour and birth in water in England and Wales", *British Medical Journal*, 310, 837, 1995.
• Paul Johnson, "Birth under water: to breathe or not to breathe", *British Journal of Obstetrics and Gynaecology*, 103, 3, 202–208, 1995.

p.307 M. Rosen, "Patient controlled analgesia", *British Medical Journal*, 289, 640–641, 1984.

p.308 Bertil Jacobson et al., "Opiate addiction in adult offspring through possible imprinting after obstetric treatment", *British Medical Journal*, 301, 1067–1070, 1990.

p.309 Michael Rosen, "Pain and its relief," in T. Chard and M. Richards (eds.), *Benefits and Hazards of the New Obstetrics*, William Heinemann, 1977.

p.310 M. B. Wingate, "Effects of epidural analgesia on fetal and neonatal status", *American Journal of Obstetrics and Gynecology*, 119, 1101–1106, 1974.
B. S. Schiffrin, "Fetal heart rate patterns following epidural anaesthesia and oxytocin infusion during labour", *Journal of Obstetrics and Gynaecology, British Commonwealth*, 79, 332, 1972.
• *Pregnancy and Childbirth*, Cochrane Database, op. cit.

p.311 Andrew Doughty, *Journal of Royal Society of Medicine*, December 1978.
• J. A. Thorp et al., "The effect of intrapartum epidural analgesia on

nulliparous labor: a randomized controlled prospective trial", *American Journal of Obstetrics and Gynecology*, 169, 851–858, 1993.
• M. Maresh, K. H. Choong and R. W. Beard, "Delayed pushing with lumbar epidural analgesia in labour", *British Journal of Obstetrics and Gynaecology*, 90, 623–627, 1983.
• C. MacArthur, M. Lewis, E. G. Knox and J. S. Crawford, "Epidural anaesthesia and long-term backache after childbirth", *British Medical Journal*, 301, 9–12, 1990. C. MacArthur, M. Lewis and E. G. Knox, *Health After Childbirth: An Investigation of Long-term Health Problems Beginning After Childbirth in 11,701 Women*, HMSO, London, 1991.
• A. D. Noble et al., "Continuous lumbar epidural using bupivicaine", *Journal of Obstetrics and Gynaecology, British Commonwealth*, 78, 559, 1971.
• Kay Standley et al., "Local-regional anesthesia during childbirth: effect on newborn behaviors", *Science*, 186, November 15, 1974.

p.312 Barbara Morgan, *Journal of Obstetric Anaesthesia*, forthcoming.
• Sheila Kitzinger, *Some Women's Experiences of Epidurals*, National Childbirth Trust, London, 1987.

p.313 Michael Rosen, op. cit.

p.314 Josephine M. Green, Vanessa A. Coupland and Jenny V. Kitzinger, "Expectations, experiences and psychological outcomes of childbirth: a prospective study of 825 women", *Birth*, 17, 1, 15–23, 1990.

p.315 Kieran O'Driscoll and Declan Meagher, *Active Management of Labour*, 3rd ed., Mosby Yearbook, Times/Mirror, London, 1993.

p.316 *Pregnancy and Childbirth*, Cochrane Database, op. cit.

p.317 R. Caldeyro-Barcia et al., "Adverse perinatal effects of early amniotomy during labor", in L. Gluck (ed.), *Modern Perinatal Medicine*, 431–439, Yearbook Medical Publishers, Chicago, 1974.

p.318 A. Huch et. al., "Continuous transcutaneous monitoring of fetal oxygen tension during

labour", *British Journal of Obstetrics and Gynaecology*, 84, Suppl. 1, 1977.
• G. C. Gunn et al., "Premature rupture of the fetal membranes", *American Journal of Obstetrics and Gynecology*, 106, 469–477, 1970.
• P. J. Steer et al., "The effect of membrane rupture on fetal heart in induced labour", *British Journal of Obstetrics and Gynaecology*, 83, 454–459, June 1976.

p.320 *Pregnancy and Childbirth*, Cochrane Database, op. cit.

p.321 Ibid.

p.322 M. S. Klein, R. C. Gaultier, J. Robbins, et al., "Relation of episiotomy to perineal trauma and morbidity, sexual dysfunction and pelvic floor relaxation", *American Journal of Obstetrics and Gynecology*, 1, 71, 3, 591–598, 1994.
• Argentine Episiotomy Trial Collaborative Group, "Routine vs. selective episiotomy: a randomized controlled trial", *Lancet*, 342, 1, 517–518, 1993.
• R. F. Harrison et al., "Is routine episiotomy necessary?", *British Medical Journal*, 288, 1971–1975, 1984.
• J. Sleep et al., "West Berkshire perineal management trial", *British Medical Journal*, 289, 587–590, 1984.
• S. Kitzinger and R. Walters, *Some Women's Experiences of Episiotomy*, 2nd ed., National Childbirth Trust, London, 1993, *available from* Sheila Kitzinger, The Manor, Standlake, Nr. Witney, Oxon OX8 7RH, UK.
S. Kitzinger and P. Simkin (eds.), *Episiotomy and the Second Stage of Labor*, ICEA, Minneapolis, 1984.

p.326 Linda Cardozo, "Is routine induction of labour at term ever justified?", *British Medical Journal*, 306, 840–841, 1993.
• "Caesarean Childbirth", Summary of a National Institute of Health statement, *British Medical Journal*, 1981.

p.327 A. W. Linston and A. J. Campbell, "Danger of oxytocin-induced labour to fetuses", *British Medical Journal*, 3, 606–607, 1974.

p.328 *Reducing the Risk*, Department of Health and Social Security, London, 1977.

p.329 Kieran O'Driscoll and Declan Meagher, op. cit.
• J. G. Thornton and R. J. Lilford, "Active management of labour: current knowledge and research issues", *British Medical Journal*, 309, 6951, 366–369, 1994.

p.331 D. A. Luthy, K. K. Shy, G. van Belle, et al., "A randomized trial of electronic fetal monitoring in preterm labor", *Obstetrics and Gynecology*, 69, 5, 687–695, 1987. D. MacDonald, A. Grant, M. Sheridan Pereira, et al., "The Dublin randomised controlled trial of intrapartum fetal heart rate monitoring", *American Journal of Obstetrics and Gynecology*, 152, 5, 524–539, 1985.
• K. J. Leveno, F. G. Cunningham, S. Nelson, et al., "A prospective comparison of selective and universal electronic fetal monitoring in 34,995 pregnancies", *New England Journal of Medicine*, 315, 10, 615–619, 1986.
• A. D. Haverkamp, M. Orleans, S. Langendoerfer, et al., "A controlled trial of the differential effects of intrapartum fetal monitoring", *American Journal of Obstetrics and Gynecology*, 134, 4, 399–412, 1979. I. M. Kelso, R. J. Parson, G. F. Lawrence, et al., "An assessment of continuous fetal heart rate monitoring in labor: a randomised trial", *American Journal of Obstetrics and Gynecology*, 131, 5, 526–532, 1978.
• S. Neldam, M. Osler, P. K. Hanse, et al., "Intrapartum fetal heart rate monitoring in a combined low- and high-risk population: a controlled risk trial", *European Journal of Obstetrics, Gynaecology and Reproductive Biology*, 23, 1–11, 1986.

p.333 D. M. Okada and A. W. Chow, "Neonatal scalp abscess following intrapartum fetal monitoring", *American Journal of Obstetrics and Gynecology*, 127, 875, 1977.

p.334 G. S. Sykes et al., "Fetal distress and the condition of newborn infants", *British Medical Journal*, 287, 943–945, October 1983. P. W. Howe, "Fetal monitoring in labour", *British Medical Journal*, 292, 6518, 427–428, February 1986.

p.335 *Pregnancy and Childbirth*, Cochrane Database, op. cit.

p.337 Ibid.
• T. Henriksen et al., "Caesarean section in twin pregnancies in two Danish counties and different section rates", *Acta Obstetrica Gynaecologica Scandinavica*, 73, 123–128, 1994.
• B. E. Chalmers, J. A. McIntyre and D. Meyer, *South African Medical Journal*, 82, 161–163, 1992.

p.338 *Pregnancy and Childbirth*, Cochrane Database, op. cit.
• Stuart Campbell, *Sharing*, Maternal Health Committee of Social Planning and Review Council of British Columbia, Summer 1979.

p.340 *Pregnancy and Childbirth*, Cochrane Database, op. cit.

p.345 Frederick Leboyer, *Birth Without Violence*, Fontana, 1977.

p.346 Hugo Lagercrantz and Theodore A. Slotkin, "The 'stress' of being born", *Scientific American*, 4, 86, 100–107, 1986.

p.353 Michel Odent, *Birth Reborn*, Fontana, London, 1986, and *Entering the World: The Demedicalization of Childbirth*, Penguin, London, 1985.
• Johnson's Baby Newsline, Autumn 1978.

p.358 Robert Hinde discovered that rhesus monkey babies separated from their mothers shortly after birth became very distressed and withdrawn. He suggested that separation from the mother might also be bad for a newborn human baby. [1]

Other research has indicated that mothers who had greater contact with their babies, and continued this contact through early childhood, produced children whose IQ, when tested at the age of five, was significantly higher than average. [2]

Those concerned about bonding at birth also advocate skin-to-skin contact between mother and child. It was suggested that the baby could become chilled, but a study of heat loss in warmed cots as compared with that in the mother's arms showed no significant difference. [3]

See 1 Robert Hinde, *Proceedings of the Royal Society*, 196, 29, 1977.

2 F. S. W. Brimblecombe, *Separation and Special Care Baby Units*, Heinemann, London, 1978.
3 C. N. Phillips, "Neonatal heat loss in heated cribs vs. mother's arms", *Journal of Obstetrical, Gynecological and Neonatal Nursing*, 6, 11–15, 1974.
• Marshall Klaus and John Kennel, *Maternal-Infant Bonding*, Mosby, 1977.

p.364 Marshall Klaus and John Kennel, op. cit.

p.366 L. Silverman, W. A. Silverman and J. C. Sinclair, *Pediatrics*, 41, 1033, 1969.

p.368 E. Jones, "Breastfeeding in the premature infant", *Modern Midwife*, 4, 1, 22–26, 1994.

p.370 P. A. and J. P. Davies, *Lancet*, 2, 1216, 1970.

p.373 *Pregnancy and Childbirth*, Cochrane Database, op. cit.
• Kevin Forbes, "Management of first trimester spontaneous abortions", *British Medical Journal*, 310, 1426, 1995.

p.376 Cicely Williams and Derrick B. Jelliffe, *Mother and Child Health*, Oxford University Press, Oxford, 1972.

p.378 Harriet Sarnoff Schiff, *The Bereaved Parent*, G. K. Hall, 1977.

p.384 H. Varendi et al., "Does the newborn baby find the nipple by smell?", *Lancet*, 344, 8, 989–990, 1994.

p.390 F. Cockburn et al., "Effect of diet on the fatty acid composition of the major phospholipids of the infant cerebral cortex", *Archives of Disease in Childhood*, 72, 198–203, 1995.

p.392 Rudolph Schaffer, *Mothering*, Fontana, London, 1977.

p.404 If a woman has never had rubella, the obstetrician may advise vaccination after delivery. Since this vaccine could affect a baby conceived within the next three months, it is vital that she does not conceive during this time. Women who are unsure about which contraceptive to use may be offered an injection of a long-acting contraceptive called Depo Provera. Those who intend to breastfeed may be reluctant to have this injection, as it introduces hormones into the bloodstream.

Glossary

Abdomen The part of the body containing the intestines, stomach, bowels, and uterus.

Abortion (Miscarriage) Either spontaneous or induced delivery of the fetus before the 28th week of development.

Abruption (Accidental haemorrhage) The peeling away of part of the placenta from the wall of the uterus during late pregnancy, which may result in bleeding.

Accelerated labour The artificial augmentation of contractions, after the cervix has started to dilate, by the injection of oxytocin through an intravenous drip. Often used to speed up a long labour.

Active birth An approach to childbirth that entails practising stretching positions and movements and being in "open" and upright positions in labour.

Active management of labour The constant monitoring and technical control of labour to limit its duration.

ALB See *Albumin.*

Albumin A protein present in all animal tissues. Albumin in the urine of a pregnant woman can be a sign of pre-eclampsia.

Alphafetoprotein (AFP) A substance produced by the embryonic yolk sac, and later by the fetal liver, which enters the mother's bloodstream during pregnancy.

Alveoli Milk glands in the breasts, which produce a flow of milk when they are stimulated by prolactin and the baby's sucking.

Amenorrhoea The absence of menstrual periods.

Amino acids The main organic chemical constituents of proteins found in all foods produced from animals, but only in limited and varying combinations in vegetables.

Ammonium chloride See *Diuretics.*

Amnesia Loss of memory, usually short term, which can be a side effect of certain drugs, especially Valium.

Amniocentesis The surgical extraction of a small amount of amniotic fluid through the pregnant woman's abdomen. This procedure is usually carried out as a test for fetal defects or maturity.

Amnion The layer of membrane immediately enveloping the fetus and the amniotic fluid inside the uterus; it is also referred to as the amniotic sac, or bag of waters.

Amniotic fluid The fluid surrounding the fetus in the uterus.

Amniotic sac See *Amnion.*

Amniotomy The surgical rupture of the amniotic sac, often done to speed up labour. Referred to as ARM (artificial rupture of the membranes).

Amytal See *Barbiturates.*

Anaemia A condition in which there is an abnormally low proportion of red corpuscles in the blood, treated by iron (Fe) supplements.

Anaesthetic Medication that produces partial or complete insensibility to pain.

Anaesthetic, general Anaesthetic that affects the whole body, with temporary loss of consciousness.

Anaesthetic, local Anaesthetic that affects a limited part of the body. See also *Caudal; Epidural; Paracervical block.*

Analgesics Painkilling agents not inducing unconsciousness.

Anencephaly The congenital absence of the brain.

Antepartum cardiotography Test to check fetal heartbeat.

Anterior position See *Occipito anterior.*

Antibacterials Chemical agents that limit the growth of, or destroy, bacteria. See also *Sulphonamides.*

Antibiotics Substances capable of destroying or limiting the growth of micro-organisms, especially bacteria.

Antibodies Protein produced naturally by the body to combat any foreign bodies, germs, or bacteria.

Anticholinergic drugs Used in the treatment of nausea and vomiting, partly by limiting the impulses through the nervous system and partly by restricting the secretion of stomach acids.

Anticoagulants Drugs that prevent the blood from clotting.

Anticonvulsants Drugs that combat convulsions, especially epilepsy.

Antihistamines Tranquillizers used in the treatment of nausea, vomiting, and certain allergies.

Apgar scale A general test of the baby's wellbeing given immediately after birth to ascertain the heart rate and tone, respiration, blood circulation, and nerve responses.

Apnoea Interrupted breathing that may occur in pre-term and low-birthweight babies.

Areola The pigmented circle of skin surrounding the nipple.

Arrhythmic contractions Irregular contractions.

ARM See *Amniotomy.*

Aspirin (Salicylate) A mild analgesic.

Bag of waters See *Amnion.*

Barbiturates Powerful and highly addictive tranquillizers.

Bearing down The pushing movement made by the uterus in the second stage of labour.

Bile pigment See *Bilirubin.*

Bilirubin Broken-down red blood cells, normally converted to nontoxic substances by the liver. Some newborn babies have levels of bilirubin too high for their livers to cope with. See also *Jaundice, neonatal.*

Birth canal See *Vagina.*

Blastocyst An early stage of the developing egg when it has segmented into a group of cells.

Blighted ovum An abnormal development of the egg in which the cells do not develop in the usual way to form a baby. It results in miscarriage.

Bradycardia A slow heart rate in the fetus and newborn baby. This is a rate of less than 120 beats a minute.

Braxton Hicks contractions (Rehearsal) Contractions of the uterus that occur throughout pregnancy, but which may not be noticed until towards the end.

Breast pump Apparatus for drawing milk from the breasts.

Breech presentation The position of a baby who is bottom down rather than head down in the uterus.

Brow presentation The position of a baby who is head down in the uterus, but with chin up, so that the brow comes through the cervix first.

Caesarean section Delivery of the baby through a cut in the abdominal and uterine walls.

Candida See *Thrush*.

Caput A small, temporary swelling on the crown of the baby's head caused by the head being pressed against an incompletely dilated cervix.

Carpal tunnel syndrome Numbness and tingling of the hands arising from pressure on the nerves of the wrist. In pregnancy it is caused by the body's accumulation of fluids.

Catheter A thin plastic tube inserted into the body through a natural channel to withdraw fluid from, or squirt fluid into, a part of the body. It can be used to draw off urine from the bladder, or to maintain a constant input of fluids into a vein, or to introduce anaesthetic into the epidural space.

Caudal (Caudal epidural block) An anaesthetic injected into the base of the spine. See also *Epidural*.

Cephalhaematoma A temporary swelling on the side of the baby's head caused by pressure during labour.

Cephalic presentation The position of a baby who is head down in the uterus. The most common presentation.

Cephalopelvic disproportion A state in which the head of the fetus is larger than the cavity of the mother's pelvis. Delivery must therefore be by Caesarean section.

Cervical dilatation See *Dilatation*.

Cervical erosion Superficial inflammation of the cervix.

Cervical incompetence A disorder of the cervix, usually arising after a previous mid-pregnancy termination or damage to the cervix during a previous labour, in which the cervix opens up too soon, resulting in repeated mid-pregnancy miscarriages. It is sometimes treated by suturing to hold the cervix closed.

Cervix The lower entrance to the uterus, or neck of the womb.

Chloasma Skin discolouration during pregnancy, often facial.

Chloral drugs Non-barbiturate hypnotic tranquillizers.

Chlorpromazine (Thorazine) A powerful sedative often used in conjunction with hypnotics, analgesics, and anaesthetics.

Chorion The outer membranous tissue that envelops the developing fetus and placenta.

Chorionic gonadotrophin See *Human chorionic gonadotrophin (HCG)*.

Chorionic villi The tiny fronds around the fertile ovum that enable it to become embedded in the uterine wall.

Chorionic villus sampling A method of screening for genetic handicap by analysis of tissue from the small protrusions on the outer membrane enveloping the embryo that later form the placenta.

Chromosomes Rod-like structures containing genes occurring in pairs within the nucleus of every cell. Human cells each contain 23 pairs. See also *Gene*.

Circumcision An operation to cut the foreskin from the penis.

Cleft palate A congenital abnormality of the roof of the mouth.

Clitoris Exquisitely sensitive small organ at the upper end of a woman's genitals, just under the pubic bone and between the folded external labia.

Club foot A congenital abnormality in which the foot is twisted out of shape.

Codeine An addictive painkilling agent derived from opium.

Colostrum A kind of milk, rich in proteins, formed and secreted by the breasts in late pregnancy and gradually changing to mature milk some days after delivery.

Conception The fertilization of the egg by the sperm and its implantation in the uterine wall.

Congenital abnormality An abnormality or deformity existing from birth, usually arising from a damaged gene, the adverse effect of certain drugs, or the effect of some diseases during pregnancy.

Contractions The regular tightening of the uterine muscles as they work to dilate the cervix in labour and press the baby down the birth canal.

Cordocentesis See *Umbilical vein sampling*.

Corpuscles Constituents of blood, divided into red and white varieties.

Corpus luteum A glandular mass that forms in the ovary after fertilization. It produces progesterone, which helps to form the placenta, and is active for the first 14 weeks of pregnancy.

Cortisone A steroid that is produced by the adrenal gland which appears in the amniotic fluid immediately before labour.

Crowning The moment when the baby's head appears in the vagina and does not slip back again.

CVS See *Chorionic villus sampling*.

Cystitis An inflammation of the bladder and urinary tract, producing a painful stinging sensation when urine is passed.

D and C The surgical dilatation (opening) of the cervix, and curettage (removal of the contents) of the uterus.

Dehydration A physical condition caused by the loss of an excessive amount of water from the body, often resulting from severe vomiting or diarrohea.

Depression, respiratory Breathing difficulties in the newborn baby.

Dextrose A solution of glucose used to supplement the level of blood sugar, usually introduced by intravenous drip.

Dextrostix A test to assess the level of sugar in the urine.

Diabetes Failure of the system to metabolize glucose, traced by excess sugar in the blood and urine.

Diastolic pressure The blood pressure between the heartbeats. See also *Systolic pressure*.

Diazepam (Valium) See *Tranquillizers*.

Dilatation The progressive opening of the cervix caused by uterine contractions during labour.

Distocia, shoulder A state in which the baby's shoulders get stuck during delivery.

Distress See *Fetal distress*.

Diuretics Drugs that increase the amount of urine excreted.

Dizygotic See *Twins*.

Doppler A method of using ultrasound vibrations to listen to the fetal heart.

Down's syndrome A severe congenital abnormality producing subnormal mentality.

Drip See *Intravenous drip*.

Dura The outer membrane protecting the spinal cord.

Eclampsia The severe form of pre-eclampsia, which is characterized by extremely high blood pressure, headaches, visual distortion, flashes, convulsions and, in the worst cases, coma and death. The condition is now rare since the symptoms of pre-eclampsia are treated immediately.

Ectopic or tubal pregnancy A pregnancy that develops outside the uterus, usually in one of the fallopian tubes. The mother has severe pain low down at one side of the abdomen at any time from the 6th to 12th week of pregnancy. The pregnancy must be surgically terminated.

EDD The estimated date of delivery.

Elective induction Induction done for convenience rather than for medical reasons. See also *Induction*.

Electrode A small electrical conductor used obstetrically for monitoring the fetal heartbeat during labour.

Electronic fetal monitoring The continuous monitoring of the fetal heart by a transducer placed on the mother's abdomen over the area of the fetal heart, or by an electrode inserted through the cervix and clipped or screwed to the baby's scalp.

Embryo The developing organism in pregnancy, from about the 10th day after fertilization until about the 12th week of pregnancy, when it is termed a fetus.

Endocrinological changes Changes in the secretion of the endocrine glands that occur in pregnancy or the four weeks after delivery (the puerperium).

Endometrium The inner lining of the uterus.

Enema The injection of fluids through the rectum to expel its contents.

Engaged (Eng/E) The baby is engaged when it has settled with its presenting part deep in the pelvic cavity. This often happens in the last month of pregnancy.

Engorgement The over-congestion of the breasts with milk. If long periods are left between feeds, or the baby is not well latched on, painful engorgement can occur. This can be relieved by putting the baby to the breast or expressing the excess milk.

Epidural (Lumbar epidural block) Regional anaesthesia, used during labour and for Caesarean sections, in which an anaesthetic is injected through a catheter into the epidural space in the lower spine.

Episiotomy A surgical cut in the perineum to enlarge the vagina.

External version (External cephalic version, or ECV) The manipulation by gentle pressure of the fetus into the cephalic position. This may be done by an obstetrician at the end of pregnancy if the baby is breech.

Face presentation The position of a baby whose face is coming through the cervix first.

Fallopian tube (Oviduct) The tube into which a ripe egg is wafted after its expulsion from the ovary, along which it travels on its way to the uterus.

False labour Braxton Hicks (rehearsal) contractions, which are so strong and regular that they are mistaken for the contractions of the first stage of labour.

Fertilization (see conception) The meeting of the sperm with the ovum or egg to form a new life.

Fetal distress A shortage in the flow of oxygen to the fetus, which can arise from numerous causes.

Fetus The developing child in the uterus, from the end of the embryonic stage, at about the 12th week of pregnancy, until birth.

FH Fetal heart.

Fibre optics The transmission of light along flexible bundles of glass. Sometimes inserted into the uterus to give a view of the fetus inside.

Fluid retention See *Oedema*.

FMF Fetal movement felt.

Folic acid A form of vitamin B essential for the production of blood cells and haemoglobin, the shortage of which may produce handicaps in the fetus.

Fontanels The soft spots between the unjoined sections of the fetal skull.

Foremilk Watery milk that accumulates in the ducts behind the nipple, which the baby takes at the beginning of a feed. It precedes the main release of milk, which is richer in calories and more satisfying.

Fraternal twins See *Twins*.

Fundal palpation Feeling through the abdominal wall for the top of the uterus to assess its height.

Fundus The upper part of the uterus.

Gamma globulin A protein-based antibody used to prevent or treat infections such as hepatitis.

Gene The part of every cell that stores genetic characteristics.

Genetic counselling Advice on the probability of recurrent hereditary abnormalities or diseases.

Gentle birth One term used for a method of delivery proposed by Frederick Leboyer in which the shock of birth upon the baby is minimized and the baby is welcomed by loving hands, skin contact, and soft lights and is able to discover itself in a warm bath.

German measles See *Rubella*.

Gestation The length of time between conception and delivery.

Glucose A natural sugar found in certain organic materials and in the blood: the main source of energy.

Glycogen The natural source of glucose; glycogen stores carbohydrate materials and is formed by the liver and muscles.

Gynaecologist A doctor who specializes in the problems of the female reproductive system.

Haemoglobin (Hb) A constituent of the red blood cells that contains iron (Fe) and stores oxygen.

Haemorrhage Excessive bleeding.

Haemorrhoids (Piles) Swelling of the veins around the rectum.

Hb See *Haemoglobin*.

HCG See *Human chorionic gonadotrophin*.

Hegar's sign The softening of the lower part of the uterus that gradually occurs during the first six weeks of pregnancy.

Hormone A chemical messenger in the blood that stimulates various organs to action.

Hormone accelerated labour See *Induction*.

Human chorionic gonadotrophin (HCG) A hormone released into the woman's bloodstream by the developing placenta from about six days after the last period was due. Its presence in the urine means that she is pregnant.

Hyaline membrane disease Respiratory distress affecting some pre-term babies, resulting from a lack of surfactant that holds the lungs open.

Hydatidiform mole A rare abnormality in which the egg fails to develop after becoming implanted in the uterine wall, so there is no baby, although the placenta and chorionic villi go on developing. If the woman does not miscarry, the growth must be removed.

Hydrocephalus A congenital abnormality in which the baby's head is swollen with fluid.

Hyperemesis gravidarum Almost continuous vomiting during pregnancy.

Hypertension (High blood pressure) In pregnancy this can reduce the fetal blood supply.

Hyperventilation Abnormally heavy breathing that flushes carbon dioxide out of the bloodstream, so that the normal chemical balance of the blood is lost.

Hypnosis A state of mental passivity with a special susceptibility to suggestion. This can be used as an anaesthetic, and can be self-induced.

Hypnotics See *Tranquillizers*.

Hypoglycaemia Low blood sugar is sometimes apparent in babies who have suffered a difficult delivery, pre-term babies, or those of diabetic mothers. It can be artificially produced by giving the mother intravenous glucose in labour, since this increases the release of insulin, which breaks the sugar down. The baby may have to be given extra sugar.

Hypotension Low blood pressure.

Hypothermia A very low body temperature, which can be fatal.

Identical twins See *Twins.*

Implantation The embedding of the fertilized ovum or egg within the wall of the uterus.

Incoordinate uterine action See *Uterine action, incoordinate.*

Induction The process of artificially starting off labour and keeping it going.

Insulin A hormone produced by the pancreas that regulates the level of carbohydrates and amino acids in the system. It may be used as a means of controlling the effects of diabetes. See also *Diabetes.*

Internal monitoring See *Electronic fetal monitoring.*

Intramuscular injection An injection into a muscle.

Intravenous drip The infusion of fluids directly into the bloodstream by means of a fine catheter introduced into a vein.

Intravenous injection An injection into a vein.

Invasive techniques Any medical technique that intrudes into the body.

Involution of the uterus The process by which the uterus returns to its normal state after pregnancy.

Jaundice, neonatal A common complaint in newborn babies, caused by inability of the liver to break down successfully an excess of red blood cells. See also *Bilirubin.*

Ketosis The accumulation of lactic acid in various body tissues and fluids, which is often indicated by acetone in the urine.

Labia The folds (or lips) of skin at the mouth of the vagina.

Lanugo The fine soft body hair of the fetus.

Lateral position Transverse lie or horizontal position of a fetus in the uterus (sometimes occurring if the mother has a large pelvis), where the presenting part is either a shoulder or the side of the head.

Laxatives Purgative drugs.

Leboyer approach See *Gentle birth.*

Let-down reflex See *Milk ejection reflex.*

Lie The position of the fetus in the uterus.

Ligament A fibrous tissue binding and connecting bones.

Lightening The engagement of the fetus in the pelvis, with its presenting part fitting securely into the pelvic inlet like an egg in an egg cup.

Linea nigra A line of dark skin that appears down the centre of the abdomen over the rectus muscle in some women during pregnancy.

Lithotomy position The position for delivery, in which the mother lies flat on her back, with her legs wide apart and raised, fixed in stirrups.

Lochia Postnatal vaginal discharge.

Longitudinal lie The position of the fetus in the uterus in which the spines of the fetus and the mother are parallel.

Long l See *Longitudinal lie.*

Low-birthweight baby A baby who at birth is below the weight of 2.5 kg (5½ lb).

Meconium The first contents of the bowel, present in the fetus before birth and passed during the first few days after birth. The presence of meconium in the amniotic fluid before delivery is usually taken as a sign of fetal distress.

Milk ejection reflex The flow of milk into the nipple.

Miscarriage See *Abortion.*

Mongolism See *Down's syndrome.*

Monilia See *Thrush.*

Monitoring See *Electronic fetal monitoring.*

Monozygotic See *Twins.*

Montgomery's tubercles Small bumps on the areola surrounding the nipple.

Morphine A narcotic opium derivative used as an analgesic.

Morula A stage in the growth of the fertilized egg when it has developed into 32 cells.

Moulding The shaping of the bones of the baby's skull as it passes through the birth canal.

Mucus A sticky secretion.

Multigravida A woman in her second or subsequent pregnancy.

Multiple pregnancy The development of two or more babies. See also *Twins.*

Mutation A damaged genetic cell. This can occur naturally or, more commonly, as an effect of outside agents, such as radiation.

Narcotic A drug that induces a state of stupor.

Nasogastric tube A pliable catheter which is passed through the nose into the stomach. Nasogastric tubes are used either for passing nourishment into the digestive tract or for draining digestive fluids.

Nembutal See *Barbiturates.*

Neural tube defects Abnormalities of the central nervous system. See also *Anencephaly; Hydrocephalus; Spina bifida.*

Nicotine A highly poisonous substance present in tobacco. During pregnancy it enters the bloodstream of a woman who smokes and may affect the efficiency of the placenta, often resulting in a low-birthweight baby.

Notochord The cells that form the primitive nervous system.

Nucleus The central part or core of a cell, containing genetic information.

Occipito anterior The position of the baby in the uterus when the back of its head (the crown or occiput) is towards the mother's front (anterior).

Occipito posterior The position of the baby in the uterus when the back of its head (the crown or occiput) is towards the mother's back (posterior).

Oedema Fluid retention, which causes the body tissues to be puffed out.

Oestriol A form of oestrogen.

Oestrogen A hormone produced by the ovary.

Os The mouth of the cervix.

Ovary One of the two female glands, set at the entrance of the fallopian tubes, which regularly produce eggs until the menopause.

Oviduct See *Fallopian tube.*

Ovulation The production of the ripe egg by the ovary.

Oxygenate To saturate with oxygen.

Oxytocin A hormone secreted by the pituitary gland that stimulates uterine contractions during labour and stimulates the milk glands in the breasts to produce milk.

Oxytocin challenge test A way of assessing the condition of the fetus and of the placenta, by which oxytocin is introduced into the mother's bloodstream and the reactions of the fetal heart to uterine contractions are recorded.

Palpation Feeling the parts of the baby through the mother's abdominal wall.

Paracervical block Regional anaesthesia sometimes used during labour, involving a series of local anaesthetic injections around the cervix.

Pelvic floor The springy muscular structure set within the pelvis that supports the bladder and the uterus, and through which the baby descends during labour.

Pelvis The pelvis is a solid ring of bone at the base of the abdomen; it shields the bladder and portions of the genital tract.

Perinatal The period from the 28th week of gestation to one week following delivery.

Perineum The area of soft tissues surrounding the vagina and between the vagina and the rectum.

PET See *Pre-eclampsia.*

Pethidine See *Analgesics.*

Phenobarbital See *Barbiturates.*

Phenothiazine Strong tranquillizers used in the treatment of nausea and vomiting. See also *Tranquillizers.*

Phototherapy Treatment by exposure to light, which may be used when a baby has jaundice.

Pituitary gland A gland set just below the brain that, among other functions, secretes various hormones controlling the menstrual cycle. In late pregnancy it releases a hormone, oxytocin, into the bloodstream, which stimulates uterine contractions and also the milk glands.

Placenta The organ that develops on the inner wall of the uterus and supplies the fetus with all its life-supporting requirements and carries waste products to the mother's system.

Placental function tests Tests to assess the condition and efficiency of the placenta.

Placental insufficiency A condition in which the placenta provides inadequate life support for the fetus, resulting in a baby at special risk.

Placental praevia A condition in which the placenta lies over the cervix at the end of pregnancy. This part of the uterus stretches in the last few weeks of pregnancy, but the placenta cannot stretch, so it may separate; the result is antepartum haemorrhage. A woman with a complete placenta praevia is delivered by Caesarean section.

Polyhydramnios An excess of amniotic fluid in the uterus.

Posterior See *Occipito posterior.*

Postmaturity The state of the fetus in an overdue pregnancy. The skin may be dry and peeling, and the fingernails may need cutting immediately after birth.

Postnatal After the birth.

Postpartum After delivery.

PP See *Presenting part.*

Pre-eclampsia (Pre-eclamptic toxaemia) An illness in which a woman has high blood pressure, oedema, albumin in the urine, and often sudden excessive weight gain. See also *Eclampsia.*

Premature See *Pre-term.*

Prenatal Before delivery.

"Prepping" Procedures carried out to prepare the woman for labour.

Presentation The position of the fetus in the uterus before and during labour.

Presenting part The part of the fetus that is lying directly over the cervix.

Pre-term A baby born before the 37th week of pregnancy and weighing less than 5½ lb (2.5 kg).

Primigravida A woman having her first pregnancy.

Progesterone A hormone produced by the corpus luteum and then by the placenta.

Progestogen A synthetic variety of the hormone progesterone used in oral contraceptives.

Prostaglandins Natural substances that stimulate the onset of labour contractions. Prostaglandin gel may be used to soften the cervix and induce labour.

Psychoprophylaxis A method of preparation for childbirth, which is centred on techniques of distraction and breathing.

Pubis The bones forming the front of the lower pelvis.

Pudendal block Injection to numb the nerves in the perineum.

Puerperium The four weeks following birth.

Purse-string (Shirodkar) suture Stitches passed through and around the cervix, and then drawn tight to support the uterus when the cervix is "incompetent".

Pyelitis An infection of the kidneys. It is treated by a course of antibiotics.

Pyridoxine Vitamin B6.

Quickening The first noticeable movements of the fetus felt by the mother.

Rectus muscle The muscles running up the centre of the abdomen.

REM Rapid eye movement in sleep, indicating mental activity.

Respiratory depression
See *Depression, respiratory.*

Rhesus factor A distinguishing characteristic of the red blood corpuscles. All human beings have either Rhesus positive or Rhesus negative blood. If the mother is Rhesus negative and the fetus Rhesus positive, severe complications and Rhesus disease (the destruction of the red corpuscles by antibodies) may occur, unless prevented by anti-D gamma globulin.

Rooting The baby's instinctive searching for the breast.

Rubella (German measles) A mild virus that may cause congenital abnormalities in the fetus if it is contracted by a woman during the first 12 weeks of pregnancy.

Sacrum The big bone at the base of the spine, forming the back of the pelvis.

Salicylate See *Aspirin.*

Scan (Screen) A way of building up a picture of an object by bouncing high-frequency soundwaves off it. The sonar or ultrasound scan is used during pregnancy to show the development of the fetus in the uterus. See also *Transducer.*

Senna Derivatives of the cassia plant, components of many laxatives.

Shirodkar See *Purse-string suture.*

Shoulder distocia See *Distocia, shoulder.*

Show A vaginal discharge of bloodstained mucus occurring before labour, resulting from the onset of cervical dilatation. A sign that labour is starting.

Small-for-dates Babies who are born at the right time but for some reason have not flourished in the uterus. See also *Placental insufficiency.*

Sonogram See *Doppler.*

Sperm (Spermatozoon) The male reproductive cell that fertilizes the egg.

Spina bifida A congenital neural tube defect in which the fetal spinal cord forms incorrectly, outside the spinal column.

Spinal anaesthesia An injection of local anaesthetic into the spinal cord.

Spontaneous abortion See *Abortion.*

Stanislavsky technique Acting exercises that increase body awareness.

Stasis of milk A reduction in the flow of breast milk with blocking of ducts.

Steroids Drugs used in the treatment of skin disorders, asthma, hay fever, rheumatism, and arthritis. Because they alter the chemical balance of the metabolism they may cause fetal abnormalities if used extensively during pregnancy.

Stethoscope, fetal A trumpet-shaped instrument placed against the pregnant woman's abdomen for the fetal heart to be heard.

Stillbirth The delivery of a dead baby after the 28th week of pregnancy.

Stool bulk producers Drugs to treat constipation.

Streptomycin A broad-spectrum antibiotic that should not be taken in pregnancy. See also *Antibiotics*.

Stress tests Tests during pregnancy that cause stress to the fetus and note fetal reactions.

Stretch marks See *Striae*.

Striae Silvery lines that sometimes appear on the skin after it has been stretched during pregnancy.

Sulpha drugs See *Sulfonamides*.

Sulphonamides Chemicals sometimes used to combat infections. See also *Antibacterials*.

Supplementary feeding Additional bottles given to a breastfed baby.

Surfactant A creamy fluid that reduces the surface tension of the lungs so that they do not stick together when deflated. Pre-term babies may have breathing difficulties if surfactant has not developed sufficiently.

Suture The stitching together of a tear or a surgical incision.

Syntocinon A synthetic form of oxytocin, which is used to induce or accelerate labour.

Systolic pressure The blood pressure built up in the arteries when the heart beats. The upper figure on any record. See also *Diastolic pressure*.

Telemetry A method of monitoring, using radio waves. See also *Electronic fetal monitoring*.

Teratogenic A general term for drugs that cause physical defects in the embryo.

Term The end of pregnancy: 40 weeks from the last menstrual period.

Termination An artificially induced abortion before the end of the 28th week of pregnancy.

Test weighing A method of assessing how much breast milk the baby is taking by weighing it immediately before and after a feeding.

Tetracycline A wide-spectrum antibiotic that should be avoided during pregnancy, because it can affect the development of the fetal teeth and bones. See also *Antibiotics*.

Thrombosis A blood clot in the heart or blood vessels.

Thrush A yeast infection that can form in the mucous membranes of the mouth, genitals, or nipples.

Thyroid gland A gland in the throat that produces hormones to control the metabolic rate.

Tochodynamometer A pressure gauge attached by a belt to the mother's abdomen in order to record her contractions.

Touch relaxation A means of stimulating release of muscular tension by resting the hands on tense areas and gently drawing out the tension.

Toxaemia See *Pre-eclampsia; Eclampsia*.

Toxoplasmosis, congenital A parasitic disease spread by cat faeces. If it crosses the placenta during the first 12 weeks of pregnancy, it can cause blindness in the baby.

Tranquillizers Drugs used to calm a state of anxiety or tension without inducing unconsciousness. Mild tranquillizers, such as Valium, may be prescribed during pregnancy, but should be avoided during labour as they can cause fetal respiratory depression. Powerful tranquillizers (along with antihistamines and hypnotics, which are sometimes used for their tranquillizing properties) should be avoided during pregnancy. See also *Barbiturates*.

Transducer An instrument that is sensitive to the echoes of very high-frequency soundwaves bounced off the developing fetus in the uterus, and that translates the information to build up an image on a television screen. This form of scan is known as ultrasound. See also *Scan*.

Transition A phase between the first and second stages of labour when the cervix is in the process of dilating to between 7 and 10 cm.

Trial of labour A situation in which, although a Caesarean section may be necessary, the mother labours in order to see if a vaginal delivery is possible.

Twins The simultaneous development of two babies in the uterus, either as a result of the production of two eggs that are fertilized independently by two sperm – dizygotic or fraternal twins – or, more rarely, as a result of one fertilized egg dividing to produce monozygotic or identical twins.

Ultrasound See *Scan; Transducer*.

Umbilical cord The cord connecting the fetus to the placenta.

Umbilical vein sampling (Cordocentesis) A fine needle is passed through the mother's abdomen into the fetal vein in the umbilical cord. The technique allows fetal blood to be tested, facilitates intra-urine blood transfusions, and enables drugs to be injected directly into the baby.

Undescended testicle A testicle that has failed to drop naturally from the lower abdomen into the scrotum.

Uterine action, incoordinate Irregular uterine contractions.

Uterine inertia Weak and ineffective uterine contractions.

Uterus (Womb) The hollow muscular organ in which the fertilized egg becomes embedded, where it develops into the embryo and then the fetus.

Vacuum extractor An instrument, used as an alternative to forceps, which adheres to the baby's scalp by suction and, with the help of the mother's bearing down efforts, can be used to suck the baby out of the vagina.

Vagina The canal between the uterus and the external genitals. It receives the penis during intercourse and is the passage through which the baby is delivered.

VE Vaginal examination.

Vernix A creamy substance that often covers the fetus in the uterus.

Vertex presentation (VX) See *Cephalic presentation*.

Vulva The external part of the female reproductive organs, including the labia and clitoris.

Water birth Birth of the baby under water.

XX/XY chromosomes The chromosomes that genetically distinguish the female and male, respectively.

Yolk sac The sac that stores the nutrients for the developing fertile egg.

Index

A

Abbreviations 40–41
Abdominal muscles 123, 126
Abdominal palpation 45
Abnormalities, congenital 11, 22, 23, 66–67, 100–101
Abortion see Termination of pregnancy
Abortion, spontaneous see Miscarriage
Abruptio placentae 137
Accelerated labour 328–329
Accidental haemorrhage 137–138
Aches and pains in pregnancy 128–129, 131–133
Active birth 180
Active Birth Movement 28, 34
Acupressure 266
Acupuncture 300–301
Admission procedures 248–249
Adrenaline 104, 346
AFP screening 220–223
Afterbirth see Placenta
AIDS and pregnancy 22–23
Alcohol 10, 104
Allergies 390
Alphafetoprotein see AFP screening
Amniocentesis 44, 221, 226–228
Amnioscope 317
Amniotic sac 68
Amniotomy 317–318
Anaemia 44, 143
Anaesthesia for Caesarean section 339 in labour 308–313
Anaesthetics 110, 308–313
Analgesics 307–308
Anencephaly 97, 221
Anomaly scan 223–224
Antenatal care 43–45
Antenatal classes 28, 155, 163, 176–182

Antenatal depression 231–233
Antenatal education 11, 12, 28, 176–182
Antenatal visits 11, 14, 15, 19, 44–49
Antepartum haemorrhage 137
Antibiotics 107–108
Anticholinergenic drugs 107
Anticoagulants 110, 309
Anticonvulsants 110
Anti-depressants 109
Antihistamines 24, 107
Antinausea drugs 107
Anxieties in pregnancy 24–30, 149–157
Apgar scale 106, 356–360
Apnoea 366
ARM (artificial rupture of membranes) 317–318
Aromatherapy 301–302
Aspirin 106
Assertiveness 48–49
Asthma 108
Augmented labour 328–329
Auscultation 333, 334
Autogenic method 180

B

Baby
appearance at birth 361–362
blood circulation 361
blood testing 334
breathing difficulties 366–368
cry 347, 393
development in uterus 10–15, 68–85
disabilities 371
growth pattern 74
journey through uterus 252–253
loss of 372
low-birthweight 366
low blood sugar 368
movements 12–15, 72, 74–75, 231
neonatal jaundice 368–370
poor temperature

Baby, cont.
control 366
position in uterus 233–234
pre-term 366
reflexes of newborn 357
sleep patterns 392–393
testing after birth 358–360
testing in uterus 220–229
worries about 155–156
Baby carrier 395
Bach Flower Remedies 303
"Back labour" 262–267
Backache 15, 119, 131
Balaskas method 180
Barbiturates 106
Bathing baby 393 immediately after birth 352–353
Bearing down 251–253
Bending 130
Bilateral episiotomy 267
Bilirubin 368–369
Birth
baby's experience 343–345
choice of venue 31–39
companion 28, 184
emergency or surprise 293–294
emotions after 381–382
"gentle" 343–353
home 37–39, 249–250, 256–261
hospital 31–37, 54–59, 247–249
hours following 353
movements in water 268–271
pool 37, 42, 267, 305
room 36–37, 183, 347–348
siblings attending 39, 73
in water 304–306
worries about 149–155
Birth control see Contraception
Birth defects see Abnormalities, congenital
Birth plan 50–53

"Birth without violence" 345
Bladder control and infections 134–135
Blastocyst 67–68
Bleeding, vaginal 136–139, 255, 372
Blighted ovum 373
Blood
baby's circulation 361
baby's, testing 334
pressure 40, 139, 310
Rhesus factor 113
Body changes during pregnancy 10–15 after giving birth 383–384, 397
Bonding 39, 75, 358, 362–364
Bottlefeeding 390–392
Bradley method 180
Bras 11, 145
Braxton Hicks contractions 14, 15, 167, 243
Breast pump 388, 389
Breastfeeding 384–390 as contraception 404 immediately after birth 358, 364, 385
Breasts
bras 11, 145
changes in early pregnancy 23
engorged 387–388
inverted nipples 135
sore and cracked nipples 388–389
tender 10, 135, 389
Breathing 201–203
breathing down your back 203
butterfly breathing 205, 207–208
for contractions 205–206
full chest breathing 203–204, 205
greeting breath 203
resting breath 203
sheep's breathing 208
upper chest breathing 204–205
Breathing difficulties in baby 366–368
Breathlessness 14, 143, 144

Breech position 32, 234
  birth in squatting
    position 273
  labour with 267,
    272–274
  Bromocriptine 390
Butterfly breathing 205,
  207–208
"Buttonhole tearing"
  322

C

Caesarean section 333,
  336–341
  for breech
    presentation 272
Calcium 98
Candida 135
Cannabis 105
Cap, contraceptive 406
Caput 362
Carbohydrates 95
Carpal tunnel
  syndrome 132
Catecholamines 241,
  346–347
Caudal anaesthesia 313
Centring down 185
Cephalic position 15
Cephalopelvic
  disproportion 32, 336,
  338
Cerebral palsy 371
Cervical cap 406
Cervical cerclage 115
Cervix
  anatomy 118
  dilation 241–242
  "incompetent" 115,
  374
  unripe 326
Checkup, postnatal 396
Chloasma 145–146
Chlorpromazine 106
Chorionic villus
  sampling 228–229
Chromosomes 65–67
Cigarettes
  see Smoking
Circumcision 364–365
Clamping the cord
  322–324, 351
Clinics, antenatal 44–49
Clitoris, anatomy 117
Clothing
  for new baby 395
  in pregnancy 134,
  144–145
Cocaine 105
Codeine 106
Coitus interruptus 404
Colostrum 14, 370, 384
Colour blindness 66–67

Comfort 144–148
  aids for birth 235
  in multiple pregnancy
  88–91
Conception 10, 18,
  67–68, 76
  after miscarriage 374,
  378–379
Condom 405
Constipation 134
  laxatives 108
Consultant units 34–35
Contraception
  after childbirth
  403–409
  breastfeeding 404
  cap 406
  coitus interruptus 404
  conceiving while
    using 20–22
  condom 405
  contraceptive implant
  409
  diaphragm 405–406
  intrauterine device 20,
  406, 408
  morning-after pill 409
  natural birth control
  404–405
  ovulation predictor
  405
  pill 20, 22, 408–409
  rhythm method 404
  spermicides 406
  sponge 406
Contraceptive implant
  409
Contractions 243–255
  Braxton Hicks 14, 15,
  167, 243
  in induced labour
  326–327
  monitoring 247–248
  pain 296–297
  practising 206, 216–219
  and relaxation 196
  sensations of 243
  simulating 216–217
  start 243
  support during
  280–283, 292–293
  timing 246
Coping with older
  children 170–173
Cord, umbilical 70
  clamping and cutting
    off 322–324
  delaying clamping
  324, 351
  prolapsed 243
Corpus luteum 11, 62
Cramps 99, 132–133
Crowning 254, 348
Crying, baby's 347, 393
Cystic fibrosis 229
Cystitis 134

D

D&C (dilatation and
  curettage) 373
Date of delivery 20,
  235–236
  chart 21
  confirmation by
    ultrasound 223
  overdue 234–237
Death of baby 375–379
Delivery
  emotions after
  381–382
  forceps 311, 334–336
  positions for 214–215
  surprise 293–294
  vacuum extraction
  335–336
Delivery room 347–348
Depression 109
  antenatal 231–233
  postnatal 360,
  381–382, 408
  respiratory see
    Breathing difficulties
    in baby
Dextrose 320
Diabetes 32, 141–143
  drugs to treat 110
Diamorphine 308
Diaphragm,
  contraceptive 405–406
Diarrhoea 15
Diazepam 105, 109, 307
Diazoxide 115
Dick-Read method 179
Diet
  balanced 96, 99–100
  in multiple pregnancy
  91
Digestive disturbances
  144
Dilatation and
  curettage 373
Disabilities 371
  mothers with 395
Discussion groups 155,
  157, 165
Diuretics 108
Dizygotic twins 86
Dizziness 10, 15, 143
Doctors, discussing
  treatment with 34–35,
  45–53
Domino scheme 35
Doula 29, 52, 184, 277
Down's Syndrome 44,
  230, 371
  testing for 221–223,
  226
Dreams in early
  pregnancy 24, 156
Drinking
  alcohol 10, 104

  milk 97
  water 386–387
Drip, intravenous 52,
  318, 320
Driving 147
Drugs 18, 110–110
  anaesthetics 110,
  308–313
  antibiotics 107–108
  anticoagulants 110,
  309
  anticonvulsants 110
  anti-depressants 109
  anti-psychotic 109
  anti-sickness 107
  diabetes 110
  fluid retention 108
  future of, in childbirth
  313
  laxatives 108
  mood-altering 105
  narcotics 307–308
  pain relief in labour
  306–313
  painkillers 106–107,
  306–313
  safety of, in
    pregnancy 100–102
  sleeping pills 106
  steroids 108
  teratogenic 101
  thyroid conditions 109
  tranquillizers 105–106,
  307
Dysfunctional labour
  276
Dyspareunia 403

E

Eclampsia 141
Egg
  development 62,
  67–68
  fertilization 62–63
Elective induction
  327–328
Electronic fetal
  monitoring 237, 249,
  330–334
Embryo development
  10, 67–85, 102
Emergency delivery
  293–294
Emotional reactions to
  pregnancy
  after delivery 381–382
  discussing with
    partner 27
  during pregnancy
  149–157, 231–233
  early on 24–27, 170
  in last weeks 231
  of partner see Partner

Emotional reactions to pregnancy, *cont.*
treating with Bach Flower Remedies 303
Engagement of baby's head 15, 41, 74
Engorgement of breasts 387–388
Entonox 308
Epidural anaesthesia 309–313 for
  Caesarean section 339
  induction with 327
Epilepsy *see* Anticonvulsants
Episiotomy 320–322
  bilateral 267
  with breech labour 267–272
  fear of 154–155
Essential oils 301–302
Estimated delivery date 20–21, 235–236
Ethanol 115
Ethical dilemmas 229–230
Examination at prenatal visit 19–20
Exercises
  abdominal muscles 123–126
  antenatal 120–133
  breathing 201–205
  feet 128
  in multiple pregnancy 90–91
  pelvic floor 119
  pelvic rocking 124, 126–127, 245, 398
  postnatal 383–384, 398–401
  posture 120–122
  relaxation 186–198
  using gravity in labour 244–245
External monitoring 331
External version 234

F

Fallopian tubes 62–63, 76–77
"False" labour 243
Father *see* Partner
Fatherhood, reacting to 27, 159–160
Fats 97
Fears during pregnancy 149–157
Feeding 384–392
  baby immediately

after birth 358, 364, 385
  baby in special care 370
Fertilization 62–63
Fetal Alcohol Syndrome 104
Fetal circulation 71
Fetal movement recording 237
Fetoscopy 229
Fetus
  blood circulation 71
  development 71–85, 102
  monitoring in labour 237, 249, 330–334
  movements in final weeks 237
  recording movements of 74–75
  testing 220–230
First stage of labour 246–251
Fluid retention 99
  drugs to reduce 108
  loss after delivery 383
Flying 147
Folic acid 97
Follicle 62
Fontanelles 251
Food
  intolerances 93–94
  poisoning 111–112
Forceps delivery 311, 334–336
Foremilk 385
Foreskin 365
Formula 390–392
Full chest breathing 203–204, 205
Fundal palpation 45
Fundus 14, 41

G

Gamma globulin 112
Gas anaesthetics 308
Genes 65–67
Genetic counselling 67, 230
Genetic disabilities, screening 220–230
Genitals
  baby's at birth 362
  female 116–119
"Gentle" birth 243–253
German measles 112, 229
Gestosis 139
Getting up in pregnancy 122
Glucose-tolerance test 142–143

GP units 35
Greeting breath 203
Grieving for lost baby 374–375, 377

H

Haemolytic jaundice 368–370
Haemophilia 67, 229
Haemorrhage 32, 103, 137–139
Haemorrhoids 133
Hair
  of baby 361
  of pregnant woman 10, 145
Haldol 106
Haloperidol 106
HCG testing 18–19, 221, 223
HDP (hypertensive disease of pregnancy) 139
Head moulding, of baby 318, 362
Headache 106, 143–144
Health service policy 42
Heartbeat, baby's 14, 333–335
  effect of amniotomy on 318
  monitoring 249
Heartburn 13, 144
Heat loss in newborn baby 350–351
Hegar's sign 19
Hereditary disease 66–67
"High risk" mothers 32, 337, 364
HIV infection and pregnancy 22–23
Home birth 37–39, 256–261
  emergency or surprise 293–294
  preparations for 42, 249–250
Homeopathy 303
Hormones, stress *see* Catecholamines
Hospital
  admission procedures 248
  antenatal clinics 44–49
  birth 31–37, 54–59
  choice of 34–35
  delivery room in "gentle birth" 347–350
  fear of 153
  medical reasons for 32–34

GP units 35
partner's support in 278–293
  when to go to 247–248
Human chorionic gonadotrophin 18–19
Husband *see* Partner
Hyaline membrane disease 367
Hyperemesis 135–136
Hypertension 139
Hyperventilation 202
Hypnosis 300
Hypnotics 106
Hypoglycaemia 320, 366, 368

I

Ibuprofen 107
Implantation 68
"Incompetent" cervix 115, 374
Incubator 366, 370
Indigestion 13, 144
Induction
  by amniotomy 317
  by sexual intercourse 168–169
  coping with 328
  elective 327–329
  procedures 324–325
  reasons for 325–326
  with epidural anaesthesia 327
Inevitable abortion 373
Infertility 68
Insomnia 148
Insulin 110, 141, 143
Intensive care *see* Special care for newborn babies
Intercourse *see* Sexual intercourse
Internal monitoring 331
Intervention in labour 306–340
Intrauterine device 20, 406, 408
Intravenous drip 52, 318, 320
Iron 45, 98, 143
Itching in pregnancy 146
IUD 20, 406, 408

JK

Jaundice 368–370
Kidney infection 134–135
Kiellands forceps 335
Kitzinger psychosexual approach 181

L

Labia 116–117
Labour
  acceleration of
    328–329
  active management of
    315–316, 329
  anxiety about 149–153
  as stimulus for baby
    345–346
  baby's experience
    343–344
  breathing 201–208
  breech baby 267,
    272–274
  comfort aids 235
  common procedures
    316–324
  drugs for pain relief
    306–313
  dysfunctional 276
  effects of orgasm on
    167–169
  emotional support
    during 28–29
  equipment 36–37, 183
  "false" 243
  first signs 242–243
  first stage 246–251
  induction 324–329
  "latent" 275
  long-drawn-out
    275–276
  lull in 292
  medical procedures
    314–341
  movements for
    208–215
  nipple stimulation
    169
  pain 296–300
  posterior baby
    262–267
  premature 115
  preparing for 233–234,
    248
  pre-term 115
  procedures 316–324
  record chart 319
  relaxation for 185–208
  second stage 251–254
  short sharp 274–275
  stages 241
  start and stop 283, 292
  support during
    277–294
  third stage 255
  transition 250–251
  understanding
    progress of 240–255
  using gravity to help
    244–245
  in water 303–304
  "wet" 243
  when to go to hospital
    247–248
Lamaze method 179
Lanugo 12–13, 72, 84,
  361
Laxatives 108
Leboyer, Dr Frederick
  345, 352
Let-down reflex
  384–385
Lifting 130
Lighting in delivery
  room 348
Linea Nigra 11
Listeriosis 111
Lithotomy position 247,
  267
Lochia 255
Loneliness 156
Losing a baby 372–379
Low birthweight babies
  366
Low blood sugar,
  babies with 368
Lung surfactant 73,
  366–367
Lying down in
  pregnancy 130–131

M

Magnesium 98
"Mask of pregnancy"
  145–146
Massage
  of baby after delivery
    350
  in relaxation exercises
    186–195
  to relieve "back
    labour" 266
  in touch relaxation
    186–195
Masturbation 117
Maternal instincts 25
Meconium 15, 360,
  367
Medical procedures in
  labour 314–341
Medical record 40–41
Medicines see Drugs
Membranes
  artificial rupture of
    317–318
  stripping 324
Menstrual cycle 62–63
Metrazinol 308
Midwives 31, 35–36, 42,
  382
Migraine, drugs for 107
Milk
  ejection reflex 384–385
  encouraging flow of
    385
expressing breast milk
  389–390
intake during
  pregnancy 97
Minerals 98–100
Miscarriage 372–375
  and choice of birth
    venue 34
Mongolian blue spot 362
Monilia 135
Monitoring see
  Electronic fetal
  monitoring
Monozygotic twins
  (identical twins) 86
Montgomery's
  tubercles 10, 23
Mood altering drugs 105
Mood changes after
  delivery 381–382
Morning sickness 10,
  11, 24
Morphine 308
Moulding see Head
  moulding
Mourning a baby
  374–377

N

Nappies 393–394
Naproxen 107
Nasal congestion 12,
  136
National Childbirth
  Trust 28, 34, 47,
  179, 414
Nausea 10–11, 24,
  135–136 (
Navel 13
NCT see National
  Childbirth Trust
Nembutal 106
Newborn reflexes 357
  in labour 344–345
Nicotine see Smoking
Nipple
  cracked 388–389
  inverted 135
  shell 135
  shield 388
  soreness 388
  stimulation during
    labour 169
Nitrous oxide 308
Noise in delivery
  room 348–350
Normacol 108
Nosebleeds 136
Notochord 69
Numbness 132
Nutrition
  during pregnancy
    93–100

O

Occipito posterior
  position see Posterior
  position
Odent approach 180
Oedema 41, 99
Oestriol 221, 223, 236
Oestrogen 22, 62, 70–71
Older children 172–173,
  364
Orgasm during
  pregnancy 167–168
Ovary 62–63
"Overdue" 234–237
Ovulation
  after childbirth 404
  cycle 63
Oxytocin 322–323
  drip 309, 325

P

Packing for hospital 235
Pain 295–296
  during intercourse
    after birth 403
  during labour
    296–297, 298–300
  during pregnancy 14,
    131–133
  fear of 151
  purposeful 299–300
  relief by acupressure
    266
  relief by acupuncture
    300–301
  relief by
    aromatherapy
    301–302
  relief by drugs 306–313
  relief by hypnosis 300
  relief by reflexology
    301
  relief by TENS 301
  relief in other cultures
    297–298
  relief using water
    303–304
Painkillers 106–107,
  306–313
Paracervical block 309
Paracetamol 107
Parenthood 396–411
Partner
  as a parent 409–411
  at the birth 28,
    277–294
  at Caesarean section
    340–341
  attending antenatal
    classes 28, 163, 165,
    181

attending antenatal clinic 162–163
attitude to childbirth 162
attitude to coming baby 159–160
emotional reactions 27, 159–163, 382
helping in the home 163
reaction to baby after delivery 360–361
reaction to second and subsequent pregnancies 170
relationship with 160, 164
relationship with parents 160
support of woman in labour 277–294
Partogram 319
Pelvic floor
after delivery 383–384
anatomy 118–119
exercises 90, 119
Pelvis 126–127
infection 318
small see Cephalopelvic disproportion
Penicillin 107
Perineum 116
Periods 62–63
after childbirth 404
missed 18, 19, 20
Pessaries 324
PET (Pre-eclamptic toxaemia) 32, 88, 139–141
Pethidine 307–308
Phenergan 308
Phenobarbital 106
Phenothiazines 107
Phototherapy 369
Physical contact at birth 350–351
Piles 133
Pill, contraceptive 20, 408–409
Pituitary gland 62, 63
Placenta 68, 70–71
assessment by ultrasound 224, 237
at end of pregnancy 236
dealing with in emergency birth 294
detachment from uterine wall after birth 255
effects of amniotomy on 318
expulsion after Caesarean section 340

insufficiency 325, 374
previa 137
retained 32, 322–323
testing by urinary oestriol test 236
Positions for delivery 214–215
Positions for labour 208–213, 219
Positions for sexual intercourse 167–169
Posterior position 233–234, 251, 262–263
forceps delivery 335
labour 262
turning baby in 234
Postnatal checkup 396
Postnatal depression 360
Postpartum period 381–384
Posture 14, 120–122, 127, 130–131
with multiple pregnancy 90
Practising for contractions 206, 216–219
Practising for pushing 217–219
Pre-eclampsia 32, 88, 139–141
Pregnancy
aches and pains 128–129, 131–133
alcohol during 104
common problems 133–144
dating 20
early signs 23
emotional reactions 24–27
exercise 127–131
finding out you are pregnant 18–20
general anaesthetic during 110
high temperature during 111
and HIV infection 22
keeping fit during 124–125
managing alone 29–30
over age of 40 32
rest and sleep during 148
second or third 170–172
sex during 166–169
smoking during 102–104
travel during 147
weekly developments 10–15
weight gain 94–95
worries 149–157

Pregnancy testing 19–20
"do-it-yourself" 19
ultrasound 223
urine 19
Premature babies 35, 366, 368
Preparation for labour 233–234, 248
Presentations for birth 263
Pressure to relieve back pain 264–266
Pre-term babies 35, 366, 368
Progesterone 11, 22, 62–63, 70–71
Progestogen 22, 115
Prostaglandin pessaries 324
Protein 95
Prozac 109
Psychoprophylaxis 179–180
Pudendal block 309
"Puppet on a string" relaxation 196–197
Pushing in labour 251–253
practising for 217–219
Pyelitis 134–135

QR

Quickening 74–75
Rapid eye movement in sleep 333, 392–393
Rectus muscle 123, 125–126
rehabilitating 125
Reflexes, baby's newborn 344–345, 357
used in labour 344–345
Reflexology 301
Relationship with baby 356–360
in special care 370–371
Relationship with future grandparents 29–30, 160
Relationship with partner 160, 164–166
after losing baby 377–378
Relaxation 185–208
autogenic method 180
Balaskas method 180
Bradley method 180
centring down 185
Dick-Read method 179

Kitzinger psychosexual approach 180
Lamaze method 179–180
psychoprophylaxis 179–180
"puppet on a string" method 196–197
Stanislavsky method 197–199
"touch" 186–196
visual imagery 199–201
REM see Rapid eye movement
Reproductive organs
female 64, 116–119
male 64
Respiratory distress 367
Responsibilities in childbearing 315
Rest 148
importance of in multiple pregnancy 88
Resting breath 203
Right to choose 314–315
Rhesus
disease 113–114, 324
factor 113
tests 14, 44
Rhythm method of contraception 404
Rooting reflex 352, 357
Rubella 112, 229

S

Salmonella 111
Salt intake in pregnancy 99
Scalp electrodes 333
Scan see Ultrasound
Screening 220–230
Second and subsequent pregnancies 170–173
Sex, baby's 65–66
Sexual characteristics of newborn 362
Sexual intercourse
after childbirth 396–397, 403
painful 403
positions 167–169
during pregnancy 166–169
Sexual organs 64, 116–119
Shaving of perineum 248
Sheath (Condom) 405
Shiatsu (Acupressure) 266
Shoes 145

Shortness of breath 144
"Show" 242
Siblings 172–173, 364
Sickness *see* Nausea
Single mothers 28–30
Sinusitis 136
Sitting 130
Skin, darkening
    145–146
Sleep 148
Sleep patterns of
    newborn babies
    392–393
Sleeping pills 106
"Small-for-dates"
    babies 366
Smallpox vaccination
    112
Smoking 102–104, 408
Soft spots on baby's
    head (Fontanelles) 251
Solid foods 387
Soya milk 390
Special care for
    newborn babies
    366–371
    with breathing
        difficulties 366–368
    with low blood sugar
        368
    with poor
        temperature control
        366
Sperm 10, 63–66
Spermicides 406
Spina bifida 97
    testing for 44, 221,
    226
Spinal anaesthesia 309
Spine, caring for your
    119–123
Spontaneous abortion
    372–375
Sport 146–147
Spotting 19, 20, 136, 167
Stanislavsky relaxation
    techniques 197–199
Start-stop labour 283,
    292
Steroids 108
Stillbirth 72, 375–378
    conceiving after
    378–379
Stitches 255, 320–322
Streptomycin 108
Stress 241, 346–347
Stretch marks 14, 146
Sucking
    for comfort 386
    inability 370
Sulphonamides
    107–108
Supplementary feeding
    387
Support in labour
    277–294

Surprise delivery
    293–294
Sweating 12
Syntocinon 320

T

Talking to your baby
    393
Taste in early
    pregnancy 10
Technology used in
    labour 315–316
Teeth of pregnant
    women 145
Telemetry 332–333
Temperature
    baby with poor 366
    in birth room 352–353
    following epidural
        311
    during pregnancy 111
TENS 301
Termination of
    pregnancy 18, 67, 112,
    227–228, 230, 372
Tests during pregnancy
    anaemia 45
    Rhesus 44
    routine 43–45
Tests on baby in uterus
    AFP screening
        220–223
    amniocentesis
        226–228
    chorionic villus
        sampling 228–229
    fetoscopy 229
    ultrasound scan
        222–226
    umbilical vein
        sampling 229
Tests on newborn
    358–360
Tetracycline 108
Thalidomide 101
Thorazine 106
Thrush 135
Thyroid condition,
    drugs to treat 109
Tiredness
    anaemia 143
    in early pregnancy 23
    in multiple pregnancy
        88–90
Tocodynamometer 331
Touch relaxation 186–196
Toxaemia 32, 88,
    139–141
Toxoplasmosis 112, 229
Tranquillizers 105–106,
    307
Transcutaneous
    Electronic Nerve

Stimulation 301
Transducer 225, 330
Transition 250–251
Travel 147
Turner's Syndrome 221
Twins 86–91
    choice of birth venue
        34
    fraternal 86
    identical 86
    position in uterus 87

U

Ultrasound scan 45, 75,
    222–226, 237
Umbilical cord *see*
    Cord, umbilical
Umbilical vein
    sampling 229
Unripe cervix 326
Upper chest breathing
    204–205
Urinary infections
    107–108, 134–135
Urinary oestriol test 236
Urination, frequent 10,
    14, 15, 134
Urine
    pregnancy test 18–19
    sugar in 142–143
Uterine stimulation 329
Uterus
    action in labour 216
    changing 10–15, 73
    implantation of egg
        10, 68
    inco-ordinate action
        276, 328
    position of baby
        233–234
    position of twins 87

V

Vaccination during
    pregnancy 112
Vacuum extraction
    335–336
Vagina 116–117
    bleeding from
        136–139, 255, 372
    colour changes 10
    discharge from 10, 12,
        135
    examination of 45, 316
    varicose veins in 133
Valium 105–106, 307
Varicose veins 133, 408
Vernix 13, 72, 362
Version 234
Vertex position 15

Visual imagery for
    relaxation 199–201
Vitamins 97
Vomiting 24, 135–136
Vulva 116, 135

W

Walking 130
Warfarin 110, 309
Water
    birth movements in
        268–271
    drinking 386–387
    use of in labour 42,
        267, 303–306
Waters breaking
    242–243
    see also Amniotomy
Weaning 387
Weight
    of baby 359, 366, 387
    gain in pregnancy
        94–95
    loss after delivery 383
Welldorm 106
"Wet" labour 243
Womb *see* Uterus
Womb, neck of
    see Cervix
Worries in pregnancy
    24–30, 149–157

XYZ

X-rays 110–111
Yeast growths 135
Zinc 98

Acknowledgments

Additional editorial assistance
Colette Connolly, Jo Evans, Samantha Gray,
Sasha Heseltine, Annabel Morgan,
Joanna Warwick, Anna Youle

Additional design assistance
Stephen Croucher, Ellen Harris, Darren Hill,
Philip Ormerod, Karl Thurston-Brown

Additional illustrations
Vanessa Luff

DTP Operator
Jason Little

Assistant for additional photography
Pauline Naylor

Black-and-white prints
Debbie Sears

Index
Sue Lightfoot

Picture research
Alison McKittrick, Damian Smith

Picture credits
CNRI: 220b; Antonia Deutsch: 407;
Sally Greenhill: 323t; National Medical Slide
Bank: 62bl; Science Photo Library, Andy
Walker, Midlands Fertility Service: 135br;
Debi Treloar: 135, 407cr.

Dorling Kindersley Limited would like to
thank all the parents and the parents-to-be who
allowed themselves and their children to be
photographed for this book. Marcia May would
especially like to thank those who so generously
agreed to share the experience of the birth of
their babies with her.

The publisher and photographer are also
deeply grateful to the nurses, doctors and
midwives involved for their warm cooperation
and advice. Special thanks go to all the staff
of the maternity ward at King's College
Hospital, London. Thanks also to Blooming
Marvellous Ltd., who kindly supplied props
for studio photography.

Parents, children and midwives
Abigail Akinola, Jane and Steve Bassett,
Amanda Browning, Stephanie Chocieszynska,
John Clarke, Rosaline Cole, Michelle
Davidson, Luke and Rufus Dye-Montefiore,
Jane Evans, Claire Farman, Jeronima Garcia,
Louise Gardner, Jayne Heaton-Harris,
Nathalie Hennequin, Sue Holt, Shoonagh
Hubble, Angela Hutcheson, Deborah Jones,
Carmel Lacy, Dave Lambert, Nicky Leap,
Rachel Lewis, Anne Magee, Stephanie
and George Marden, Pauline and Clifton
McDonald, Linda Miller, Lucinda Montefiore,
Julia Morrissy-Swan, Damilola Mercy
Oye-Akinola, Susan Ray, Becky Reed,
Alison Retout, Adrian Richardson, Simone
and Ricardo Roberts, Hugo Robins, Imogen
Poppy Robins, Lisa Scott, John Stewart,
Polly and Lucy Stewart, Julia Terrila and
Isaac Acheampong and their baby Una,
Max and Sophie Toocaram, Mr. and Mrs.
Trew and Patsy Tummings.